PLANT-DERIVED ANTICANCER DRUGS IN THE OMICS ERA

Biosynthesis, Functions, and Applications

PLANT-DERIVED ANTICANCER DRUGS IN THE OMICS ERA

Biosynthesis, Functions, and Applications

Edited by

Deepu Pandita, MPhil

Anu Pandita, MSc

APPLE ACADEMIC PRESS

First edition published 2024

Apple Academic Press Inc.
1265 Goldenrod Circle, NE,
Palm Bay, FL 32905 USA

760 Laurentian Drive, Unit 19,
Burlington, ON L7N 0A4, CANADA

CRC Press
2385 NW Executive Center Drive,
Suite 320, Boca Raton FL 33431

4 Park Square, Milton Park,
Abingdon, Oxon, OX14 4RN UK

Library and Archives Canada Cataloguing in Publication

CIP data on file with Canada Library and Archives

Library of Congress Cataloging-in-Publication Data

CIP data on file with US Library of Congress

ISBN: 978-1-77491-265-2 (hbk)
ISBN: 978-1-77491-266-9 (pbk)
ISBN: 978-1-00337-741-2 (ebk)

About the Editors

Deepu Pandita, MPhil
Senior Lecturer, Government Department of School Education, Jammu, Union Territory of Jammu and Kashmir, India

Deepu Pandita is working as a Senior Lecturer in the Government Department of School Education, Jammu, Union Territory of Jammu and Kashmir, India. Deepu Pandita has more than 19 years of teaching experience and earned her Master of Botany (MSc) at the University of Kashmir, Jammu and Kashmir, India, and Master of Philosophy (MPhil) in Biotechnology from the University of Jammu, Jammu and Kashmir, India. Deepu Pandita has a number of international and national courses to her credit. Deepu Pandita has qualified for fellowships including JRF NET and SRF from the Council of Scientific & Industrial Research (CSIR), New Delhi, India; Biotechnology Fellowship, Government Department of Science and Technology, Jammu & Kashmir, India; and IAS-INSA-NASI Summer Research Teacher Fellowship, India. Deepu Pandita has presented her research work at both the national and international conferences and was awarded a Best Oral Presentation Award in an International Conference on Biotechnology for Better Tomorrow, a Women Researcher Award, and Research Excellence Award from two professional associations in India. Deepu Pandita is a life member of various scientific societies. Deepu Pandita acts as a reviewer (18 journals), associate editor and editor of a number of international journals. Deepu Pandita has published a number of editorials, 40 book chapters (Springer, Elsevier, CRC, etc.), 20 reviews, and research articles in various journals of national and international repute like *Cells* (MDPI) (IF=7.666), *Frontiers in Plant Sciences* (IF=6.627), and *Frontiers in Physiology* (IF=4.566) and has currently various books in the process of production.

Anu Pandita, MSc
Dietician, Vatsalya Clinic, New Delhi, India

Anu Pandita is working as a Senior Dietician at Vatsalya Clinic, Krishna Nagar, New Delhi, India. Previously she worked as a Lecturer at the Bee Enn College of Nursing, Talab Tillo, Jammu, India, and Dietician at the Ahinsa Dham Bhagwan Mahavir Charitable Health Centre, New Delhi, India. Anu Pandita has done her MSc internship and a course in the Dietetics Department of PGI, Chandigarh, India. Anu Pandita has taken a case study at the Pediatric Gastroenterology Ward at Nehru Hospital PGI, Chandigarh, India, on a patient suffering from chronic liver disease. She earned a certificate for a course on food and nutrition as well. She has a number of trainings, refresher courses, and workshops to her credit. Anu Pandita is a life-time member of the Indian Dietetic Association and Indian Science Congress Association, Kolkata, India. Anu Pandita has presented her research work at both the national and international conferences. Anu Pandita has published various book chapters in Springer, CRC press, etc. and has a number of review and research articles in various journals of national and international repute, including *Cells* (MDPI) (IF=7.666) and *Frontiers in Physiology* (IF=4.566). She currently has various books in the process of production.

Contents

Contributors

Ahmad Ali
University Department of Life Sciences, University of Mumbai, Vidyanagari, Mumbai, India

María Uxua Alonso-Fresan
Centro de Investigación y de Estudios Avanzados en Salud Animal (CIESA), Facultad de Medicina Veterinaria y Zootecnia (FMVZ), Universidad Autónoma del Estado de México (UAEM), Toluca, Estado de México, México

Sarafraz Arqum Shah
Department of Radio-diagnostics, Maharishi Markandeshwar University, Mullana Ambala, Haryana, India

Muhammad Arslan Akhtar
Institute of Plant Breeding and Biotechnology, MNS University of Agriculture Multan, Old Shujabad Road, Multan, Pakistan

S. Ruth Assumi
Division of System Research and Engineering, ICAR Research Complex for NEH Region, Meghalaya, India

Yumna Baqi
Department of Saidla, Aligarh Muslim University, Aligarh, India

Alberto Barbabosa-Pliego
Centro de Investigación y de Estudios Avanzados en Salud Animal (CIESA), Facultad de Medicina Veterinaria y Zootecnia (FMVZ), Universidad Autónoma del Estado de México (UAEM), Toluca, Estado de México, México

Hebert Jair Barrales-Cureño
Instituto de Investigaciones Químico-Biológicas, Universidad Michoacana de San Nicolás de Hidalgo, Morelia, Michoacán, México

Pooja Bhadrecha
University Institute of Biotechnology, Chandigarh University, Punjab, India

Lekha Bhagtaney
Caius Research Laboratory, St. Xavier's College (Autonomous), Mumbai, India

Ambika Chaturvedi
Dayalbagh Educational Institute, Department of Botany, Dayalbagh, Agra, India

Salvador Chávez-Salinas
División de Ingeniería en Biotecnología, Universidad Politécnica del Valle de Toluca, Toluca, Estado de México, México

José María Eloy Contreras-Ortiz
Centro de Investigación y de Estudios Avanzados en Salud Animal (CIESA), Facultad de Medicina Veterinaria y Zootecnia (FMVZ), Universidad Autónoma del Estado de México (UAEM), Toluca, Estado de México, México

Nilanjana Das
Post Graduate Department of Biotechnology, St. Xavier's College (Autonomous), Kolkata, West Bengal, India

Jordi Orlando González-Osuna
División de Ingeniería en Biotecnología, Universidad Politécnica del Valle de Toluca, Toluca, Estado de México, México

Younis Ahmad Hajam
Department of Life Sciences and Allied Health Sciences, Sant Baba Bhag Singh University, Jalandhar, Punjab, India

Braulio Edgar Herrera-Cabrera
Colegio de Postgraduados, Campus Puebla. Puebla, State of Puebla, Mexico

Khanmi Kasomva
Functional Genomics Laboratory, School of Biotechnology, Jawaharlal Nehru University, Delhi, India

Zulqurnain Khan
Institute of Plant Breeding and Biotechnology, MNS University of Agriculture Multan, Multan, Pakistan

Bushra Hafeez Kiani
Department of Biological Sciences (Female Campus), International Islamic University, Islamabad, Pakistan

Rajesh Kumar
Department of Biosciences, Himachal Pradesh University, Shimla, Himachal Pradesh, India

Luis Germán López-Valdez
Laboratorio de Productos Naturales, Área de Química, Universidad Autónoma de Chapingo, Texcoco, Estado de México, México

Gonzalo Guillermo Lucho-Constantino
Universidad Tecnológica de Gutiérrez Zamora. Gutiérrez Zamora, State of Veracruz, Mexico

Mubasshira Mohammed Mazhar-Ul-Haque
Caius Research Laboratory, St. Xavier's College (Autonomous), Mumbai, India

Sana Nafees
All India Institute of Medical Sciences, New Delhi, India

Huda Nafees
Department of Saidla, Faculty of Unani Medicine, Aligarh Muslim University (A.M.U), Aligarh, Uttar Pradesh, India

S. Nizamudeen
Government Unani Medical College, Chennai, Tamilnadu, India

Rajiv Ranjan
Dayalbagh Educational Institute, Department of Botany, Dayalbagh, Agra, India

César Reyes
División de Procesos Naturales. Universidad Intercultural del Estado de Puebla, Puebla, México

Aryadeep Roychoudhury
Post Graduate Department of Biotechnology, St. Xavier's College (Autonomous), Kolkata, West Bengal, India

Pooja Saraswat
Dayalbagh Educational Institute, Department of Botany, Dayalbagh, Agra, India

Onur Sercinoglu
Gebze Technical University, Faculty of Engineering, Department of Bioengineering, Kocaeli, Turkey

Muhammad Shan
Institute of Plant Breeding and Biotechnology, MNS University of Agriculture Multan, Old Shujabad Road, Multan, Pakistan

Aishwarya Sharma
Department of Biosciences, Division Zoology, Career Point University, Hamirpur, Himachal Pradesh, India

Priya Sundarrajan
Department of Life Science and Biochemistry and Caius Research Laboratory, St. Xavier's College (Autonomous), Mumbai, India

Esvieta Tenorio-Borroto
Centro de Investigación y de Estudios Avanzados en Salud Animal (CIESA), Facultad de Medicina Veterinaria y Zootecnia (FMVZ), Universidad Autónoma del Estado de México (UAEM), Toluca, Estado de México, México

Fulden Ulucan-Karnak
Ege University, Institute of Health Sciences, Department of Medical Biochemistry, Izmir, Turkey

Juan Carlos Vázquez-Chagoyan
Centro de Investigación y de Estudios Avanzados en Salud Animal (CIESA), Facultad de Medicina Veterinaria y Zootecnia (FMVZ), Universidad Autónoma del Estado de México (UAEM), Toluca, Estado de México, México

Zeynep Yilmaz-Sercinoglu
Marmara University, Faculty of Engineering, Department of Bioengineering, Istanbul, Turkey

Fabiola Zaragoza-Martínez
Centro de Investigación y de Estudios Avanzados del Instituto Politécnico Nacional, Mexico City, Mexico

Abbreviations

ACEA	anticancer activity enrichment analysis
ACS	American Cancer Society
ADME/T	adsorption, distribution, metabolism, excretion, and toxicity
ADR	anthracyclines-like doxorubicin
ANOVA	analysis of variance
APCI	atmospheric pressure chemical ionization
APIs	active pharmaceutical ingredients
ATP	Artemisinin
BAM	business activity monitoring
BLASTN	nucleotide basic local alignment search tool
BLASTP	protein basic local alignment search tool
CADD	computer-aided drug design
CAP	Contig Assembly Program
CATCH	Cas9-assisted targeting of chromosome
CaUGT2	*C. amada* and glucosyltransferase gene
CDK	cyclin-dependent kinase
CHMP	Committee for Medicinal Products for Human Use
CHO	Chinese hamster ovary
CIESA-UAEM	Centro de Investigación y Estudios Avanzados en Salud Animal
CISMR	CRISPR-mediated isolation of specific mega base-sized regions
CMap	connectivity map
CNV	copy number variation
COSTREL	super combinatorial change of transplastomic beneficiary lines
COX	cyclooxygenase
COX2	cycloxygenase 2
CP	coat protein
CPT	camptothecin
CRAM	challenge response authentication mechanism
CRISPR	clustered regular short palindrome repeats

CrSTR	strictosidine synthase
CrTDC C.	roseus, tryptophan decarboxylase
Cu/ZnSOD	copper/zinc superoxide dismutase
CURS	curcumin synthases
CYP	Cytochromes P450
DAT	deacetylvindoline 4-O-acetyltransferase
DBAT	deacetylbaccatin III-10-O-acetyltransferase
DCS	diketide-CoA synthase
DESI	desorption electrospray ionization mass spectrometry
DLA	Dalton's lymphoma ascites
DME	Dulbeco's Modified Eagle's
DMS	differential mobility spectrometry
DMSO	dimethylsulfoxide
DNA	deoxyribonucleic acid
DW	dry weight
EAC	Ehrlich ascites caecinoma
EGCG	Epigallocatechin-3-gallate
EGR-1	epidermal growth receptor 1
EI	electron impact
EMA	European Medicines Agency
ER	endoplasmic reticulum
ESI	electrospray ionization
FBS	fetal bovine serum
FDA	food and drug administration
FT-ICR-MS	Fourier transform ion cyclotron resonance mass spectrometry
FW	fresh weight
G10H	geraniol 10-hydroxylase
GC	gas chromatography
GGPP	geranylgeranyl pyrophosphate
GSH	glutathione
HCA	N-nitroso and amines which are heterocyclic in nature
HCC	hepatocellular carcinoma
HDAC	histone deacetylase
HDR	homology-coordinated fix
HeLa	cervical papilloma
hERG	human ether-a-go-go-related gene
HILIC	hydrophilic-interaction liquid chromatography

HPLC-MS	HPLC-mass spectroscopy
HPV	human papilloma virus
HR	homologous recombination
HuH-7	human hepatocarcinoma
IMS	ion mobility spectroscopy
LBDD	ligand-based drug design
LC	liquid chromatography
LOX	lysyl oxidase
LPS	lipopolysaccharide
mAbs	monoclonal antibodies
MALDI	matrix-assisted laser desorption ionization
MAPK	mitogen-activated protein kinases
MAQ	mapping and assembly with quality
MARS	MS-assisted resolution of signals
MD	molecular dynamics
MEP	methylerythritol-phosphate
MM/PBSA	molecular mechanics/Poisson Boltzmann surface area
MMP	matrix metalloproteinases
MnSOD	manganese superoxide dismutase
MRS	magnetic resonance spectroscopy
mTOR	mechanistic target of rapamycin
NAFLD	non-alcoholic fatty liver disease
NCAM	neural cell adhesion molecule
NCED1	9-cis-epoxycarotenoid dioxygenase-1
NGS	new generation sequence techniques
NGSEP	next generation sequencing eclipse program
NMR	nuclear magnetic resonance
NOS	nitric oxide synthase
ORF	open reading frame
PAH	hydrocarbons which are polycyclic aromatic
PAL	phenylalanine ammonia lyase
PAM	pair adjacent protospacer
PDGFR	platelet-derived growth factor
PgSS1	overexpression of squalene synthase 1
PSA-NCAM	polysialic acid neural cell adhesion molecule
PTF	phyllanthi tannin fraction
QOL	quality of life
QTOF-MS	quadrupole time of flight mass spectrometry

RAD-SEQ	restriction site-associated DNA sequencing analysis
RMSD	root mean square deviation
RNA	ribonucleic acid
RNPs	ribonucleoproteins
ROS	reactive oxygen species
RPLC	reversed-phase liquid chromatography
RS	reactive species
RSM	response surface methodology
SAM	software asset management
SBDD	structure-based
SBVS	structure-based virtual screening
SFCMS	supercritical fluid chromatography mass spectrometry
SFN	sulforaphane
SNV	single-nucleotide variants
STR	strictosidine synthase
STS	stilbene synthase
T4SSs	type IV secretion system
TACE	trans-arterial chemoembolization
TBLASTN	protein-nucleotide 6-frame translation
TBLASTX	nucleotide 6-frame translation-nucleotide 6-frame translation
TCM	traditional Chinese medicine
TE	transposable element
TK	tyrosine kinase
TMV	tobacco mosaic virus
TNBC	triple negative breast cancer
TXS	taxadiene synthase
UPLCMS	ultrahigh performance liquid chromatography mass spectometry
USM	Unani system of medicine
VEGF	vascular endothelial growth factor
VEGFR1	vascular endothelial growth factor receptor-1
VFU	vertical farming units
VS	virtual screening
WHO	World Health Organization
ZOOM	zillions of oligos mapped

Preface

This book unveils the nature's Pharmacy of cancer killers and provides insights into the OMICS-Driven plant-derived anticancer drugs.

Cancer involves the unbeatable proliferation of cells and is the second most leading cause of death in humans in around 112 countries. By the year 2030, the deaths due to this disease alone are estimated to be 11.5 million (World Health Organization (WHO)). The scenario of cancer epidemics revealed almost 19.3 million patients and 10 million deaths in 2020. The fight with the cancer is going on but the heterogeneous nature of cancer makes it difficult to handle. The current cancer treatment includes conventional as well as advanced promising techniques of surgery, chemotherapy, radiotherapy, and immunotherapy alone or in combination. The anticancer therapy and oncogenic drugs are costly, inefficient and unsafe with many side-effects and resistance to chemotherapy and radiation therapy is observed in highly metastatic and aggressive malignancy patients, whereas the anticancer compounds derived from plants are easily accessible, non-toxic, and harmless with negligible antagonistic impacts, and neutralizes the impact of this dreaded disease on the human body. The novel therapeutic drugs are needed to fight this irrepressible and complicated disease. The imminent substitution is plant metabolite-based progression of drug discovery and drug designing.

The dawn of human existence states utilization of plants for medical purposes and are the backbone of medicine and fountains and wellsprings of drugs even in the contemporary times. According to the WHO, approximately 80% of human populace depends on the natural treatment method. Approximately 3000 plant species are gifted with valuable drug source and pharmaceutically active compounds with a potential to treat cancer syndromes. Secondly, the most therapeutic agents or molecules for cure to cancer are plant-based. Plant based biologically active compounds or lead molecules are bestowed with the potential as the potent anticancer drug molecules such as, artemisinin, betulinic acid, camptothecin (CPT), cyclopamine, curcumin, vincristine, docetaxel, epigallocatechin gallate, flavopiridol, glucoraphanin, homoharringtonine, irinotecan, ingenol mebutate, vinblastine, vincristine, paclitaxel, podophyllotoxins, resveratrol and several other anticancer compounds from nature's arsenal, are potentially safe, powerful alternative means that effectively fight against cancer. These plant secondary metabolites or chemotherapeutic compounds, are the basis of anticancer activity by protecting the cell from reactive oxygen species (ROS) and oxidative damage, activation of DNA repair pathways, modulating several molecules, activation of antimitotics, topoisomerase inhibitors, angiogenesis inhibitors, histone deacetylases inhibitors, and mitotic kinase inhibitors, trigger apoptosis and hinder proliferation of cancer cells and interfere with intracellular signaling pathways in cancer cells.

The chapters in this book explain the different traditional medicinal systems that offer alternative prevention and treatment of cancer, provide an up-to-date review of efficient antitumor/anticancer novel lead drug molecules beneficial in cancer drug discovery, and present new research arenas, such as genomics, metabolomics, bioinformatics, and genome editing of anticancer plants in general. The bioinformatics-based approaches aid in the identification of potential anticancer drug candidates and molecular targets in a fast and cost-effective mode. The computer-aided drug design (CADD) and discovery by Structure-based drug design (SBDD) and ligand-based drug design (LBDD) candidates is based on data-driven modelling and prediction of specific small molecule target protein interactions. Traditional biotechnology and the new generation genome editing tools, namely, clustered regularly interspaced short palindromic repeats (CRISPR)/Cas, zinc finger nucleases (ZFNs), transcription activator-like endonuclease (TALENs) have designed proficient plants via knock-out, knock-in, point-mutation, gene expression fine-tailing, and target-mutagenesis with enhanced secondary metabolites of desired biomedical importance, the knowledge about which can be gained through the genomics and metabolomics of desired plants. The prospects of CRISPR/Cas, ZFNs and TALENs in anticancer medicinal plants will also be deliberated in this book.

Few Lines on the Omics of Anti-Cancer Plants

In fields of green, a secret lies,
Of genes and proteins, that mesmerize,
From roots to leaves, and every stem,
A story of life, in plant omics, we condemn.
In nature's garden, a wonder unfolds,

Of plants with power, that science beholds,
From cancer to inflammation too,
Anti-cancer plants, hold a clue.

Omics, a science of the whole,
A field of study, that's vast and bold,
From genomics, to proteomics too,
And metabolomics, a journey anew.

From DNA, we read the code,
Of every trait, that life bestows,
And then we move, to the proteins they make,
The workhorses of life, in every cell they take,
From structure to function, we delve deep,
Their roles in life, we begin to reap.
With every cell, and every gene,
A world of data, is waiting to be seen,
With tools so sharp, and knowledge profound,
The mysteries of life, we begin to unbound.

With plant omics, we begin to explore,
The molecules and genes, that these plants implore,
From alkaloids to polyphenols too,
A treasure trove, of cancer-fighting brew.

From genomics, we unravel the code,
Of every gene, that's waiting to unfold,
that these plants bestowed,
A blueprint of life, that's written in DNA,
The roadmap of health, in every way,
And then we look, at the proteins they make,
The enzymes and receptors, that never forsake,
From photosynthesis, to defense against pests,
From apoptosis to angiogenesis,
A world of wonder, that science never misses.

With metabolomics, we explore the small,
The molecules, that fight it all,
The metabolites, that drive the rules,
From sugars to secondary metabolites,

A treasure trove, of plant insights,
From curcumin to resveratrol,
A treasure trove, of plant insights on the whole,
From energy production, to signalling too,
A story of life, that's forever new.

And then we delve, into the epigenetic realm,
Of histones and modifications, that overwhelm,
From gene expression, to developmental cues,
A story of life, that's waiting for you.

In plant omics, we find the key,
To sustainable agriculture, and biodiversity,
we explore, the mysteries, one by one,
In omics of anti-cancer plants,
We find the key to health, that enchants,
A world of wonder, that's waiting to be seen,
In the fields of green, where life reigns supreme.

CHAPTER 1

Evaluation of Extracts from *Curcuma longa* and *Zingiber officinale* as Growth Inhibitors of HeLa and HuH-7 Cell Lines

JORDI ORLANDO GONZÁLEZ-OSUNA[1], ALBERTO BARBABOSA-PLIEGO[2], ESVIETA TENORIO-BORROTO[2], SALVADOR CHÁVEZ-SALINAS[1], MARÍA UXUA ALONSO-FRESAN[2], JOSÉ MARÍA ELOY CONTRERAS-ORTIZ[2], JUAN CARLOS VÁZQUEZ-CHAGOYAN[2], LUIS GERMÁN LÓPEZ-VALDEZ[3], CÉSAR REYES[4], BRAULIO EDGAR HERRERA-CABRERA[5], FABIOLA ZARAGOZA-MARTÍNEZ[6], GONZALO GUILLERMO LUCHO-CONSTANTINO[7], and HEBERT JAIR BARRALES-CUREÑO[8]

[1]*División de Ingeniería en Biotecnología, Universidad Politécnica del Valle de Toluca, Toluca, Estado de México, México*

[2]*Centro de Investigación y de Estudios Avanzados en Salud Animal (CIESA), Facultad de Medicina Veterinaria y Zootecnia (FMVZ), Universidad Autónoma del Estado de México (UAEM), Toluca, Estado de México, México*

[3]*Laboratorio de Productos Naturales, Área de Química, Universidad Autónoma de Chapingo, Texcoco, Estado de México, México*

[4]*División de Procesos Naturales, Universidad Intercultural del Estado de Puebla, Puebla, México*

[5]*Colegio de Postgraduados, Campus Puebla, Puebla, State of Puebla, Mexico*

[6]*Centro de Investigación y de Estudios Avanzados del Instituto Politécnico Nacional, Mexico City, Mexico*

Plant-Derived Anticancer Drugs in the OMICS Era: Biosynthesis, Functions, and Applications.
Deepu Pandita, Anu Pandita (Eds.)

[7]*Universidad Tecnológica de Gutiérrez Zamora, Gutiérrez Zamora, State of Veracruz, Mexico*

[8]*Instituto de Investigaciones Químico-Biológicas, Universidad Michoacana de San Nicolás de Hidalgo, Morelia, Michoacán, México*

ABSTRACT

The objective of this study was to evaluate the potential to inhibit the cell proliferation of *Curcuma longa* and *Zingiber officinale* extracts, at different doses, in two cancer cell lines: human hepatocarcinoma (HuH-7) and cervical papilloma (HeLa). The extracts of *C. longa* and *Z. officinale* have a promising antiproliferation capacity. The inhibitory effects of the extracts were demonstrated at 72 h, with curcumin-achieving values of 66% and 78% for HeLa and HuH-7, respectively. On the other hand, gingerol reached values of inhibition of 60% (HeLa) and 75% (HuH-7). It is important to emphasize that the inhibition of lymphocytes isolated from peripheral blood was around 17.8%. The quantification of inhibitory capacity of curcuminoids and gingerols applied to the cell lines HeLa and HuH-7 was determined through cell viability assays (MTS) at 24, 48, and 72 h after each treatment. Finally, the morphological changes caused by apoptosis and necrosis were determined by ethidium bromide and acridine orange staining at 72 h of exposition. The results proved the capacity of growth inhibition of human hepatocarcinoma (HuH-7) and carcinoma uterine cervix (HeLa) cell lines, with the secondary metabolites curcumin and gingerol, when added extracts of *C. longa* and *Z. officinale*, respectively.

1.1 INTRODUCTION

Cancer is basically a disease of accelerated cell divisions, resulting in the growth of tumors. One characteristic is their ability to develop in any part of the body and they can migrate in a process known as metastasis (Malcom, 2001). There are various factors that induce cellular alterations, such as environmental conditions, xenobiotic substances, types of foods, and genetic or immune deficiencies of the own (Ames and

Gold, 2000). The lung, prostate, stomach, liver, and colorectal cancer are the most common types of cancers in men, while lung, breast, uterine, stomach, and colorectal cancer are the most common in women (Colder et al., 2006). More than 50% of deaths caused by cancer could be prevented by modifying or avoiding key risk factors, especially tobacco consumption (Flay et al., 2006). According to statistics provided by the World Health Organization, it is estimated that tobacco consumption is linked to 20% of cancer deaths worldwide, therefore is considered as the main preventable cause of cancer in the world. On the other hand, one-fifth of reported cases are often due to chronic diseases such as the human papillomavirus which is closely linked to uterus neck cancer and hepatitis B which is related to hepatic cancer (OMS, 2014). Besides avoiding exposure to tobacco smoke in the air and carcinogenic food consumption, the regular consumption of chemopreventive compounds is a promising approach, particularly antioxidant substances of plant origin, which have proved to be particularly encouraging as potential chemoprotective agents (Menon and Sudheer, 2007). The extracts of *Curcuma longa* and *Zingiber officinale* are chemopreventive models that have the potential of being a viable alternative for killing cancer cells and shrinking tumors, as well as cancer prevention because of their ability to inhibit antioxidant properties that have shown in experimental trials. *C. longa* is an herbaceous perennial plant with roots or shriveled tubers with an oblong palmate structure, brown color on the outside, and orange intense color inside it. The plant reaches 2 m high, with long, lanceolate, and petiolate leaves with a uniform light green all over (Cos, 2014). The flowers of *C. longa* are opaque yellow flowers prone white; stem bracts are present in groups from three to five flowers. The inflorescence is tinged reddish-purple, and it is more intense in the upper part of the endings. There is no seed formation; therefore, *C. longa* reproduce vegetatively by root cuttings. Turmeric is a very interesting plant in gastronomy for its medicinal properties, food, and from cosmetic perspective (Cos, 2014). In the Indian medicinal system, the ground rhizomes of turmeric are used to cure stomachache, as a blood purifier, carminative, appetizer, and tonic. Curcumin is also used as anticancer drug, dermatitis, AIDS, and to decrease the cholesterol level (Singh, 2002). Curcumin is the main curcuminoid of the popular Indian spice curcumin, a member of the ginger family (Zingiberaceae). Ginger (*Z. officinale*) is an important species in various types of Asiatic cuisine.

Ginger has a long history of medicinal use. Ginger is an integral part of different systems of folk medicine in China and India and is used to treat headaches, colds, rheumatoid arthritis, chronic bronchitis, muscular pains, and fever (Ali et al., 2008). The commercial ginger consists of thick and scaly plant rhizomes (underground stems); the rhizomes are 7–15-cm long and 1–1.5-cm thick and laterally compressed. The lateral branches emerging obliquely from the rhizome are 1–3 cm long and end in scars or buds without developing (Govindarajan, 1982). The ginger is used to treat dyspepsia, flatulence, abdominal discomfort, and nausea. It is recommended to use as carminative, diaphoretic, antispasmodic, and expectorant and stimulates peripheral blood circulation, astringent, appetite stimulant, anti-inflammatory agent, diuretic, and digestive agent (Chrubasik et al., 2005). Derivatives include sesquiterpenes such as zingiberene (12.24%), curcumene (4.18%), β-sesquifelandrene (6.45%), and β-bisabolene (5.63%); these molecules are responsible for aroma and form an important part of volatile fraction. On the other hand, the compounds present at lower concentrations include monoterpenes derivatives such as β-pinene (1.49%), β-elemene (0.14%), farnesene (0.33%), α-phellandrene (0.21%), myrcene (1.6%), β-pinene (0.26%), and sabinene (0.11%). Nonvolatile phytochemicals that are found in the ginger consist of bioactive chemical compounds dominated by gingerols, shogaoles, paradoles, and zingerones; these molecules are responsible of the stinging sensation in the mouth (Ekundayo, 1988). The main pharmacological activity of the ginger is due to the presence of gingerol and shogaol; the relative proportions of gingerols, shogaols, and paradoles in ginger extracts are determined by different factors that include geographical origin, maturity of rhizomes, and by the extraction method (Keum et al., 2002).

1.2 MATERIALS AND METHODS

1.2.1 CELL LINES

Cell lines of human hepatocarcinoma (HuH-7) and carcinoma uterine cervix (HeLa) were used, which were kindly donated by Centro de Investigación y Estudios Avanzados en Salud Animal (CIESA-UAEM). One of the main features is their capacity to proliferate in growing media chemically defined that contain selenium traces instead of serum.

1.2.2 CULTURE MEDIA

The cell lines were grown with Dulbeco's Modified Eagle's Medium-High Glucose (DME, Gibco) (Yang and Xiong, 2012) and it was enriched with 2% of fetal bovine serum (FBS) (SFB, Atlanta Biologica) and added with 1% of penicillin/streptomycin (GibcoLife Technologies).

1.2.3 MAINTENANCE OF THE CELL LINES

The growth media culture was renewed each 30 days. In order to maintain the cells suspended in a submerged culture, these cells were placed in culture bottles with 4 mL of medium volume. The inoculated bottles with HeLa and HuH-7 cell lines were placed at 37°C with 5% of CO_2 added with an automatic incubator. Every 24 h, the culture appearance was analyzed under a microscope for avoiding potential and undesirable contamination. At the end of the culture, the cells were removed with trypsin and 5% of these cells were kept and used for a new inoculum.

1.2.4 CELL LINES CRYOPRESERVATION

The cell lines were preserved in liquid nitrogen. Freezing of the cell lines was done by a slow protocol with 90% of FBS and 10% of dimethylsulphoxide (DMSO). This solution was kept at 4°C for avoiding toxicity. To withdraw the cells from the monolayer structure, first the culture medium was removed and washed with PBS. Then 1 mL of trypsin was added and incubated at 37°C by 5 min in order to take off the cells. After 0.95 mL of suspended cells was centrifuged for 5 min at 2100 rpm, the trypsin was removed, and the cells were resuspended with 1 mL of freezing solution and deposited in cryovial tubes. The freezing process was performed through slow changes of temperature in an ultrafreezer: –20°C for 1 h, –80°C for 24 h, and the last step was performed into the nitrogen liquid. From unfreezing the cells, a cryovial tube was taken and placed in a water bath at 30°C. Finally, 10 mL of culture media was added and then centrifuged for 5 min at 2100 rpm to eliminate the DMSO.

1.2.5 VEGETATIVE MATERIAL

The plant material used consisted of capsules that contain fine powder made by rhizomes, facilitating their process. The ginger and turmeric materials were obtained from health food stores without specifying trademark.

a) Plant extracts preparation

For the extraction of active substances, the solvents used were acetone (70%), petroleum ether (15%), and ethyl alcohol (10%). The vegetative powder was submerged in test tubes with the solvent for a 72-h period. Later, the mixture was filtered with a filter paper, and the aqueous phase was placed at 37°C in a furnace until the solvents evaporate. The retained mass was resuspended in PBS and filtered with acrodiscs of 22 µm in order to withdrawing all suspended particles; finally, the extracts were conserved in vials at 4°C.

b) Bioactive extracts quantification

In order to determine the concentration of active compounds, a curve pattern was performed in a spectrophotometer UV (EPOCH 1209284). To achieve this, the quantitative determination of standard gallic acid and curcumin was performed at 750 nm (Odomosu et al., 2015).

1.2.6 CELL CULTURES

For the assays, we used well cultures of 96 microplates, each assay consisted of 15,000 HuH-7 and HeLa cells, respectively. On the well suspensions were added the extract doses of *C. longa* and *Z. officinale* (Table 1.1) and trypan blue in order to assess the cell viability with MTS. The cells were taken from monolayer structure, leaking previously by trypsin; these cells were centrifuged at 2100 rpm by 5 min.

TABLE 1.1 Cell Viability Treatments and Doses.

Treatments and doses					
Treatments	**Doses (µg/mL)**				
Control –	–	–	–	–	–
Control +	40	40	40	40	40
Curcuma longa	5	15	25	35	50
Zingerber officinale	5	15	25	35	50

1.2.7 FLUORESCENCE STAINS

After 24 h of culture, the specific extract doses were added to HuH-7 and HeLa cell lines (Table 1.1); for positive control treatment, raloxifene was used. In order to determine cell inhibition, a differential staining with acridine orange and ethidium bromide was used, using the protocol reported by McGahon et al. (1995). Before every staining, the cell suspension was centrifuged at 2100 rpm by 5 min and 8 μL of fresh medium was added to it.

1.2.8 CYTOTOXICITY ASSAYS WITH LYMPHOCYTES

Lymphocytes from peripheral blood were isolated through differential centrifugation using Ficoll-Hipaque gradients (Hystopaque-1077, Sigma) at 1500 rpm, 30 min at room temperature, and washed twice with DME (Sigma-Aldrich) at 1500 rpm for 10 min. The initial viability was determined by the exclusion method using trypan blue (Sigma-Aldrich). For the cytotoxicity assay, 10,000 lymphocytes were used by triplícate probes in wells with 100 μL of volume; the tests included all extract concentrations probed (Table 1.1) with their respective controls. All the assays were performed at 37°C, with humid atmosphere and 5% of CO_2; besides the specific extract concentrations, the lymphocyte suspensions were supplemented with 2% of bovine fetal serum. The cytotoxicity assays were performed in MTS viability and a spectrophotometer UV–vis (EPOCH 1209284) at 490 nm through software Gen5.

1.2.9 STATISTICAL ANALYSIS

To establish significant statistical differences between extracts treatments, we used the Student's *t* test to determine significant differences between two independent experiments and two-way analysis of variance. The analysis was performed using the Software Prism 6 v6.01 (GraphPad). The significant differences were conducted at $P < 0.001$ and $P < 0.0001$.

1.2.10 EQUITOXIC DOSES IC_{50}

IC_{50} was estimated via the classic Hill equation (O'Connor et al., 2014):

$$\text{Vial [Extract]} = \text{Vial}_{\infty} + \frac{\text{Vial}_0 - \text{Vial}_{\infty}}{1 + \left(\frac{\text{Extract}}{\text{IC}_{50}}\right)^{\beta}} \tag{1.1}$$

where Vial (Extract) is the viability measured at a particular extract concentration, $Vial_\alpha$ corresponds to nonliving cells, $Vial_0$ is the cell viability in absence of extracts, and β refers to the slope factor or Hill coefficient, considering the extract concentration.

1.2.11 SPECIFIC CELL DEATH RATE

For the purpose of estimating the specific death rate of cell lines, we considered a reaction of first-order kinetic, then:

$$\frac{dN}{dt} = -KdN \quad (1.2)$$

Integrating:

$$N = Noe^{-Kdt} \quad (1.3)$$

$$\ln N = \ln No - Kdt \quad (1.4)$$

$$\ln\left(\frac{N}{No}\right) = -KdN \quad (1.5)$$

1.3 RESULTS

1.3.1 C. LONGA EXTRACT TREATMENTS

The cell viability assay (MTS) was determined once applied every dosage extract of *C. longa* on HuH-7 and HeLa cell line cultures (Table 1.1). In general terms, it was noted that with the increase of dosing in the extracts of *C. longa* on HuH-7 cell line cultures, the viability diminishes. For example, with 5 μg/mL of extract, the cell viability of the HuH-7 cell line was around 67%, 65.8%, and 65.8% in 24, 48, and 72 h, respectively. However, at the highest extract doses (50 μg/mL), the cell viability was 23.9%, 23.9%, and 21.2%, respectively (Fig. 1.1).

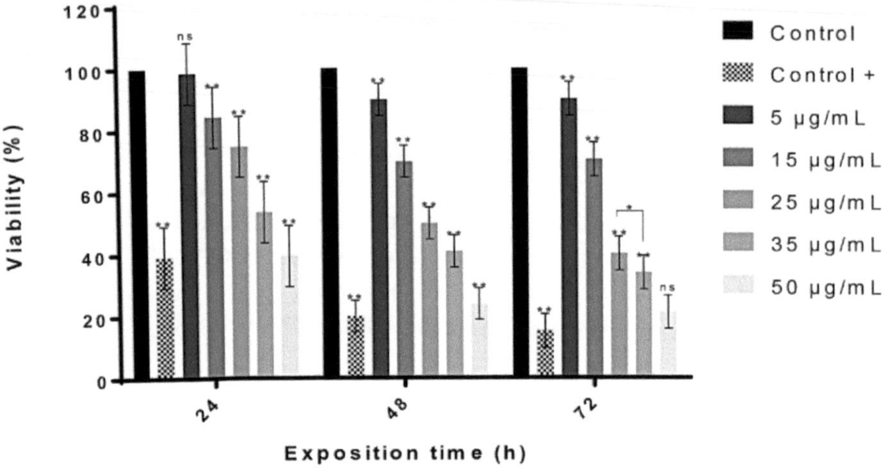

FIGURE 1.1 Viability of HuH-7 cell line at different concentrations of *C. longa* extracts. Significant difference (**P* = 0.0001, ***P* < 0.001). Error bars indicate standard deviation (*n* = 3).

This behavior also was observed in the HeLa cell line, at every curcumin concentration tested. At the lowest concentration (5 μg/mL) of *C. longa* extracts, in the same periods of incubation, the cell viability was kept at 100%, 85.5%, and 86.4%, respectively. On the other hand, when high extract doses (50 μg/mL) were used, the cell viability was kept at 75.4% (24 h), 34.5% (48 h), and 34% (72 h), respectively (Fig. 1.2).

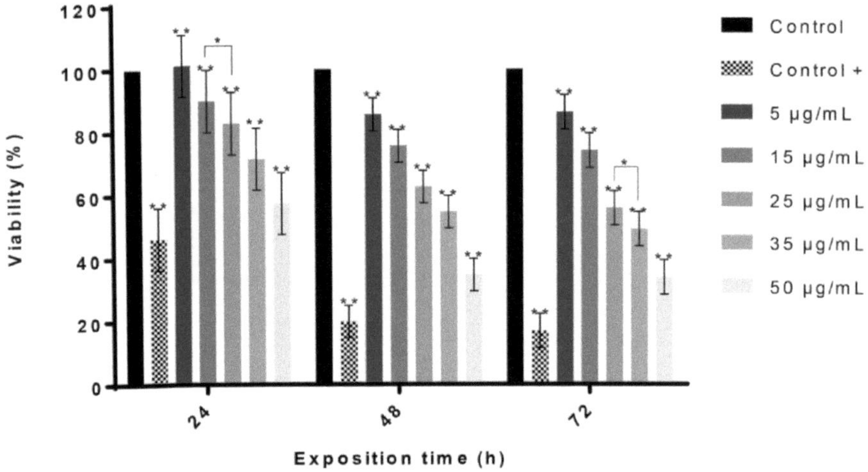

FIGURE 1.2 Viability of HeLa cell line at different concentrations of *C. longa* extracts. Significant difference (**P* = 0.0001, ***P* < 0.001). Error bars indicate standard deviation (*n* = 3).

In the meantime, the exact toxicity of *C. longa* was evaluated through its exposition on lymphocyte suspensions. Figure 1.3 shows that the reduction of cell viability was less than 20% in 24 h of exposition when the highest concentration of *C. longa* extract was used (50 μg/mL), suggesting that the toxicity of these compounds was minimal when compared with HuH-7 and HeLa cell lines. Figure 1.4 shows the IC_{50} values for HUH-7 cell line when exposed through 24, 48, and 72 h to different concentrations of *C. longa* extracts; these IC_{50} values correspond to 42.6, 42.3, and 20.6 at 24, 48, and 72 h, respectively. In the meantime, the IC_{50} values for HeLa cell line were 90.4, 300, and 385 for 24, 48, and 72 h, respectively.

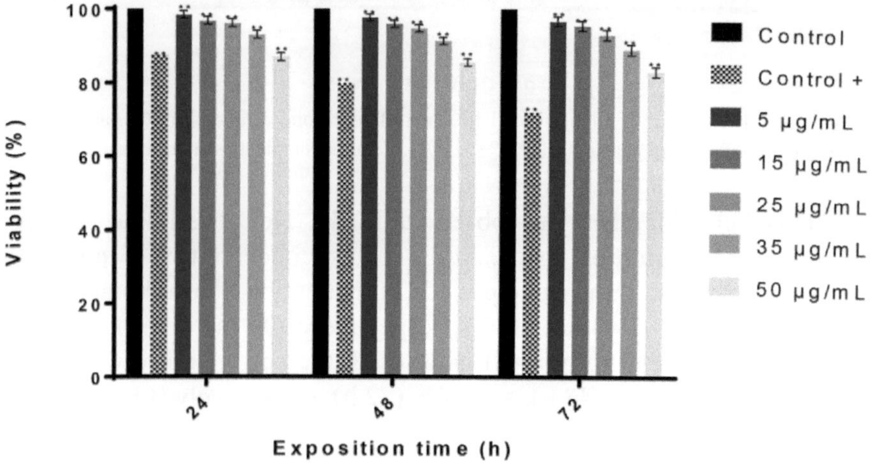

FIGURE 1.3 Viability of lymphocytes at different concentrations of *C. longa*. Significant difference (*$P = 0.0001$, **$P < 0.001$). Error bars indicate standard deviation ($n = 3$).

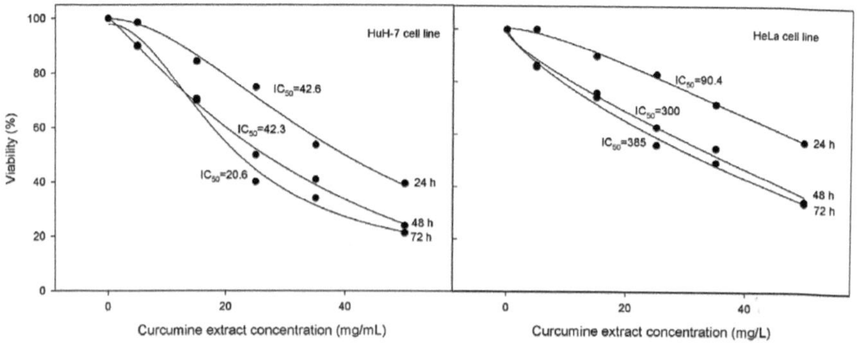

FIGURE 1.4 IC_{50} estimation for HuH-7 and HeLa cell lines when exposed at different exposition times of *C. longa*.

The specific death rate (K_d) of the cell lines exposed to every concentration of *C. longa* extracts was time-dependent to the exposition and extracts concentration. For example, for HUH-7 cell line (Fig. 1.5a), exposed at 50 μg/mL, the K_d values reached up to 0.038 h^{-1} at 24 h of exposition, but when the time of exposition was extended at 72 h, the K_d was only 0.024 h^{-1}. For HeLa cell line, at the same time and extracts concentration of *C. longa* extracts, the K_d was 0.018 h^{-1} (24 h) and 0.018 h^{-1} (72 h), indicating less tolerance.

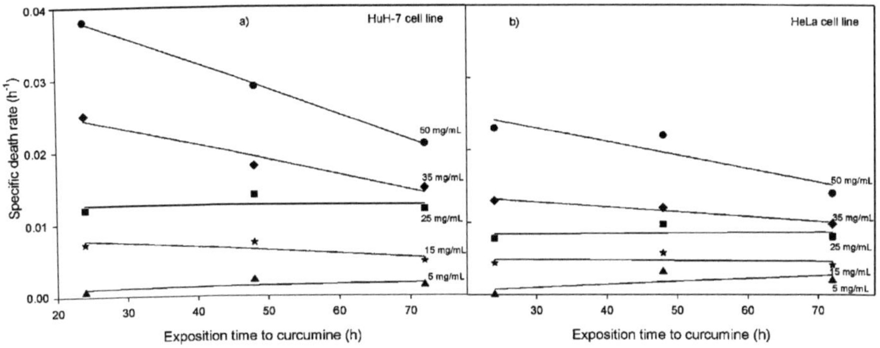

FIGURE 1.5 Specific death rate of (a) HuH-7 cell line and (b) HeLa cell line when was exposed at different times and concentrations of extracts of *C. longa*.

According to the morphological characteristics of HuH-7 and HeLa cell lines, the cells were classified into necrotic, apoptotic, and viable cells at 78 h of exposition with different extracts concentrations of *C. longa*. For HuH-7 cell line, at 5 μg/mL, the number of necrotic cells was 14%, but with 50 μg/mL, the necrotic cells significantly increase (53%); the percentage of apoptotic cells increased by 28% and 53%, respectively (Fig. 1.6).

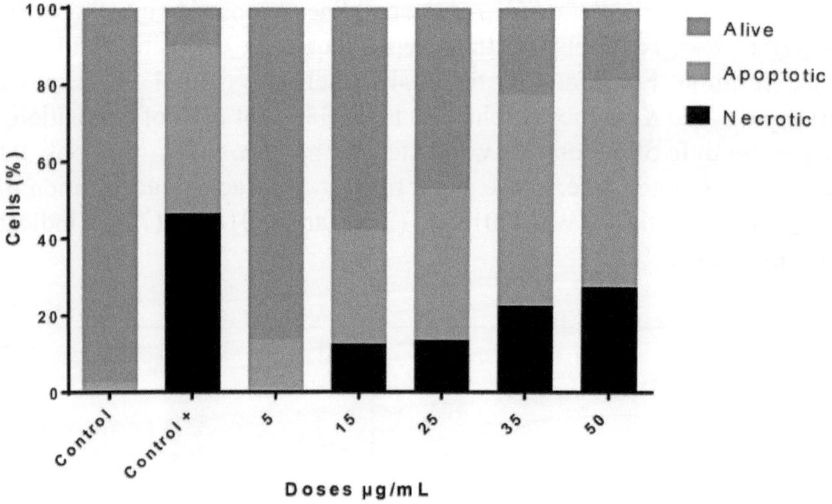

FIGURE 1.6 Relationship between apoptotic, necrotic, and alive cells of HuH-7 cell line at different extract doses of *C. longa.*

For HeLa cell line, with the same extract concentrations, the necrotic cells increase from 6% (5 µg/mL) to 45% (50 µg/mL) and the presence of apoptotic cells was 30% and 45%, respectively (Fig. 1.7).

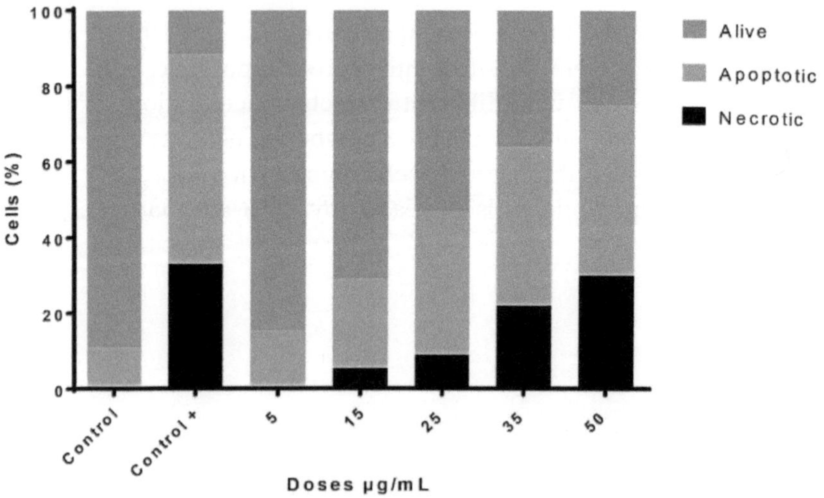

FIGURE 1.7 Relationship between apoptotic, necrotic, and alive cells of HeLa cell line at different extract doses of *C. longa.*

The morphological appearance of both cell lines was the chromatin condensation and loss of the characteristic morphology when observed with ethidium bromide and acridine orange staining; furthermore, the cell lines were unable to retain its current monolayer structure.

1.3.2 TREATMENTS WITH Z. OFFICINALE EXTRACT

For the analysis of the extracts' effect of *Z. officinale* on HuH-7 and HeLa cell lines, the same procedure was used as described for *C. longa* extracts. In the case of HuH-7 cell line, a greater inhibition was noticed when an extract concentration of 50 μg/mL (25% of viability) was added, in contrast at 5 μg/mL, the viability was around 77.8% (Fig. 1.8).

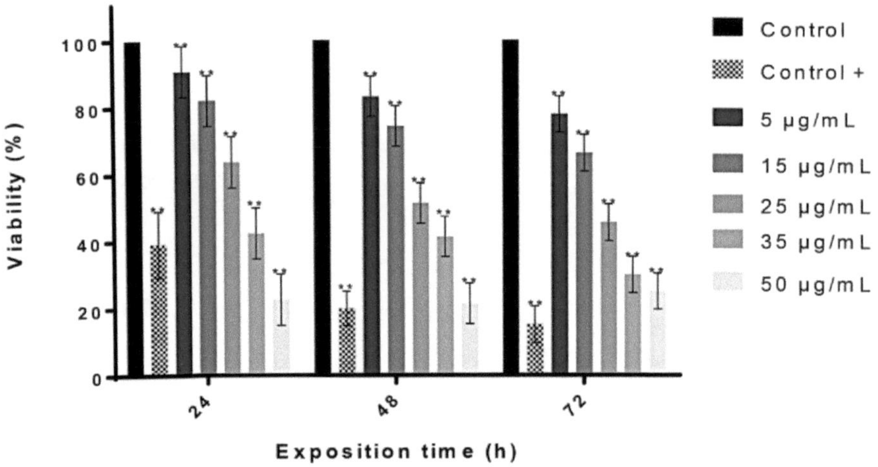

FIGURE 1.8 Viability of HuH-7 cell line at different concentrations of *Z. officinale* extracts. Significant difference (*P = 0.0001, **P < 0.001). Error bars indicate standard deviation (n = 3).

On the other hand, the inhibitory effect of HeLa cell line was slightly less, as the viability percentage was 40% with 50 μg/mL, while at 5 μg/mL, the cell viability was maintained at 91.2% (Fig. 1.9).

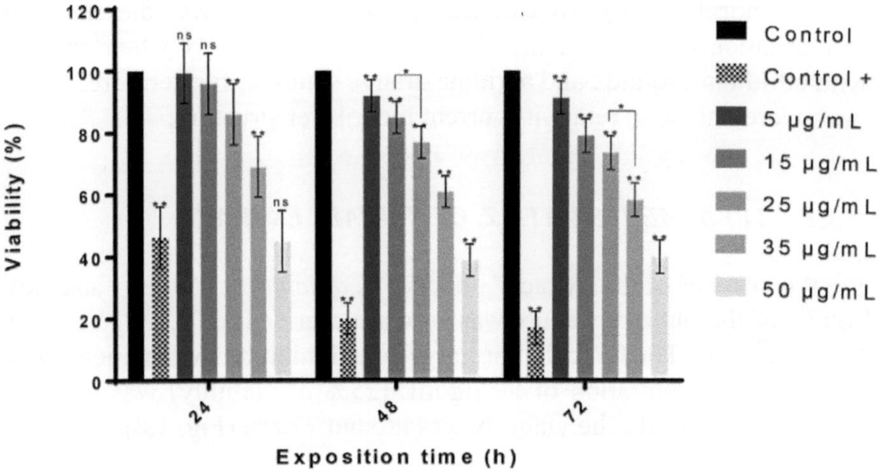

FIGURE 1.9 Viability of HeLa cell line at different concentrations of *Z. officinale* extracts. Significant difference (*$P = 0.0001$, **$P < 0.001$). Error bars indicate standard deviation ($n = 3$).

The toxicity evaluation of *Z. officinale* extracts remained up to 82% in all the treatments tested; the major toxic effect was achieved with 50 μg/mL (Fig. 1.10).

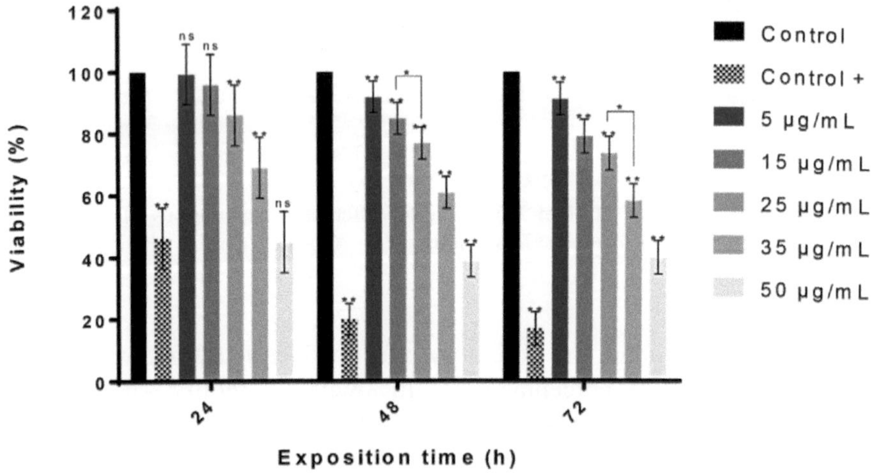

FIGURE 1.10 Viability of lymphocytes at different concentrations of *Z. officinale*. Significant difference (*$P = 0.0001$, **$P < 0.001$). Error bars indicate standard deviation ($n = 3$).

This indicates that if the extracts of *Z. officinale* were used in therapeutic treatments; they would have slight adverse effects in human cells. The morphological characteristics of HuH-7 and HeLa cell lines exposed to *Z. officinale* extracts showed chromatin condensation, loss of normal morphology, and inability to retain their current monolayer structure. Figure 1.11a shows the IC_{50} values of HUH-7 cell line exposed to *Z. officinale* extracts at 24 h (IC_{50} = 97.4), 48 h (IC_{50} = 101), and 72 h (IC_{50} = 440). On the other hand, the IC_{50} values for HeLa cell lines were 44.4, 60, and 80, at 24, 48, and 72 h, respectively (Fig. 1.11b).

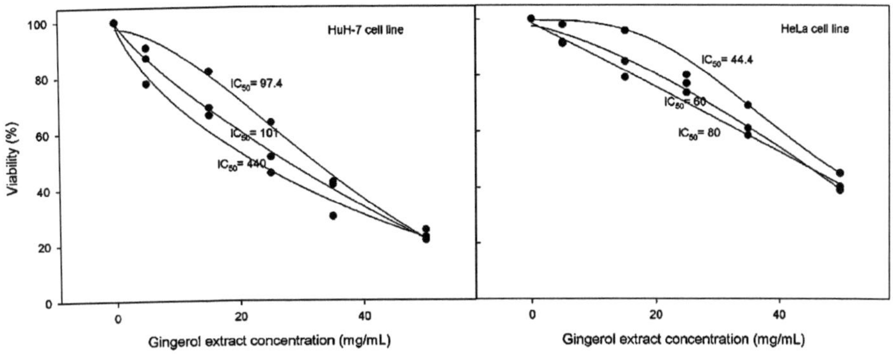

FIGURE 1.11 IC_{50} estimation for HuH-7 and HeLa cell lines when exposed at different exposition times of *Z. officinale*.

Finally, the K_d for HUH-7 cell line exposed to 50 μg/mL *Z. officinale* extracts were 0.06 h^{-1} at 24 h and 0.025 h^{-1} at 72 h of exposition (Fig. 1.12a). For HeLa cell line, K_d was slightly lower at 50 μg/mL, for example, K_d was around 0.038 h^{-1}, 0.022 h^{-1}, and 0.019 h^{-1} at 24, 48, and 72 h of exposition, respectively (Fig. 1.12b).

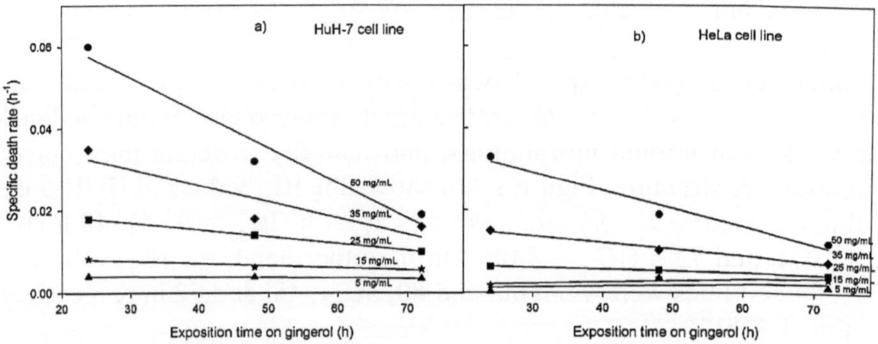

FIGURE 1.12 Specific death rate of (a) HuH-7 cell line and (b) HeLa cell line when exposed at different times and concentrations of extracts of *Z. officinale*.

The quantification of necrotic cells for HuH-7 cell line with 50 μg/mL of extract dose was approximately 26%, apoptotic cells of 44% and 40% of viable cells, the complete results are shown in Figure 1.13.

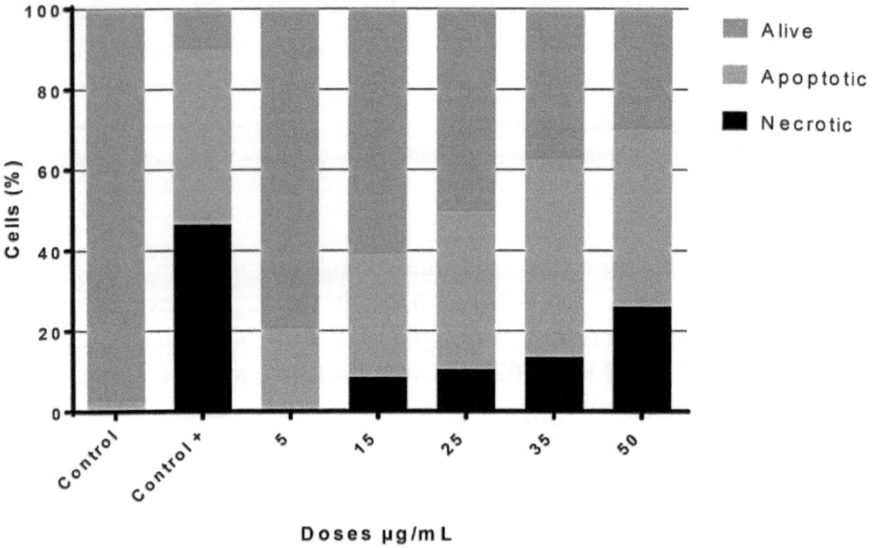

FIGURE 1.13 Relationship between apoptotic, necrotic, and alive cells of HuH-7 cell line at different extract doses of *Z. officinale*.

Finally, for HeLa cell lines with 50 μg/mL of dose extract of *Z. officinale*, the percentage of necrotic cells was around 26%, apoptotic cells were 48%, and viable cells were 26% (Fig. 1.14). We conclude that the extract of *Z. officinale* was more effective against HeLa cell line than for HuH-7 cell line.

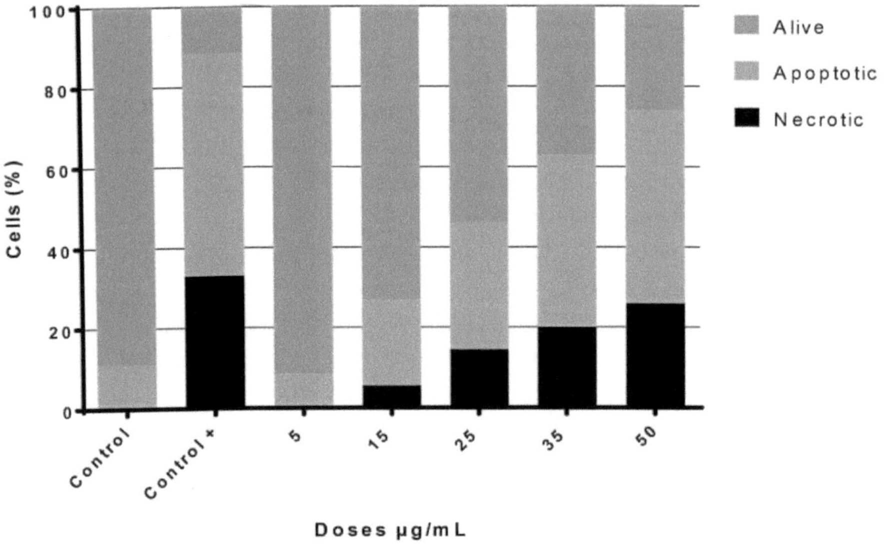

FIGURE 1.14 Relationship between apoptotic, necrotic, and alive cells of HeLa cell line at different extract doses of *Z. officinale*.

1.4 DISCUSSION

In the current investigation, the capacity of reducing cell proliferation was proved on tumor cell lines HuH-7 and HeLa, using extracts from *C. longa* and *Z. officinale* at different exposition times and dosage strengths, such variables being fundamentals in growth inhibition of tumor cell lines (Anand et al., 2008; Yang et al., 2006; Keum et al., 2002). The loss of cell viability depends on the extract concentration and exposure time; thus, it has been shown that adding these vegetable extracts causes cell death through the activation the apoptosis signaling (Anand et al., 2008; Yang et al., 2006; Keum et al., 2002). In previous studies, it was shown that curcumin, in combination with commercial Taxol (paclitaxel), increases its effectiveness. As reported by Dang et al. (2015), using treatment of 5 µL of paclitaxel with 10 µL of curcumin for 24 h obtain a cell viability of 45% ($P < 0.01$) of HeLa cell line. According to Gupta and Panda (2002), who obtained 28% of inhibition in the HeLa cell line at 10 μM of concentration, previous results showed that curcumin inhibits cell cycle progression in G2-M phase by means of decreasing Cdc2, a molecule that induces apoptosis. This event is characterized by the collapsing of the mitotic spindle, presence of tiny microtubules, and rarely, the metaphase induced that the chromosomes misaligned. This phenomenon can be explained by the fact of the curcumin causes the depolymerization of the microtubules. For example, at 100 μM the tubulin assembly reduced 59%. The curcumin disturbs the dynamic of the microtubules, by reducing the GTPasa activity, inducing aggregation of tubulin dimers and its depolymerization in the interphase (Gupta and Panda, 2002).

Yan et al. (2010) report that the treatment of 100 mg/kg of curcumin before the administration of docetaxel, a drug similar to taxol, increases the anticancer effect in rodents. At low curcumin concentrations, it was possible to detect apoptotic cells showing a size reduction, the chromatin distributed in the nuclear membrane with different shapes and sizes; moreover, the cells showed a denser cytoplasm, compared with control treatments. Programmed cell death or apoptosis is intrinsically linked to the mitochondria; this phenomenon occurs due to the deprivation of growth factors that induce the inactivation of caspase activity or activated in response by lethal stimuli, such as DNA damage, oxidative stress, hypoxia, chemotherapeutic drugs, reduction of the mitochondrial membrane potential (ΔΨm), and the cytochrome c releasing, which is a characteristic marker of apoptosis (Jian-Ye et al., 2015).

According to the results published by Chakraborty et al. in 2012, the bioactive 6-gingerol, derived from the *Zingiber* sp. extract, the equitoxic dose (IC_{50}) was determined in HeLa cell line at values around 126.89 and 114.58 μg/mL at 24 and 48 h, respectively ($P < 0.05$). In these treatments, it was observed: dose-dependent chromatin condensation, cell fragmentation, and reduction of mitochondrial membrane potential. The ginger extract contains a great number of polyphenols and flavones; these compounds have activity against cancer (Chakraborty et al., 2012). The *Zingiber* sp. extract has the potential as an agent against hepatic inflammation, because 6-gingerol molecule inhibits IL-6, IL-8, and SAA1 in HuH-7 cell line when stimulated by cytokines; the mechanism includes the suppression of COX2 receptors via NF-kB signaling; this anti-inflammatory activity avoids insulin or resistance, which is related to type 2 diabetes (Roufogalis, 2014).

With the results achieved during this investigation, the optimal inhibitory dose was determined for every extract treatment: for curcumin extracts, these doses were 35 and 50 μg/mL for HuH-7 and HeLa cell lines, respectively. In the case of *Z. officinale* extracts, they were obtained the same inhibitory concentrations for both of cell lines. In all the evaluations proved, the lymphocytes kept viability at values more than 80%. The efficiency of extract combinations for HeLa cell line, the inhibition was greater with the extract treatments of *Z. officinale* and *C. longa*. Thus, here we demonstrated that the extracts proved could be used to protect the health and these compounds can be added to the list of natural and chemical products normally used against cancer. The anticancer compounds include coumarins, diterpenes, dithiolethiones, indoles, isothiocyanates, lactones, organosulphides, and phenols. The compounds with chemoprevention properties against cancer are subdivided into blocking agents and suppression agents; their mode of action during carcinogenesis is to prevent that carcinogen substances alter DNA sequence or cause mutations (Hayes et al., 1999). The removal capacity of xenobiotic agents is normally achieved by increasing the expression levels of detoxification system and antioxidant capacity in the tissues, although alterations in the pharmacokinetics of the xenobiotics serve as body protectors from carcinogenesis and tumorigenesis. These cell responses could be a result of cellular adaptation, oxidative stress, and for the stimulation of apoptosis or cellular differentiation (Hayes et al., 1999).

Hepatic cell carcinoma is associated with hepatitis virus B or C infection; the genesis of hepatocellular carcinoma is triggered by the oxidative stress generated by these viruses (Hagen et al., 1994). The somatic cells are different to tumoral cells in their metabolism; somatic cells obtain their energy through the aerobic oxidation of the glucose, which is the oxidative phosphorylation in the mitochondria. In the case of tumoral cells, the production of energy depends basically on the glycolysis, despite the rich presence of oxygen (Annibaldi and Widman, 2010), although the molecular mechanisms in tumoral cells remain largely unknown in these molecular actions behind the nature of immortality (Warburg, 1956). In this context, it is widely accepted that the increase of the glycolysis activity in tumoral cells is a key process for maintaining the phenotype. The oxidative stress plays a key role in different malignant diseases, such as atherosclerosis, diabetes, and viral infections (Behrend et al., 2003). The reactive oxygen species (ROS) can cause DNA oxidation and damage both proteins and tumor suppressor genes, causing the increase of expression levels of proto-oncogenes; it has been shown that the oxidative stress induces the malignant transformation of cells *in vitro* (Bohr et al., 1999). Dröge (2002) associated the diseases with oxidative stress, including diabetes mellitus and cancer; these conditions show a pro-oxidant action on the redox state and an alteration in the mechanism of glucose elimination, which suggests that the muscle mitochondria is the primary site of intense production of ROS. Patients with cancer reduced their capacity of glucose elimination, glycolytic activity, and lactate production. Therefore, there is a pro-oxidative shift and this change is mediated by the increase of energetic substrate availability in the mitochondria.

The oxidative inflammatory conditions are typically associated with an excessive stimulation of NAD(P)H by citokines, including other factors (Dröge, 2002). Wei et al. (1998) argue that such ROS produced by mitochondria itself are the main substances that cause their own damage. The oxygen consumption by the cells is around 85% for ATP production; however, during the process of oxidative phosphorylation, about 0.4–4% of oxygen is converted in superoxide radicals (O_2) and then turned into H_2O_2 by the action of manganese superoxide dismutase (MnSOD) or copper/zinc superoxide dismutase (Cu/ZnSOD), and subsequently transformed into water by glutathione peroxidase, being this one quite important as an antioxidant. Considering that mitochondria are the only organelles, besides the cell nucleus, that has its own DNA; the main difference between them is that the nuclear DNA is protected by histones besides possessing repair mechanisms; this property causes for mitochondrial DNA to become susceptible to damage by free radicals (Wei et al., 1998). The processes of DNA repairing and its instability, ruptures of the DNA chain, and presence of alkali labile sites, purine, and pyrimidine oxidases are the main causes of genetic mutations on oxidative damage to DNA (Breen and Murphy, 1995). Due to the multiple DNA modifications produced by ROS, it is hard to establish the frequency and specificity of such mutations induced by oxygen radicals. Some of these modified bases have mutagenic properties; therefore, if they are not repaired, they may lead to a process of carcinogenesis.

Studies show that the four bases are modified by ROS, mainly modify the base pairs guanine–cytosine; nevertheless, the base pairs adenine–cytosine mutations are extremely rare (Retel et al., 1993). Higher level of modified bases in cancer tissue due to the great amount of H_2O_2 produced is a feature of human cancer cells. Samali et al. (1999) define the apoptosis as a type of cell death mediated by caspases and the cells have the following morphological characteristics: nuclear and cytoplasmic condensation, chromatin excision, apoptotic body apparition, maintenance of the plasmatic membrane structure intact, exposure on their surface molecules that conveys addressing toward phagocytosis. More specifically, the molecular definition of apoptosis covers the proteolytic activity of certain caspases (caspase-2, -3, -6, -7, -8, -9, and -10); these enzymes mediate the process of apoptotic cell death. The apoptotic cells can display a variety of signals of recognition which are detected by the phagocytes and are then eliminated.

Recent evidence suggests that some apoptotic cells may secrete chemotactic factors that cause local accumulation of macrophages. The content released by necrotic cells includes molecules acting as signals in order to promote inflammation. On the contrary, the absorption of apoptotic bodies abolishes the secretion of inflammatory mediators from activated macrophages. Therefore, a critical component of all definitions of apoptosis and autophagy is their anti-inflammatory performance. An essential element of oncosis is its inflammatory nature (Shi et al., 2003).

1.5 CONCLUSION

In this investigation, the capacity of growth inhibition of human hepatocarcinoma (HuH-7) and carcinoma uterine cervix (HeLa) with the secondary metabolites curcumin and gingerol was proved when added extracts of *C. longa* and *Z. officinale*, respectively. The extract of *C. longa*, when added at dose of 35 μg/mL, was optimal against cell line HuH-7 proliferation, and for HeLa, the optimal results were achieved at doses of 50 μg/mL. In the meantime, the extract of *Z. officinale*, the best inhibitory effect was obtained in doses of 50 μg/mL for both cell lines. However, the effectiveness of these extract doses was knowing the best when comparing with the rest of the treatments.

KEYWORDS

- ***Curcuma longa***
- **curcumin**
- **extracts gingerol**
- **HeLa cell line**
- **HuH-7 cell line**
- ***Zingiber officinale***

REFERENCES

Ali, B. H.; Blunden, G.; Tanira, M. O.; Nemmar, A. Some Phytochemical, Pharmacological and Toxicological Properties of Ginger (*Zingiber officinale* Roscoe): A Review of Recent Research. *Food Chem. Toxicol.* **2008,** *46,* 409–420.

Ames, B. N.; Gold, L. S. Paracelsus to Parascience: The Environmental Cancer Distraction. *Mutar. Res.* **2000,** *447,* 3–13.

Anand, P.; Sundaram, C.; Jhurani, S.; Kunnumakkara, A. B.; Aggarwal, B. B. Curcumin and Cancer an "Old Age" Disease With an Age Old Solution. *Cancer Lett.* 2008, *267,* 133–164.

Annibaldi, A.; Widmann, C. Glucose Metabolism in Cancer Cells. *Curr. Opin. Clin. Nutr. Metab. Care* **2010,** *13,* 466–470.

Behrend, L.; Henderson, G.; Zwacka, R. M. Reactive Oxygen Species in Oncogenic Transformation. *Biochem. Soc. Trans.* **2003,** *31* (6), 1441–1444.

Bohr, V. A.; Dianov, G. L. Oxidative DNA Damage Processing in Nuclear and Mitochondrial DNA. *Biochimie* 1999, *81* (1–2), 155–160.

Breen, A. P.; Murphy, JA. Reactions of Oxyl Radicals With DNA. *Free Radic. Biol. Med.* 1995, *18* (6), 1033–1077.

Chakraborty, D.; Bishayee, K.; Ghosh, S.; Biswas, R.; Mandal, S. K.; Khuda-Bukhsh, A. R. [6]-Gingerol Induces Caspase 3 Dependent Apoptosis and Autophagy in Cancer cells: Drug DNA Interaction and Expression of Certain Signal Genes in HeLa Cells. *Eur. J. Pharmacol.* **2012,** *694,* 20–29.

Chrubasik, S.; Pittler, M. H.; Roufogalis, B. D. Zingiberis Rhizoma: A Comprehensive Review on the Ginger Effect and Efficacy Profiles. *Phytomedicine* **2005,** *12,* 684–701.

Colder, C. R.; Lloyd-Richardson, E. E.; Flaherty, B. P.; Hedeker, D.; Segawa, E.; Flay, B. R. The Natural History of College Smoking: Trajectory of Daily Smoking During the Freshman Year. *Addit. Behav.* **2006,** *31* (12), 2212–2222.

Cos, S. P. Cúrcuma I (*Curcuma longa* L.). *Serie Botánica* **2014,** *7* (2), 84–99.

Dang, Y. P.; Yuan, X. Y.; Tian, R.; Li, D. G.; Liu, W. Curcumin Improves the Paclitaxel-Induced Apoptosis of HPV-Positive Human Cervical Cancer Cells Via the NF-κB-p53-Caspase-3 Pathway. *Exp. Ther. Med.* **2015,** *9* (4), 1470–1476.

Dröge, W. Free Radicals in the Physiological Control of Cell Function. *Physio. Rev.* 2002, *82* (1), 47–95.

Ekundayo, O. Composition of Ginger (*Zingiber officinale* Roscoe) Volatile Oils From Nigeria. *Flavour Fragr. J.* **1998,** *3,* 85–90.

Flay, B. R.; DuBois, D.; Allred, C. G.; Berbaum, M. The Positive Action Program. Social and Character Development Research Program Biannual Meeting; Arlington, VA 2006; pp 19–20.

Govindarajan, V. S. Ginger Chemistry, Technology, and Quality Evaluation: Part 2. *Crit. Rev. Food Sci. Nutr.* **1982,** *17,* 189–258.

Gupta, K.; Panda, D. Perturbation of Microtubule Polymerization by Quercetin Through Tubulin Binding: A Novel Mechanism of its Antiproliferative Activity. *Biochemistry* **2002,** *41,* 13029–13038.

Hagen, T. M.; Huang, S.; Curnutte, J.; Fowler, P.; Martinez, V.; Wehr, C. M.; Ames, B. N.; Chisari, F. V. Extensive Oxidative DNA Damage in Hepatocytes of Transgenic Mice With Chronic Active Hepatitis Destined to Develop Hepatocellular Carcinoma. *Proc. Natl. Acad. Sci. USA* **1994,** *91,* 12808–12812.

Hayes, J. D.; Ellis, E. M.; Neal, G. E.; Harrison, D. J.; Manson, M. M. Cellular Response to Cancer Chemopreventive Agents: Contribution of the Antioxidant Responsive Element to the Adaptive Response to Oxidative and Chemical Stress. *Biochem. Soc. Symp.* **1999,** *64,* 141–168.

Keum, Y. S.; Kim, J.; Lee, K. H.; Park, K. K.; Surth, Y. J.; Lee, J. M.; Lee, S. S.; Yoon, J. H.; Joo, S. Y.; Cha, I. H.; Yook, J. I. Induction of Apoptosis and Caspase-3 Activation by Chemopreventive [6]-paradol and Structurally Related Compounds in KB Cells. *Cancer Lett.* **2002,** *177,* 41–47.

Malcom, R. A. Cancer. In *Encyclopedia of Life Sciences*, 2001.

McGahon, A. J.; Martin, S. J.; Bissonnette, R. P.; Mahboubi, A.; Shi, Y. F.; Mogil, R. J.; Green, R. D. The End of the (Cell) Line: Methods for the Study of Apoptosis in Vitro. *Methods Cell Biol.* **1995,** *46,* 153–185.

Menon, V. P; Sudheer, A. R. Antioxidant and Anti-inflammatory Properties of Curcumin. *Exp Med. Biol.* **2007,** *595,* 105–125.

O'Connor, M.; Lee, C.; Ellens, H.; Bentz, J. A Novel Application of t-Statistics to Objectively Asses the Quality of IC50 Fits for p-Glycoprotein and Other Trasnsporters. *Pharmacol. Res. Perspect.* **2014,** *3* (1), 1–16.

Odumosu, P.; Ojerinde, S.; Egbuchiem, M. Polyphenolic Contents of Some Instant Tea Brands and Their Anti-Oxidant Activities. *J. Appl. Pharm. Sci.* **2015,** *5* (9), 100–105.

Organización Mundial de la Salud [OMS]. 10 Datos Sobre el Cáncer [Online] 2014. http://www.who.int/features/factfiles/cancer/es/. Accessed 10 may 2016.

Retel, J.; Hoebee, B.; Braun, J. E.; Lutgerink, J. T.; Van den Akker, E.; Wanamarta, A. H.; Joenje, H.; Lafleur, M. V. Mutational Specificity of Oxidative DNA Damage. *Mutat. Res.* **1993,** *299,* 165–182.

Roufogalis, B. D. *Zingiber officinale* (Ginger): A Future Outlook on Its Potential in Prevention and Treatment of Diabetes and Prediabetic States. *New J. Sci.* **2014,** *55* (6), 2129–2136.

Samali, A.; Zhivotovsky, B.; Jones, D.; Nagata, S.; Orrenius, S. Apoptosis: Cell Death Defined by Caspase Activation. *Cell Death Differ.* 1999, 6, 495–496.

Shi, Y.; Evans, J. E.; Rock, K. L. Molecular Identification of a Danger Signal That Alerts the Immune System to Dying Cells. *Nature* **2003,** *425,* 516–521.

Singh, Y. N. Therapeutic Potential of Kava in the Treatment of Anxiety Disorders. *CNS Drugs* 2002, *16* (13), 731–743.

Warburg, O. On Respiratory Impairment in Cancer Cells. *Science* **1956,** *124,* 269–270.

Wei, Y. H.; Lu, C. Y.; Lee, H. C.; Pang, C. Y.; Ma, Y. S. Oxidative Damage and Mutation to Mitochondrial DNA and Agedependent Decline of Mitochondrial Respiratory Function. *Ann. N. Y. Acad. Sci.* **1998,** *854,* 155–170.

Yan, Y. D.; Kim, D. H.; Sung, J. H.; Yong, C. S.; Choi, H. G. Enhanced Oral Bioavailability of Docetaxel in Rats by Four Consecutive Days of Pretreatment With Curcumin. *Int. J. Pharm.* **2010,** *339,* 116–120.

Yang, J. H.; Hsia, T. C.; Kuo, H. M.; Chao, P. D.; Chou, C. C.; Wei, Y. H.; Chung, J. G. Inhibition of Lung Cancer Cell Growth by Quercetin Glucuronides Via G2/M Arrest and Induction of Apoptosis. *Drug Metab. Dispos.* **2006,** *34,* 296–304.

Yang, Z.; Xiong, H. R. Culture Conditions and Types of Growth Media for Mammalian Cells in Biomedical Tissue Culture. InTechOpen, 2012; pp 1–18.

CHAPTER 2

Role of Herbal Medicines in Liver Cancer

S. NIZAMUDEEN[1], YUMNA BAQI[2], and SARAFRAZ ARQUM SHAH[3]

[1]*Government Unani Medical College, Chennai, Tamil Nadu, India*

[2]*Department of Saidla, Aligarh Muslim University, Aligarh, Uttar Pradesh, India*

[3]*Department of Radio-Diagnostics, Maharishi Markandeshwar University, Mullana, Ambala, Haryana, India*

ABSTRACT

Cancer is defined as uncontrolled cellular growth anywhere in the body which is considered to be unnatural, as the normal cellular physiology is disrupted and spreads throughout the body via bloodstream. According to WHO estimates in 2020, cancer is the foremost cause of mortality, which accounts for nearly 10 million deaths globally. Various types of reactive species are considered to be potent oxidizing agents, with capability of damaging DNA and other biomolecules, and can stimulate the progression of malignancy, which becomes the major reason for the increased risk of cancer development. Many studies proposed that lower antioxidant activity increases the risk of cancer. Consequently, the use of antioxidants can avert the growth of malignant cells or cause the destruction of cancer-developing cells. It has been revealed that grains, vegetables, fruits, and medicinal plants possess a protective effect against the development of several diseases including cancer. This protection is mainly attributed due to the phytochemicals present in them. Many of the medicinal plants have potential hepatogenic/hepatoprotective properties and prevent

Plant-Derived Anticancer Drugs in the OMICS Era: Biosynthesis, Functions, and Applications.
Deepu Pandita, Anu Pandita (Eds.)

hepatotoxicity produced by hepatotoxicants. Many of the medicinal plants possess versatile immunomodulatory, antioxidant, and phagocytic activities and accordingly may be beneficial in liver diseases. Recently, number of phytomedicines is the area of interest and being used for the prevention, management, and treatment of various hepatic diseases. Many experimental studies of these plant-derived phytochemicals and their formulation encompass hepatogenic/hepatoprotective effects in liver diseases or reduce hepatotoxicity caused by hepatotoxic agents such as chemicals, drugs, pollutants, and infections.

2.1 INTRODUCTION

Cancer is a Latin word for "crab;" it is an abnormal cell growth with undefined boundary and it has the tendency to rapidly proliferate in an uncontrolled fashion and some can rapidly metastasized to other parts of the body. Cancer cells can grow from any tissue which is named after the origin of its growth and its characteristic features. Cells become cancerous because of the accumulation of defects or mutations in their DNA.

Global cancer estimates in 2020 suggest that there were 19.3 million newly diagnosed cases with a mortality of 10 million cases. CA breast in female is the most common form of cancer with 11.7% of total cases, closely followed by CA lung 11.4%, colorectal carcinoma 10.0%, prostate cancer 7.3%, CA stomach 5.6%, and liver cancer 4.7%. Among all the cancers, the mortality of carcinoma lung is leading with 18.0% of the total cancer deaths, followed by colorectal carcinoma 9.4%, liver cancer (8.3%), CA stomach 7.7%, and female CA breast 6.9%. In India, 2020 estimates suggest that the incidence of cancer in male was 679,421 (i.e., 94.1/100,000) and female patients was 712,758 (i.e., 103.6/100,000). One in 68 males (lung cancer), 1 in 29 females (breast cancer), and 1 in 9 Indians will develop cancer during their lifetime (0–74 years of age). Incidence and mortality of CA lung are the most common to occur in men, that is, 1 in 68 males, and CA breast is the most common to occur in females, that is, 1 in 29 followed by CA prostate, colorectal carcinoma, and liver cancer (GCS, 2020; Kooti et al., 2017; Shu-Yi et al., 2013).

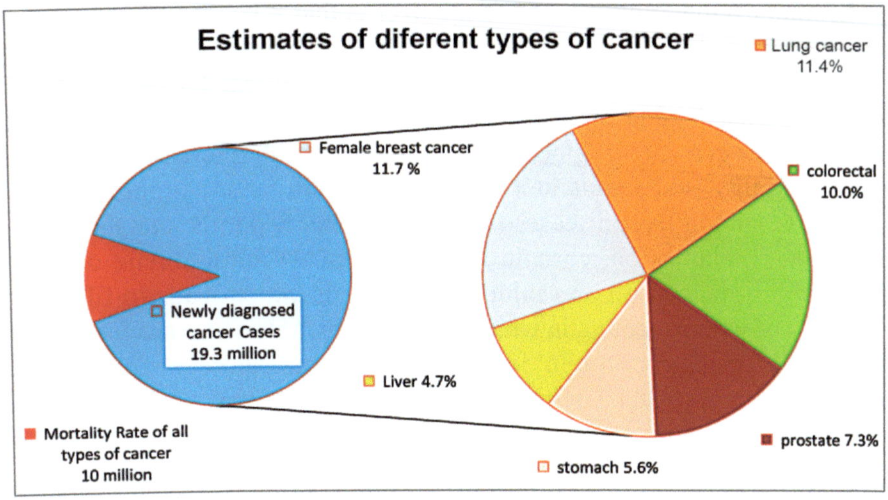

FIGURE 2.1 2020 global estimates.

Medicinal plants produce a number of biochemical compounds; the secondary metabolites of these compounds do not play a direct role in plant's growth. The important constituents of these secondary metabolites are alkaloids, terpenoids, flavonoids, pigments, and tannins. These secondary metabolites encompass many of the biological properties such as anti-inflammatory and anticancerous, as a contraceptive and diverse effect on hematopoietic cells, lipids, and the cardiovascular system (Kooti et al., 2017). Medicinal plants and herbs are used since the evolution of mankind since few decades' medicinal plants' derivatives and their phytochemical compounds are being very well recognized for treatment cancer cells. Many of the scientific clinical studies have been reported for the advantageous effects of medicinal herbs along with conventional therapeutics on increasing immune response and reducing the growth of cancer cells which can increase the survival rate and quality of life (QOL) in cancer patients (Shu-Yi et al., 2013).

2.2 LIVER CANCER

Liver is the largest exocrine and endocrine gland of the human body, which weighs about 1.5 kg in an adult; it plays a pivotal role in metabolism of carbohydrates, proteins, fats, and secrete bile which regulates many enzymatic actions for the metabolism of intestinal lipids and its absorption.

The major remarkable feature of the liver is that it has the competence to regenerate up to 75% of parenchymal tissues in a few weeks after damage to the liver cells (Wallace et al., 2018). The "Global burden of disease 2010 estimate" suggests that hepatic diseases represent 1.03 million per year causing a major global health burden, with increased morbidity and mortality, and stands in a row with the 14th most common cause of death. Common liver diseases like chronic viral hepatitis, metabolic liver diseases, malnutrition, chronic alcohol abuse, or autoimmune disorders lead to constant insult and injury to liver cells which leads to fibrosis, a process of wound healing in which the parenchymal tissues are enclosed by extracellular matrix protein deposits and undergo rigorous structural and functional modification with succeeding complications, such as cirrhosis of liver/hepatocellular carcinoma (Marra et al., 2014; Wallace et al., 2018; Yang et al., 2018). Globally, chronic liver diseases represent a major health concern, diseases like chronic viral hepatitis, metabolic disorders, malnutrition, alcohol abuse, or autoimmune diseases induce chronic liver injury with succeeding complications such as cirrhosis of liver or hepatocellular carcinoma (Giannitrapani et al., 2014). And global scenario, the "global burden of disease 2010 study," represents that liver disease is the 14th most common cause of death with morbidity and mortality of 1.03 million per year globally (Yang et al., 2018). In India, among general population, the prevalence of liver disease was found to be around 9–32%. Rural areas are more prevalent for liver disease in India than urban areas due to lack of awareness on health education and advanced medical facilities. WHO in May 2014 published its estimates on mortality due to liver diseases in India, which indicates that death due to liver disease has reached around 216,865, that is, 2.44% of total deaths (Unnati et al., 2018). Recent scenario in 2020 projected that there is a steep rise in deaths due to liver disease making it to stand on the 12th leading cause of death (Murray et al., 2020).

2.3 RISK FACTORS OF LIVER CANCER (SINGAL AND EL-SERAG, 2015)

- Hepatitis B or hepatitis C virus infection
- Chronic alcohol abuse
- Nonalcoholic fatty liver disease (NAFLD)
- Smoking, obesity, diabetes type I, or type II.

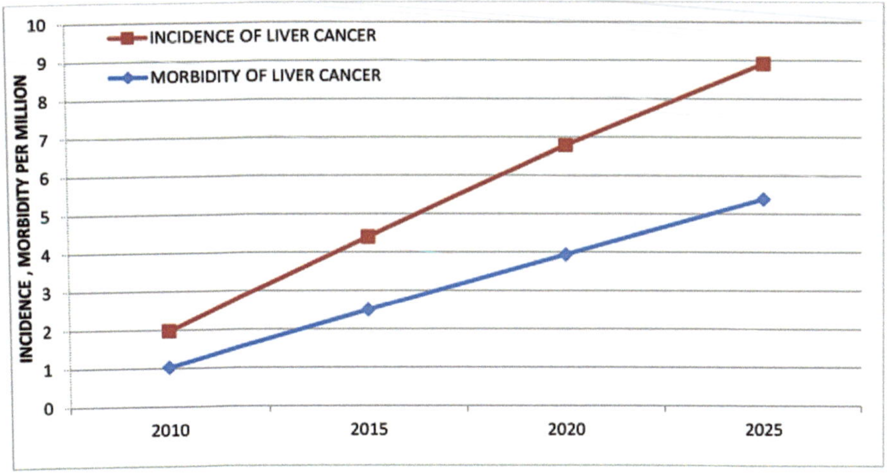

FIGURE 2.2 Liver cancer incidence and morbidity rate per million.

2.4 LIVER CANCER TYPES

1. **Hepatocellular carcinoma/Hepatoma**: According to the American Society of Clinical Oncology, hepatocellular carcinoma (HCC) is the most common form of liver cancer and accounts for about three-fourths of all liver cancer cases, that is, 75% of all liver cancer types. HCC mainly targets hepatocellular cells which occur due to Hepatitis B or Hepatitis C virus infection or liver cirrhosis caused by chronic alcohol abuse. It is more prevalent in men than women; in 2021, nearly 42,230 US adults are likely to be diagnosed with liver cancer. HCC may start as a solitary growing tumor which perhaps spreads all through the hepatic cells at more advanced stages or it illustrates as multiple small tumors. The second type of liver cancer is more common and is associated with cirrhosis of liver (Balogh et al., 2016).

2. **Fibrolamellar HCC**: **Fibrolamellar HCC** is an uncommon type of hepatocellular carcinoma that is usually much more responsive to treatment than other types of liver cancer. The management of fibrolamellar HCC is similar to HCC. The incidence of **fibrolamellar HCC** is common in women younger than age 35. According to the American Cancer Society, nearly 1% of all HCC are fibrolamellar HCC (Torbenson, 2012).

3. **Cholangio-carcinoma (bile duct cancer)**: The carcinoma which originates from the tube-like structures called bile ducts, which carry the bile from the hepatic cells into the gallbladder, is called cholangio-carcinoma; this form of carcinoma accounts for about 10–20% of all liver cancers. The cancer which begins inside the ducts is called intrahepatic bile-duct cancer; the cancer which begins outside the bile ducts is called extrahepatic bile-duct cancer (Buettner et al., 2017).
4. **Angiosarcoma**: It accounts for about 1% of all types of liver cancer; it can also be called colangio-carcinoma. Angiosarcomas take its root from the hepatic blood vessels and grow very rapidly; mostly angiosarcomas are diagnosed at an advanced stage where it becomes a difficult task in the management and treatment of angiosarcoma (Cao et al., 2019).
5. **Secondary liver cancer**: A study in 2016 published by *SAGE Journal* states that secondary liver cancers are much more common than primary liver cancer, as metastasis in liver develops when primary cancer spreads to the liver from other parts of the body. Most of the liver metastases instigate from colon or colorectal cancer. More than 50% of diagnosed patients with colorectal cancer probably grow secondary liver cancer (EASL Clinical Practice Guidelines, 2018).

2.5 STAGES OF LIVER CANCER (AMERICAN JOINT COMMITTEE ON CANCER, 2017)

Stage I: One tumor is found in the liver only.

Stage II: One tumor is found, but it has spread to the blood vessels, or more than one tumor is present, but they are all smaller than 3 cm.

Stage III: In Stage III liver cancer, there is more than one tumor and one of them at least is larger than 5 cm, or cancer cell has moved beyond the liver to large blood vessels, another organ and tissues, or the lymph nodes.

Stage IV: Cancer cells have spread to other tissues in the body, such as the lungs or bones, as well as lymph nodes.

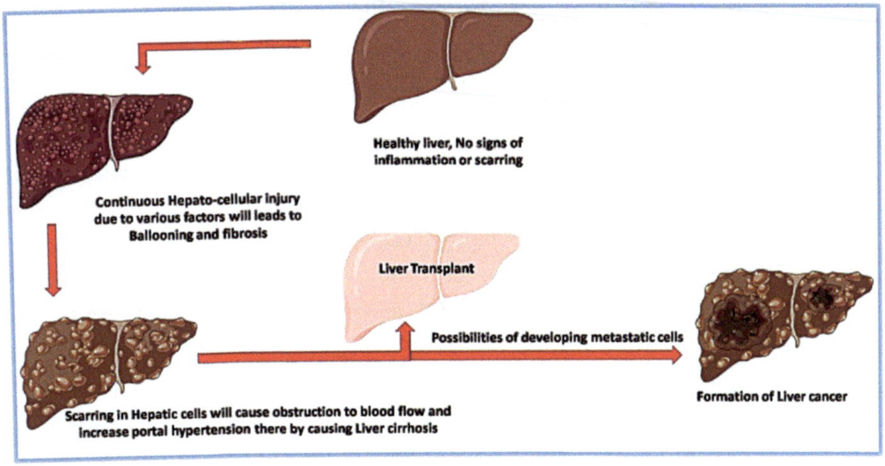

FIGURE 2.3 Stages in the formation of liver cancer.

2.6 MANAGEMENT OF LIVER CANCER

Over the last decade, the mortality and morbidity of HCC is increasing steadily. The available clinical therapeutic management for HCC is not much flourished, as the steep raise in HCC may indicate less efficacy of available therapeutic approaches, since the past decade, the advanced surgical treatment and locoregional therapies have enhanced the survival rate for a short term; the major concern is the recurrence of disease which still remains to be a big setback. At earlier stages of the disease, patients may have higher possibility of curative response to diverse treatment options (Forner et al., 2017). Well-defined staging of HCC is imperative in considerable prognostic approaches which levy best treatment options for the patient, namely, in absence of cirrhosis in HCC, hepatic resection remains an important treatment modality (Alex et al., 2002).

Some of the surgical managements for liver cancer are described below:

1. **Liver transplantation:** Transplantation of liver is considered to be the best remedial treatment of choice in patients with decompensative cirrhosis. Pragmatically, it has been observed that tumor number and size, are rough criteria of the disease prognosis. In recent advancement, the succeeding molecular marker studies or gene signature studies will expound biology of tumor, which

will be helpful in including the list of eligibility criteria for liver transplantation (Bhoori et al., 2017).

2. **Surgical abscission:** This is the therapeutic option being used in many patients with single nodule, very well liver function, and no cirrhosis, as this approach will be difficult in treating with cirrhosis which will increase the risk of hepatic decompensation. The surgical outcome relays on presence or absence of portal-hypertension, abiding liver function, size of resected segment, and volume of remnant liver after resection. The patients who opt to go for surgical resection may have almost 70% of 5-year increased life expectancy, but also they have a high possibility of recurrence. Although the rate of recurrence depends upon the microscopic vascular invasion into hepatocytes, more than 30% of HCC patients do not have any evidence of macroscopic vascular invasion. Recurrence of tumor, to develop within 2 years after surgery, is mostly associated with local invasion into tissues and intrahepatic metastasis. Recurrence of tumor lately after 2 years of surgery is due to de-novo tumor formation. In the recent scenario, surgical segmental resection is preferred in patients with early-stage disease of CA liver with normal liver function. However, the option for surgical resection must be considered against the therapeutic availability and the rate of response with other local ablative therapies like radiofrequency ablation (Barbier et al., 2013).

3. **Radio-embolization**: Recently, a restorative treatment option for intermediate-stage HCC has emerged, known as radio-embolization or selective internal radiation therapy. The role of radio-embolization in liver disease associated to segmental resection is yet to be more analyzed. In radio-embolization, the implantable radioactive microspheres are administered into the arteries supplying the tumor/cancer cells so that the radioactive microspheres will reach the tumor nodules and being treated regardless the number, size, or location of tumor. At present, the microspheres coated with Y90 b-emitting isotope are the most accepted radio-embolization technique used in HCC (Mazzaferro et al., 2013).

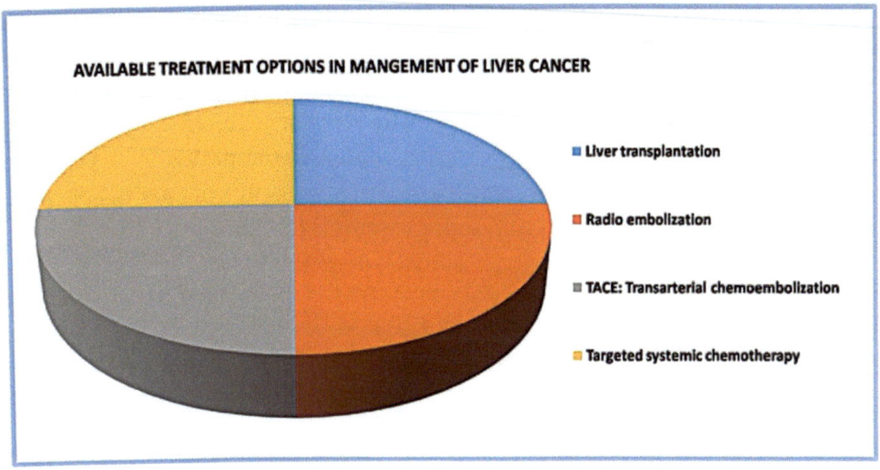

FIGURE 2.4 Available treatment options for the management of liver cancer.

4. **TACE:** Transarterial chemoembolization is measured as a standard treatment protocol used in patients suffering through intermediate-stage HCC. Those patients having compensated liver function, with large solitary nodule or multifocal hepatocellular carcinoma with no evidence of vascular invasion or extrahepatic spread, are categorized as candidates for TACE. The use of TACE as standards of care for the management of intermediate-stage HCC is relied on the manifestation of improved survival rate in comparison with the other best supportive care or suboptimal treatment (Forner et al., 2012). Intermediate-stage HCC comprises a heterogeneous population in patients with variable burden of tumor and function of liver. However, the menace in TACE-associated complications may be higher in patients with more severe disease, those who require nonselective embolization along with portal venous thrombosis and poor residual function of liver. The ultimate TACE procedures must allow the utmost and persistent concentration of chemotherapeutic agent in the tumor, with minimal exposure into systemic circulation combined with calibrated tumor vessel obstruction (Ishizawa et al., 2008).
5. **Targeted systemic chemotherapy**: The genetic alterations play a major key role in hepatocarcinogenesis; these genetic alterations will disrupt multiple signaling cascades in normal physiological

growth of the cells and apoptosis leading to uncontrolled progressive growth of the hepatic cells. A systemic targeted therapy targets on the crucial steps of the carcinogenic pathways, controlling widespread systemic toxicity. The currently approved drug for the treatment for HCC is sorafenib, which corresponds to a paradigm shift in the systemic treatment of HCC, and various other novel molecular therapies are under research (Chiang et al., 2008).

Medicinal plants and herbs may become the possible approach for the management and treatment of liver diseases, liver fibrosis, and HCC. In China, Japan, and other parts of Asia, these medicinal plants and herbs are already considered as official drugs. Diverse chemically activated fibrosis rat models were deliberately designed by targeting the rat liver system to instigate the preventive and therapeutic effects of precise herbal extracts on fibrosis of liver.

2.6.1 ASTRAGALUS

Katira manifests that it may help to reduce the side effects of platinum-based chemotherapy components such as cisplatin and carboplatin. Both of them are considered as efficacious chemotherapy agents for mesothelioma. Patients with *Astragalus* ingestion had enhanced physical function and improvement in appetite, and they experienced less fatigue, pain, nausea, and vomiting.

2.6.2 GINGER

According to a review paper published in the *British Journal of Anaesthesia* in 2000, this herb is recognized for its anticancer and anti-inflammatory properties in laboratory studies. It also suppresses the chemotherapy-related vomiting and nausea. It was advised that ginger must be purely avoided before and after surgery. It elevates bleeding and should be prohibited by patients with a low platelet count.

2.6.3 ALOE VERA

In 2011, a review paper published in the Cochrane database systematic proclaims that the use of *Aloe vera* during chemotherapy reduced mouth sores in some patients.

2.6.4 TURMERIC

Turmeric is a common herb being used since decades; its bioactive compound curcumin has been proven for many medicinal properties like anti-inflammatory property. A study published in the *Journal of Cancer Chemotherapy and Pharmacology* in 2011 innovated that extract of curcumin may be safe to add with the chemotherapeutic agent gemcitabine in treating pancreatic carcinoma.

2.6.5 MORINGA TREE

A test tube study published by *Journal of Experimental Therapeutics* in 2000 in oncology found that a compound from a Moringa tree has shown to be useful in killing ovarian cancer cells. Another study done by Michelle et al. (2021) suggested that the use of Moringa may reduce cancer symptoms like sore throat, fever, breathlessness, cough, and joint pain.

2.6.6 ALLIUM SATIVUM

Previous studies that the *Allium sativum* belongs to the Aparagales order, which comes from the Amaryllidaceae family; it is a thick stem 40-cm plant which is permanent; the part of this plant grows under the earth, is divided into several membranes, and covered in separate septae. The leaves are chlorophyll filled that appear dark but are thin while the flowers of this plant do not grow large and are attached to the end of stem.

Literature shows that this plant exhibits the property to reduce carcinogenesis in many organs while the compounds have been proven to be effective on breast and prostate carcinoma. Its role in other carcinomas is still not clear. It is believed to have cytotoxic effect on cancer. The compound allicin is extracted from *A. sativum*; when undergoes mixing with enzyme, it is converted to another. The compound allicin acts to inhibit the growth of malignant cells (Kooti et al., 2017).

2.6.7 AMMI MAJUS

Few studies have stated that another annual plant *Ammi majus*, which belongs to Apiaceae family, grows up in damp land. Its impact with ethanol was studied; this compound was also toxic for malignant cells. Studies revealed that phenol is a major compound that causes cell toxicity and thus impacts cell lineages and induces apoptosis. Psoralens are stated as the most vital compound responsible for its anticarcinogenic property (Kooti et al., 2017).

2.6.8 *NIGELLA SATIVA*

Another flower from Ranunculaceae family yields black seed. It is an annual flower that can be found in southwest Asia. The plant is stated to exhibit antioxidants property on liver. A study found apoptotic effect on renal carcinoma. This compound was compared with dinitroquinone and thimoquinone, in the property of inhibiting carcinoma cell growth on colorectal carcinoma. It is also said to cause programmed cell death in an alcoholic extract of this plant. The mechanism and impact of black beans were proved in breast carcinoma treatment (Kooti et al., 2017).

TABLE 2.1 Traditional Hepatoprotective Medicines.

S. no.	Traditional drugs	Scientific name	Action	Reference
1.	Garlic	*Allium sativum*	Prevention of antioxidant glutathione (GSH) depletion	Sabayan et al. (2007)
2.	Tea plant	*Camellia sinensis*	Inhibit hepatocellular apoptosis	Xu et al. (2007)
3.	Fennel seeds	*Nigella sativa*	Scavenger of superoxide, hydroxyl radicle	Abdel et al. (2013)
4.	Basil plant	Occimum basilicum	Decrease AST, ALP, SGOT levels	Liu et al. (2013)
5.	Cape jasmine	*Gardenia jasminoides*	Antioxidant	Tseng et al. (1995)
6.	Common madder	*Rubia cordifolia*	SGOT, SGPT, SALP level decrease	Rao et al. (2006)
7.	Long pepper	*Piper longumlinn*	Anti-inflammatory, hepatoprotective, hypocholestrolemic	Gupta et al. (2003)
8.	Indian barberry	*Berberis aristata*	Reduce serum and lipid peroxides	Brijesh et al. (2010)
9.	Giloy	*Tinospora cordifolia*	Antifibrolytic, immunomodulatory activity	Varsha et al. (2011)
10.	Green chiretta	*Andrographis paniculata*	Protective activity against paracetamol-induced toxicity and increased excretion of xenobiotics from liver	Varsha et al. (2011)

2.7 CHALLENGES IN LIVER CANCER

Patients who are often diagnosed with liver cancer carcinoma in advanced stages, that is, HCC, are mainly due to its poor prognosis. Mostly are of the HCCs, for which the best treatment is chemotherapy with immunotherapy. Patients can use natural compounds which may provide lower systemic toxicity and lesser adverse effects. Advancements in management and treatment of carcinoma can show the way to a better prognosis for a better result and to improve the basic QOL and life expectancy. For early stage, patients of only 5–15% are eligible for surgical removal due to diminished hepatic regenerative capacity.

2.8 USE OF MEDICINAL PLANTS FOR MAINTAINING LIVER HEALTH

Over hundred decades, people have the faith in food as medicine. Numerous categories of medicinal plants and food plants have chemopreventive properties to prevent carcinogen-induced neoplasia. They are classified as citrus fruits, cruciferous vegetables, caraway (*Carum carvi*) seed oils, and *Allium* species (Wattenberg et al., 1990).

Patients who have liver disease are not advisable to take Solanaceae family, that is, nightshade plants; Solanaceae family has more than 2800 plants. Familiar nightshade plants are ground cherries (any of the genus *Physalis*), eggplant, mandrake (*Mandragora officinarum*), peppers, pimentos (*Capsicum annuum*), potatoes, tobacco, tomatillos (*Physalis carpa*), and tomatoes. Many in-vivo animal studies revealed that the use of nightshades resulted in hepatotoxicity, amyloidosis, and moderate necrosis in liver (Aguilar et al., 2013).

TABLE 2.2 Traditional Plants Used in Hepatic Disorders.

S. no	Botanical name	Family	Local name
1.	*Abrus precatorius* Linn.	Fabaceae	Gunj
2.	*Aegle marmelos* Linn.	Rutaceae	Bael
3.	*Asparagus racemosus* Wild.	Asparagaceae	Satawar
4.	*Berberis aristata* DC	Berberidaceae	Dar hald
5.	*Mentha arvensis* Linn.	Lamiaceae	Pudina

TABLE 2.2 *(Continued)*

S. no	Botanical name	Family	Local name
6.	*Ocimum sanctum* Linn.	Lamiaceae	Kali tulas
7.	*Terminalia chebula* Retz.	Combretaceae	Hirda
8.	*Apium graveolens* L.	Apiaceae	Karafs
9.	*Terminalia chebula* Retz.	Combretaceae	HalilehSiah
10.	*Rheum palmatum* L.	*Rheum palmatum* L.	RevandChini
11.	*Cichorium intybus* L.	Asteraceae	Kasni
12.	*Linum usitatissimum*	Linaceae	Katan
13.	*Curcuma zedoaria*	Zingiberaceae	Zaranbad

TABLE 2.3 Common Plant Foods Containing Antioxidants for Liver Health (Gunjan et al., 2011; Ghorbani et al., 2005; Dolatkhahi et al., 2014; Mardaninejad et al., 2013; Guan et al., 2015).

S.no	Common name	Botanical name	Main active element	Action
1.	Beets	Beta vulgaris	Betaine	Chloretic
2.	Broccoli	*Brassica oleracea*	Diindolylmethane, glucoraphanin	Antiviral, anticancer
3.	Sweet potato	*Ipomoea batatas*	Beta carotene, fiber	Attenuating liver injury
4.	Cabbage	*Brassica oleracea*	Glucosinolates	Countering alcohol, hangover
5.	Banana	*Musa acuminata*	Pectin	Relieving cirrhosis
6.	Cherry	*Prunu savium*	Methyl jasmonate	Antioxidant activity
7.	Fig	*Mora ceaeficus*	Fumaric acid, ficin	Antifatty liver action
8.	Lemon	*Citrus limon*	Naringin, citric acid	Decreasing liver damage
9.	Papaya	*Carica papaya*	Lycopene, danielone	Antioxidative activity
10.	Pomegranate	*Punica granatum*	Punicalagins	Anticancer
11.	Watermelon	*Citrullus lanatus*	Citrulline, lycopene	Antitoxic, hypoglycemic
12.	Barley	*Hordeum vulgare*	Caffeic acid, *p*-coumaric acid	Antifatty liver action
13.	Maize	*Zea mays*	Lutein, linolic acid	Antioxidant activity
14.	Brown rice	*Oryza sativa*	Anthocyanins, tocopherols	Anti-inflammatory
15.	Oat	*Avena sativa*	Ergothioneine	Antioxidant activity

2.9 CONCLUSION AND FUTURE PERSPECTIVE

A substantial confirmation has emphasized the medical applications of Unani medicine in therapy of liver cancer. Unani herbal medicines can improve the prognosis and outcome measures of liver cancer whereby these herbal drugs may target multifactorial components through multiple signaling pathways, which may be helpful to reduce symptoms of liver cancer. Moreover, current treatment regimens, like chemotherapy, radiotherapy, TACE, and so on, may lead to dose-dependent toxicities with substantial side effects. Several herbal medicines are abundant in potential phytochemicals and bioactive compounds which can specifically target any one of the malignancy pathways, which can take us through to develop target-based drug design molecules to develop anticancer drug therapies. In recent scenario, computational drug designing and targeting have given a wide spectrum of hope to pipeline the anticancer drugs to go for further clinical in-vitro and in-vivo studies, though many in-vitro and in-vivo clinical trials on herbal-based anticancer drug therapy for liver cancer are being explored, still the validation of these drugs with human clinical trial is a challenging task as the risk of toxicity due to herbal medicines has yet to be completely explored. The use of herbal medicines may increase the life expectancy, thereby reducing the mortality rate due to liver cancer.

KEYWORDS

- **cancer**
- **liver**
- **herbs**
- **management**
- **hepatoprotective properties**

REFERENCES

Abdel-Wahab, W. M. Protective Effect of Thymoquinone on Sodium Fluoride-Induced Hepatotoxicity and Oxidative Stress in Rats. *J. Basic Appl. Zool.* **2013,** *66,* 263–270.

Aguilar-Santamar´ıa, L.; Herrera-Arellano, A.; Zamilpa A.; et al. Toxicology, Genotoxicity, and Cytotoxicity of Three Extracts of Solanumchrysotrichum. *J. Ethnopharmacol.* **2013,** *150* (1), 275–279.

American Joint Committee on Cancer. Liver. In *AJCC Cancer Staging Manual,* 8th ed.; Springer: New York, NY, 2017; p 287.

Balogh, J.; Victor III, D.; Asham, E. H.; Burroughs, S. G.; Boktour, M.; Saharia, A.; Monsour Jr, H. P. Hepatocellular Carcinoma: A Review. *J. Hepatocell. Carcinoma* **2016,** *3,* 41.

Barbier, L.; Fuks, D.; Pessaux, P.; Muscari, F.; Le Treut, Y. P.; Faivre, S.; Belghiti, J. Safety of Liver Resection for Hepatocellular Carcinoma After Sorafenib Therapy: A Multicenter Case-Matched Study. *Ann. Surg. Oncol.* **2013,** *20* (11), 3603–3609.

Beetroot in Uganda, [Online] 2019. travelguide.com/beetrootinuganda.html.

Befeler, A. S.; Adrian Biscegelle, A. Hepatocellular Carcinoma; Diagnosis and Treatment. *Gastroenterology* **2002**, *122* (6),1609–1619.

Bhoori, S.; Schiavo, M.; Russo, A.; Mazzaferro, V. First-Line Treatment for Hepatocellular Carcinoma: Resection or Transplantation? *Transplant Proc.* **2007,** *39,* 2271–2273.

Brijesh Tiwari, K.; Khosa, R. L. Evaluation of the Hepatoprotective and Antioxidant Effect of Berberisaristata against Experimentally Induced Liver Injury in Rats. *Int. J. Pharmacy Pharmaceutical Sci.* **2010,** *2* (1), 92–99.

Buettner, S.; van Vugt, J. L.; IJzermans, J. N.; Koerkamp, B. G. Intrahepatic Cholangio Carcinoma: Current Perspectives. *OncoTargets Ther*. **2017,** *10,* 1131.

Calle, E. E.; Rodriguez, C.; Walker-Thurmond, K.; Thun, M. J. Overweight, Obesity, and Mortality From Cancer in a Prospectively Studied Cohort of U.S Adults. *N. Engl. J. Med.* **2003,** *348,* 1625–1638.

Cao, J.; Wang, J.; He, C.; Fang, M. Angiosarcoma: A Review of Diagnosis and Current Treatment. *Am. J Cancer Res.* **2019,** *9 (*11), 2303.

Chaudharia, G. M.; Mahajanb, R. T. Comparative Antioxidant Activity of Twenty Traditional Indian Medicinal Plants and its Correlation With Total Flavonoid and Phenolic Content, 2014.

Chiang, D. Y.; Villanueva, A.; Hoshida, Y.; Peix, J.; Newell, P.; Minguez, B.; LeBlanc, A. C.; Donovan, D. J.; Thung, S. N.; Solé, M.; et al. Focal Gains of VEGFA and Molecular Classification of Hepatocellular Carcinoma. *Cancer Res.* **2008,** *68,* 6779–6788.

Daily Monitor, Natural Remedies and Cancer: What's the Truth? 2019.

Dolatkhahi, M.; Dolatkhahi, A.; Bagher Nejad, J. Ethno Botanical Study of Medicinal Plants Used in Arjan–Parishan Protected Area in Fars Province of Iran. *Avicenna J. Phytomed.* **2014,** *4,* 402–412.

European Association for the Study of the Liver. EASL Clinical Practice Guidelines: Management of Hepatocellular Carcinoma. *J. Hepatol.* **2018,** *69* (1), 182–236.

Forner, A.; Llovet, J. M.; Bruix, J. Chemoembolization for Intermediate HCC: Is There Proof of Survival Benefit? *J. Hepatol.* **2012,** *56,* 984–986.

Ghorbani, A. Studies on Pharmaceutical Ethnobotany in the Region of Turkmen Sahra, North of Iran (Part 1): General Results. *J. Ethnopharmacol.* **2005,** *102,* 58–68.

Giannitrapani, L.; Soresi, M.; Bondi, M. L.; et al. Nanotechnology Applications for the Therapy of Liverfibrosis. *World J. Gastroenterol.* **2014,** *20,* 7242–7251.

Global Cancer Statistics (GCS). GLOBOCAN Estimates of Incidence and Mortality Worldwide for 36 Cancers in 185 Countries, 2020.

Guan, Y. S.; Qing, H. Plants Consumption and Liver Health, Department of Oncology, West China Hospital, Sichuan University, China, 2015.

Gupta, A. K. Quantitative Analysis of Medicinal Aromatic Plants (III), 2003; pp125–129.

Ishizawa, T.; Hasegawa, K.; Aoki, T.; Takahashi, M.; Inoue, Y.; Sano, K.; Imamura, H.; Sugawara, Y.; Kokudo, N.; Makuuchi, M. Neither Multiple Tumors Nor Portal Hypertension are Surgical Contraindications for Hepatocellular Carcinoma. *Gastroenterology* **2008,** *134,* 1908–1916.

Kashaw, V.; Nema, A. K.; Agarwal, A. Hepatoprotective Prospective Of Herbal Drugs and Their Vesicular Carriers– A Review. *Int. J. Res. Pharmaceutical Biomed. Sci.* **2011,** (2), 360–374

Kodi, P.; Mwangi, M. E.; Kiplagat, C. P.; Karuiki, T. S. Ethnobotanical Survey of Antimalarial Medicinal Plants Used in Butebo County, Eastern Uganda. *Eur. J. Med. Plants* **2017,** *21* (4), 1–22.

Kooti, W.; Servatyari, K.; Behzadifar, M.; Majid Asadi-Samani, M.; Sadeghi, F.; Marzouni, H. Z. Effective Medicinal Plant in Cancer Treatment, Part 2: Review Study, 2017.

Liu, Y.; Flynn, T. J.; Ferguson, M. S.; Hoagland, E. M. Use of the Combination Index to Determine Interactions Between Plant-Derived Phenolic Acids on Hepatotoxicity Endpoints in Human and Rat Hepatoma Cells. *Phytomedicine* **2013,** *20,* 461–468.

Mardaninejad, S.; Janghorban, M.; Vazirpour, M. Collection and Identification of Medicinal Plants Used by the Indigenous People of Mobarakeh (Isfahan), Southwestern Iran. *J. Herbal Drugs* **2013,** *4,* 23–32.

Marra, F.; Tacke, F. Roles for Chemokines in Liver Disease. *Gastroenterology* **2014,** *147,* 577–594.

Mazzaferro, V.; Sposito, C.; Bhoori, S.; Romito, R.; Chiesa, C.; Morosi, C.; Maccauro, M.; Marchianò, A.; Bongini, M.; Lanocita, R.; Civelli, E.; Bombardieri, E.; Camerini, T.; Spreafico, C. Yttrium-90 Radioembolization for Intermediate-Advanced Hepatocellular Carcinoma: A Phase 2 Study. *Hepatology* **2013.**

Michelotti, G. A.; Machado, M. V.; Diehl, A. M. NAFLD, NASH, and Liver Cancer. *Nat. Rev. Gastroenterol. Hepatol.* **2013,** *10,* 656–665.

Murray, J. L.; Lopez, A. L. Alternative Projections of Mortality and Disability by Cause 1998–2020: Global Burden of Disease Study. *Lancet* **1997,** *349,* 1498–1504.

Nadkarni, K. M.; In *Indian Materia Medica*; Dr. KM Nadkarni's Indianmateriamedica: With Ayurvedic, Unani-Tibbi, Siddha, Allopathic, Homeopathic, Naturopathic and Home Remedies, Appendices and Indexes, 1st ed.; Popular Prakashan, 1996; vol 1, 487–507.

Rao, G. M.; Rao, C. V.; Pushpangadan, P.; Shirwaikar, A. Hepatoprotective Effects of Rubiadin, a Major Constituent of Rubiacordifolia Linn. *J. Ethnopharmacol.* **2006,** *103,* 484–90.

Sabayan, B.; Foroughinia, F.; Chohedry, A. A Postulated Role of Garlic Organosulfur Compounds in Prevention of Valproic Acid Hepatotoxicity. *Med. Hypotheses* **2007,** *68,* 512–514.

Singal, A. G., El-Serag, H. B. Hepatocellular Carcinoma From Epidemiology to Prevention: Translating Knowledge Into Practice. *Clin. Gastroenterol. Hepatol.* **2015,** *13* (12), 2140–2151.

Singh, D.; Gupta, R.; Saraf, S. A. Herbs-are They Safe Enough? An Overview. *Crit. Rev. Food Sci. Nutr.* **2012,** *52* (10), 876–898.

Tiwari, A. K. Revisiting "Vegetables" to Combat Modern Epidemic of Imbalanced Glucose Homeostasis. *Pharmacogn. Mag.* **2014,** *10* (2), S207–S213.

Torbenson, M. Fibrolamellar Carcinoma: 2012 Update. *Scientifica* **2012.**

Traka, M. H.; Mithen, R. F. "Plant Science and Human Nutrition: Challenges in Assessing Health-Promoting Properties of Phytochemicals. *Plant Cell.* **2011,** *23* (7), 2483–2497.

Tseng TH, Chu CY, Huang JM, Shiow SJ, Wang CJ. Crocetin protects against oxidative damage in rat primary hepatocytes. *Cancer Lett.* **1995,** *97*, 61–67.

Unnati, P.; Patel, G.; Patel, D.; Patel, S.; Patel, M.; Dass, E. A Prospective Study of Liver Cirrhosis: An Overview, Prevalence, Clinical Manifestation and Investigations in Patients Admitted to the Medicine Ward in a Rural Teaching Hospital. *Int. J. Sci. Res.* **2018,** *7,* 2016–2018.

Wallace, K.; Burt, A. D.; Wright, M. C. Liver Fibrosis. *Biochem. J.* **2008,** *411,* 1–18.

Wattenberg, L. W. Inhibition of Carcinogenesis by Naturally Occurring and Synthetic Compounds. *Basic Life Sci.* **1990,** *52,* 155–166.

Xu, C.; Shu, WQ.; Qiu, ZQ.; Chen, J. A.; Zhao, Q.; Cao, J. Protective Effects of Green Tea Polyphenols Against Subacute Hepatotoxicity Induced by Microcystin-LR in Mice. *Environ. Toxicol. Pharmacol.* **2007,** *24,* 140–148.

Yang, J.; Zhang, Y.; Luo, L.; Meng, R.; Yu, C. Global Mortality Burden of Cirrhosis and Liver Cancer Attributable to Injection Drug Use, 1990–2016: An Age-Period Cohort and Spatial Autocorrelation Analysis. *Int. J. Environ. Res. Public Health* **2018,** *15,* 170.

Yin, S. Y.; Wei, W. C.; Jian, F. Y.; Yang, N. S Therapeutic Applications of Herbal Medicines for Cancer Patients, 2013.

Whitmer, M. Herbal Medicine and Cancer, February 10, 2021.

CHAPTER 3

Unani Approaches of Anticancer Plants Against Cancer

SANA NAFEES[1] and HUDA NAFEES[2]

[1]*All India Institute of Medical Sciences, New Delhi, India*

[2]*Department of Saidla, Faculty of Unani Medicine, Aligarh Muslim University, Aligarh, UP, India*

ABSTRACT

On a global scale, cancer is one of the foremost causes of morbidity and mortality. Currently, there are more than 100 different forms of cancer, each with its own etiology and natural history. Hippocrates (460–370 BC), a Greek physician, is credited with coining the term cancer, because of the morphological resemblance of the cut surface of a hard malignant tumor, veins extended on all the sides of the tumor as finger like projections that looks like the crab's feet. Hippocrates used the term karkinos (carcinos), Greek word (καρκίνος) for crayfish or crab. In Unani terminology, it is defined as *Sartan* an Arabic word which literally means crab. Hippocrates stated that a person is healthy if all the humors of the body are in equilibrium, and if any of the humor is not in balance or if any of the humor is too much or too little, then disease will occur. Cancer was thought to be caused by an excess of black bile in body sites. *Al Razi* described the majority of malignancies cancers known at his time and advised the removal of black bile from the organ by emesis and purgation, as well as the use of cold-tempered foods and drugs. *Sartan* is the hard inflammation (*Warm-e-Salabat*), its tributaries and lesions filled with the *Madda-e-Saudavia* (morbid melancholic

Plant-Derived Anticancer Drugs in the OMICS Era: Biosynthesis, Functions, and Applications.
Deepu Pandita, Anu Pandita (Eds.)

humor) having characteristic pain, burning sensation with pulsation and rapidly increasing in size due to accumulation of excess morbid matter. In Unani System of Medicine (USM), the diseases are caused by the derangement and pathophysiological changes in temperament of certain bodily parts or organs, which can be treated or cured using medications and nondrug elements. Because of the limited success of current clinical therapies including immunomodulation, radiation, and surgery that is evident by high morbidity and mortality rates. Therefore, there is urgent demand for novel and better treatment resources, particularly new chemotherapeutic drugs for cancer management. The principal line of treatments for the patients of cancer (*Sartan*) are: (1) Correction in the temperament (*Taadil-e-Mizaj*) and (2) Evacuation of Morbid matter (*Tanqia-e- Mawad*). Plants used for *Taadil-e-Mizaj* such as *Lactuca sativa (*Kahu), Brassica oleracea (karamkalla), *Linum usitatissimum (*Alsi/Katan), and the drugs used for the *Tanqia-e-Mawad are Borago officinalis* (Gaozaban), *Althaea officinalis* (Khitmi), *Lavandula stoechas* (Ustukhuddus), *Cichorium intybus* (Kasni), etc. Hence this chapter will present discussion of cancer and plant-based approach toward cancer treatment based on the traditional USM.

3.1 INTRODUCTION

Globally, cancer is the leading cause of morbidity and mortality and at present there are more than 100 different types of cancer, which are differentiated on the basis of their etiology, origin, and natural history. Since current chemotherapeutic agents have low selectivity and there is a limited success of other clinical therapies that includes surgery, radiation, and immunomodulation, therefore new and better treatment resources, particularly new chemotherapeutic drugs for cancer management, are urgently needed (IARC, 2014; Jemal et al., 2011). For thousands of years, nature has provided medicinal substances, and an astounding amount of recent medicaments that have been extracted from natural sources, playing a significant and important role in treating ailments (Cragg and Newman, 2001). The search for new remedies has always been a part of traditional medicinal plant knowledge. The traditional medicinal plants are frequently in use because they are less expensive, more readily available, and easy consumable in any form whether in raw or in formulation form. A number of chemical constituents are present in these medicinal plants due to these chemical constituents they exhibit significant pharmacological activities (Park and Pezzutto, 2002). The medicinal plants are commonly referred to as "Chemical Goldmines" as they encompass natural compounds and are safe to use for both animals and humans. It is not possible to synthesize all these compounds in laboratories. There are many plant secondary metabolites which are commercially valuable and are used in a number of pharmaceutical products. Since the dawn of civilization, the plants have long served as a source of health treatment for humans. More than 80,000 plant species of 250,000 higher plant species are in use as therapeutic agents (Thomas, 1997).

Herbal plants have long been proven to be good and dependable sources for developing new and novel anticancer drugs (Schwartsmann et al., 2002). Natural products and their derivatives are increasingly being used worldwide for the new drug development of chemotherapeutic regimes as they are less toxic as compare to their synthetic counterparts (Newman et al., 2003; Srivastava et al., 2006; Gupta et al., 2010). Plants and their derivatives account for more than 60% of chemotherapeutic agents as the phytocompounds have antiproliferative and antimetastatic activities (Sun et al., 2009).

The "Unani System of Medicine (USM)" was known from the ancient times and considered as one of the oldest systems of medicine, and continues till date because many productive and efficient compounds and drugs have been developed from plants, animals, and mineral resources. Hippocrates, the father of medicine, practiced medicine about 2400 years ago, yet his medicine incorporated elements of ancient Egyptian medicine and also major Mesopotamian traditions. As people become aware of the natural benefits of medications derived from plants, demand of herbal treatments are increasingly popular across worldwide and also they are less expensive than contemporary pharmaceutics; hence, they become the preferred choice of an average person. According to WHO an estimate of around 80% of world inhabitants depend on the use of medicinal flora to cater their primary health care needs (Hussain et al., 2017).

3.2 ANCIENT TRADITIONAL KNOWLEDGE ABOUT CANCER (SARTAN)

Hippocrate (460–370 BC), a Greek physician was the first to whom credited has been given for coining the term cancer. He used the word *Karkinos* (carcinos) which is the "Greek" term (καρκίνος) used for crayfish or crab because of the physical appearance of a solid malignant tumor's cut surface, veins exposed on all sides and finger like projections that resembles to the crab feet. Later, a Latin word cancer was translated by "Celcus" (ca. 25 BC–50 AD) from the Greek word *Karkinos*. Another Greek physician, Galen (130–200 AD) coined the term "oncos" to describe tumor, a Greek name that means swelling. Malignant tumors are still described using Hippocrates' and Celsus' crab analogy (Hussain et al., 2017). In Unani classical text, cancer is defined by the name of *Sartan*, which is an Arabic word meaning crab and was derived from "karkinos" means crab, an ancient Greek word (καρκίνος) (Ahmed et al., 2016). According to Hippocrate, a person is healthy if all the four humors, that is, *Dam, Balgham, Safra,* and *Sauda* are in equilibrium and if there is any imbalance in these four humors then disease will occur. Cancer was believed to be caused by an excess accumulation of Sauda, that is, Black bile in the body of an individual (ACS, 2014). He also specified that cancer is one of the nontreatable diseases (Tabri, 2010). This "Hippocratic" concept of cancer was accepted and understood by Galen and he disseminated this concept in his medical curriculum, and it remains an incontrovertible norm for nearly a thousand years during the Middle Ages.

Al Razi also known as Rhazes (860–930 AD), *Al Zahrawi* (Abucalsis 936–1013 AD) and *Ibn Sina* (Avicenna 980–1037 AD), were the Arab Muslim scholars who were well versed about the disease. Majority of malignancies described by *Razi* known at his time, he advised emesis and purgation to remove black bile from the organs, and he also advise to use foods and drugs having cold temperament. The Andalusian Scholar named Abulcasis, who was the first to perform surgery of a malignant tumor of breast, and he proposed that "cancer" can only be treated by the surgical mode of treatment in its early stages, if there is possible of total removal. Ibn Sina also deduced that an accumulation of excess black burnt bile causes cancer, which is particularly difficult to treat. He also distinguished benign tumor and malignant tumors by observing several signs and symptoms such as pain which is throbbing in nature, rapid growth of tumors as well as observed that malignant tumors leave "crab-like tracks," these malignant tumors are most commonly seen in hollow organ. He also stated that cancer frequently affect tendons, lymph nodes, and muscles (Said et al., 2011). For the first time, Abulcasis specifically identified kidney cancer and was made the distinction in between acute renal inflammatory conditions and cancer. All eminent Arab scholars including

Al Razi, *Al Zahrawi,* and *Ibn Sina,* realized that the chances of curing cancer are increased if it is detected in early stages. According to Avicenna and Rhazes (Rhazes, 925; Sina, 1992], malignant tumors are difficult to treat. According to them, a cancerous tumor is harmful and grows in size over time, spreading its roots into the tissues. The first and the foremost strategy for treating cancer should be to hinder or to stop the growth of the malignant lesion. *Ibn Sina* or Avicenna was the first who documented the treatment of cancer by surgical removal of minor and accessible tumors that were not adjacent to vital organs in his book *Canon of Medicine*. He recommended doing a radical excision to remove all diseased tissues, as well as veins or done amputation in the tumor's direction. Secondly, in order to strengthening the immune system, Avicenna advised the patient to eat a balanced and nutritious diet to purify the body from excess black bile. He also tried the first pharmacological treatment of cancer with plant drug namely *Cichorium intybus* (*Kasni*) that was later discovered by *Ibn al Baitar* as potent anticancer drug that might be used to treat a variety of tumors and neoplastic illness (Said et al., 2011; Rhazes, 925; Sina, 1992; Baitar, 1874; Saad et al., 2005; Saad et al., 2008; Khan, 2006).

3.3 ETIOPATHOGENESIS OF SARTAN (CANCER) IN UNANI SYSTEM OF MEDICINE (USM)

Sartan is a melancholy inflammation caused by increased black bile (*Sauda*) combustion, which produces more intrinsic heat and hence becomes pathological. According to Avicenna, cancer is caused by the combustion of pure yellow bile, black bile mixed with yellow bile or pure black bile and having characteristic of hard inflammation (*warm e salabat*) with lesions and tributaries filled with *madda e saudavia* known as morbid melancholic humor (Maseehi, 1995). Cancer usually occurs in the persons who are obese and fatty and because of this it commonly occurs in females and have high incidence in females than males specifically in those organs which are hollow and where the morbid matter, that is, *Madda Saudavia* can easily accumulate for, for example, breasts, cervix, uterus, etc. Morbid *sauda* considered as the main cause of cancer (Maseehi, 1995; Rushd, 1980; Zohar, 1986; Sina, 2010; Razi, 1997), this morbid *Sauda* is formed by the combustion *Sauda* known as *Sauda e Ahtraqi* (Maseehi, 1995), combustion of blood known as *Dam e saudavi* changes the blood color from red to black and while palpation no sign of hyperaemia, despite that the quantity is more than that of hyperaemia, that is, *Imtila-e-Dam.*

The characteristic features of cancer are pain, pulsation, and burning and the size of tumor increases very rapidly because of the excess accumulation of the matter which is morbid and also swelling. The newer vessels are blackish or greenish in color and resembling crab-walking legs are produced by cancer. Neovascularization in malignant lesions resembles crab legs that penetrate deep into the epidermis and subcutaneous tissue before hardening. The malignant organs veins dilated and filled with cancerous material and becomes hardened (Tabri, 1995). Cancer is a condition that is primary in origin that does not happen as a result of another diseases condition. It lies latent at first, then manifests clinically as a tumor and swelling with following sign and symptoms (Sina, 1992). Extreme hemorrhage, severe pain, and cancer recurrence are the three most serious side effects of surgical ablation (Rhazes, 925). According to *Ibn Rushd* also known as Averroes, the ailment is caused by a disturbance in the quality, that is, *Kaifiyat* and also in Quantity, that is, *Kamiyat* of melancholic bile or when both will occur. The change in normal black bile constituents may be due to substances stimulated by the excessive and prolonged consumption of *barid*, that is, cold and y*abis*, that is, dry foods, as well as the preponderance of hot and dry" (*Har khushk)* or "cold and dry" (*Sard khushk*), alteration in temperament of gastrointestinal organs, or it can be due to factors which are external like environment and occupation, or both or it may be related to genetic factors (Rushd, 1980). Cancer is caused by abnormal humors, which can be ulcerative or nonulcerative. Ulcerative cancer is caused by the combustion of abnormal black bile, whereas the combustion of normal black bile can cause nonulcerative cancer (Rushd, 1980). The lesions that are ulcerative in nature have a strong sensation and their ulcer's edges are thick, lustreless, dark red, and averted from outside. Malignancy frequently affects nerves, veins, arteries, oesophagus, and larynx (Qamri, 2008). Initially it begins as a little circular abscess with an earthy hue, small in size and in consistency it is hard and eventually develops into a large abscess (Maseehi,1995; Samarqandi, 2010). Its size varies from the size of a gram up to the size of the watermelon (Qamri, 2008). It is a strong solid tumor with deep roots in the organs. *Sartan* is more common in women because of their soft bodies which easily receive morbid stuff, whereas men firm bodies hardly accept these morbid substances making it less common in men than women (Qamri, 2008).

3.4 SITES OF SARTAN

According to Unani classical literature, *sartan* is most commonly occurs in organs which are hollow in nature or *Aza-e-Ratab* such as *Pistan* (Breast), *Halaq* (Throat), *Aalat-e-Tanaffus* (Respiratory organs), *Reham* (Uterus), *Amma* (Intestine), *Dahan* (Mouth), *Asaab* (Nerves), *Ahleel* (Urethra), *Unq* (Neck), and *Ain* (Eyes).

3.4.1 PREVENTION OF SARTAN

In traditional USM, classical literature emphasizes that s*artan* can be prevented by adhering the principles of *Asbab-e-Sitta Zarooriyah* (six prerequisites of healthy living) for restoring the healthy lifestyle and improving the quality of life of the patients. These are as follows:

1. *Hawa* (Air): Air should be fresh and pollution free air for breathing and also should avoid exposure to excessive cold and excessive hot air.
2. *Makool o Mashrroob* (Food and Drink):
   - (i) Avoid junk and smoked food, preserved foods, alcohol, and also carbonated drinks, etc.
   - (ii) Do not use excessive nonvegetarian diet.
   - (iii) Stop chewing of tobacco and stop smoking.
   - (iv) Avoid diets that are responsible for producing black bile such as dried and salted meat, red meat, fish, etc.
   - (v) Increase consumption of turmeric, tomatoes, broccoli, garlic, flax seeds, spinach, walnuts, etc.
   - (vi) Take diets that are soft and are easily digestible.
   - (vii) Take diets that are rich in fiber approximately 20–30 g/day.
3. *Harkat o sukoon Badani* (bodily movement and repose): A person should do exercise daily for about 30–45 min at least 5 days in a week and also avoid sedentary lifestyle.
4. *Harkat o Sukoon Nafsani* (psychic movement and repose): should avoid extreme emotions such as anger, fear, sadness, and also avoid anxiety and stress and lead a spiritual peaceful life.
5. *Naum o yagza* (sleep and wakefulness): sleep should be for 6 to 8 h.

6. *Ihtibas o Istifragh* (retention and evacuation): should ensure proper evacuation, urination, perspiration, and menstruation. Avoid constipation, avoid dehydration, and ensure retention of electrolytes and minerals.

3.4.2 MANAGEMENT OF SARTAN IN USM

***Usool-e-Ilaj* (Principles of treatment):** The goal of cancer treatment can be achieved by the restoration of humoral balances with the help of Mizaj, that is, Temperament and Islah-e-Jigar. This can be accomplished by using emetics, laxatives, purgatives, diuretics, enemas, and bloodletting, to eliminate excess and unhealthy humors from the body. Cancer prevention is best achieved by a well-balanced (qualitative and quantitative) diet and regular exercise. "Unani physicians" stressed that *Tabiyat* which is also called physis/nature is the finest healer, and it is the physician's role to assist nature/physis in healing process.

The occurrence of disease is due to the pathological changes in the temperament in certain body part or organ, can be cured or treated using medications and nondrug factors. In USM, there is a correlation between temperament and other factors which are nondrug like diet, environment, mental state, etc., which affect the temperament directly or indirectly. The USM promotes the use of these no drug components on a regular and substantial basis. In USM, the patients of cancer can be treated on the principles which are: (1) *Taadil-e-mizaj,* that is, correction of temperament and (2) *Tanqia-e-mawad,* that is, cleansing of morbid matter. In USM, it has been mentioned that cancer is caused by when the imbalance in black bile, that is, *Sauda* occur, having dry and cold temperament and in USM treatment is done by *Ilaj-bil-zid* therefore, in this treatment can be done by giving the drugs and food which are having Hot and Mosit, that is, *Har Ratab* temperament are used. Moreover, the drugs focus should be done on diet the *Latif* (Light), *Saaleh* (healthy), and easily digestible diets are used (Shamsi et al., 2016; Baghdadi, 2004; Samarqandi, 2010).

3.4.3 TREATMENT OF SARTAN IN TRADITIONAL USM

In USM, the principal mode of treatments are as follows:

1. *Ilāj bi'l-Tadbīr* (Regimenal therapy).
2. *Ilāj bi'l-Ghidhā* (Dietotherapy).

3. *Ilāj bi'l-Dawā* (Pharmacotherapy).
4. *Ilāj bi'l-Yad* (Surgery).

In the management of *sartan,* the first and the foremost step is to clean the body from the black bile by evacuation and by using regimental methods or by using medications. Avicenna mentioned that the medications used for the treatment of cancer have four purposes these are:

1. Cancer lesion should be completely arrested.
2. Arrest the progress of the lesion.
3. To stop the ulceration.
4. If ulceration occurs then the healing of ulcers.

"Galen" in his book entitled *Methods of Treatment* stated that the treatment can be achieved by the removal of black bile, that is, *Sauda* from the body as it is the main cause of causing cancer by using suitable purgatives, following purgation the formation of black bile in the body should be avoided if at all possible, and if not possible then black bile should be deflated at regular intervals from the body (Said et al., 2011; Shamsi et al., 2016).

Unani physicians Avicenna and Galen both said emphatically that malignancies that form inside the body and are not visible to human sight should be treated. The removal of morbid material which is black bile or *Sauda* should be accomplished initially through continuous purging or venesection, that is, *Fasd*, with the consumption of foods which are highly nutritious having cold temperament and balanced foods so that they produce normal blood in patients and in this way the patients can be treated safely (Razi, 1997).

3.4.4 UNANI MEDICINAL PLANTS AS ANTICANCEROUS AGENTS

According to Avicenna and Rhazes, treatment of disease can be done on three basis, first done by using physiotherapy and diet, secondly by using drugs, and lastly by surgery. The drugs used are categorized into single (*Mufrad*) and compound formulations (*Murakkab*). First, treatment of the disease should start with single drug to avoid drug–drug interaction and if this not works, then second option will be the use of compound formulations and if it fails too then lastly the only choice is the surgery. Nowadays, researchers have emphasized and mentioned herbal-based treatments are among the greatest choices for management and prevention of cancer. This is mainly because of the presence of a wide range of bioactive chemical compounds present in plants which exerts their effects in diseases including cancer. These phytochemical substances are found naturally, economical, and easier to take orally than synthesized drugs, and also these natural drugs are having minimal- or low-side effects and having rich physiologically active properties in comparison to that of synthetic chemotherapeutic agents (Zaid et al., 2012; Ahmad et al., 2016; Seca and Pinto., 2018; Lichota and Gwozdzinski, 2018).

Some of the Unani drugs having anticancerous effect on the basis of basic Unani principle, that is, *Munzij-e-Sauda* and *Mushil-e-Sauda* described in classical literature have been mentioned in Table 3.1. Table 3.2 describes the anticancerous studies on Unani antcancerous drugs as well as those drugs that do not have *Munzij-e-Sauda* and *Mushil-e- Sauda* activity; however, they have been explored for anticancerous activity either in vitro or in vivo.

TABLE 3.1 Unani Anticancerous Drugs (*Munzij-e-Sauda and Mushil-e-Sauda Advia*).

Unani drugs	Scientific name	Temperament and degree	Other uses	References
Aftimoon	(*Cuscuta reflexa*)	Hot 2° and dry 2°	Anti-inflammatory, deobstruent, anthelmintic	Ghani, 2010; Baitar, 1999; Hakeem, 1999
Bisfayej	(*Polypodium vulgare* L.)	Hot 2° and dry 3°	Exhilarant, carminative	Ghani.,2010; Hakeem.,1999
Gaozaban	*Borago officinalis*	Hot 1° and moist 1°	Exhilarant, cardiotonic	Rafeequddin, 1985; Kabeeruddin,2010
Ustukhuddus	*Lavandula stoechas*	Hot 1° and dry 2°	Antioxidant, sedative, anticonvulsive	Hakeem,1999; Kabeeruddin, 2010
Kharbaqsiyah	*Helliborous niger*	Hot 3° and dry 3°	Anti-inflammatory, strengthening of teeth	Ghani,2010; Baitar,1999
Turbud	*Ipomoea turpethum*	Hot 1° and moist 1°	Digestive, carminative	Hakeem,1999; Kabeeruddin, 2010
Shahm e Hanzal	*Citrullus colocynthis*	Hot dry 3°	Strong purgative	Ghani, 2010
Habbul Neel	*Ipomoea hederacea*	Hot dry3°	Purgative, anthelmintic	Ghani, 2010; Baitar, 1999

TABLE 3.1 *(Continued)*

Unani drugs	Scientific name	Temperament and degree	Other uses	References
Saqmonia	*Convolvulous scammonia*	Hot 3° and dry 2°	Purgative	Hakeem, 1999; Kabeeruddin, 2010
Sibr	*Aloe barabadensis*	Hot 2° and dry 2°	Anti-inflammatory, laxative, purgative	Hakeem, 1999; Kabeeruddin, 2010
Ghareeqoon	*Polyporus officinalis*	Hot 1° and dry 2°	Purgative, deobstruent	Ghani, 2010
Habbul Ghar		Hot and dry 3°	Anticonvulsive, antiparalysis	Hakeem, 1999; Kabeeruddin, 2010
Banslochan	*Bambusa arundinacea*	Cold and dry 3°	Astringent, exhilarant	Ghani, 2010
Nilofar	*Nymphaea alba*	Cold and moist 2°	Cardiotonic, brain tonic	Ghani, 2010
Methi	*Tigonella foenumgraecum*	Hot and dry 2°	Anti-inflammatory	Ghani, 2010
Banafsha	*Viola odorata*	Cold and moist 1°	Antipyretic, antioxidant	Hakeem, 1999; Kabeeruddin, 2010
Guggul	*Commiphora mukul*	Hot 3° and dry 2°	Carminative, anti-inflammatory	Ghani, 2010; Hakeem, 1999

3.5 MECHANISM OF ACTION OF ANTICANCEROUS PLANTS

The exact mechanism of action of Unani medicine is not fully understood; however, their actions are because of the fact that Unani drugs contain thousands of pharmacologically active phytocompounds that act in different ways. The pathogenesis of cancer includes uncontrolled proliferation of a normal cell, which results in variabilities and changes at genetic level caused by both external (radiation, chemicals, tobacco, smoking, food, air, drinking water pollutants, infectious agents, and certain metals) and internal (immune system disorder, genetic mutations, and hormonal disorders) factors (Krishnamurthi, 2007). In "OMICS" concerning new era, however has discovered that there is a dysregulation of about 500 different genes (Vogelstein, 2004). Variabilities in genes include mutations in DNA repair genes (p21, p22, p27, p51, p53), oncogenes/biological accelerators (MYC, RAF, Bcl-2, RAS), tumor suppressor genes (p53, NF1, NF2, RB), and cell growth metabolism genes. For the treatment of cancer multiple targets drugs are favorably used like sorafenib, imatinib, and lapatinib. Sorafenib acts by inhibiting multiple protein kinases that comprises

TABLE 3.2 Anticancerous Studies on Unani Medicinal Plants.

Unani drugs	Part used	Nature of study	Type of cancer suppressed	Phytochemical	References
Aftimoon (Cuscuta Reflexa)	Whole plant	In vivo	Ehrlich ascites carcinoma (EAC) cell line	Amarbelin, cuscutin, coumarin, dulcitol, kaempferol, β-sitosterol, stigmasterol, myricetin, oleanolic acid, quercetin.	Chatterjee et al., 2011
Gaozaban (*Borago officinalis)*	Flower	In vitro	Acute promyelocytic leukemia (HL-60), Human cancer cell lines: liver (HPG2), prostate (LNCaP), and colon (HT-29)	Rosmarinic acid, phenols	Baena et al (2016) Karimi et al., 2017
Ustukhuddus (Lavandula stoechas	Aerial parts	In vitro	HepG2 cells lines	Alpha-fenchone, 1,8-cineole, triterpenes	Siddiqui et al., 2020
Halela Zard (Terminalia chebula	Leaf gall	In vitro	MCF-7 (human mammary gland adenocarcinoma) and A-549 (human lung cancer) BRL3A, MCF-7, and A-549 cells	Phenols, flavanoids	Shankara (2016)
Ajwain Desi (Pimpinella anisum)	Seeds Oil	In vitro	MCF-7 (human mammary gland adenocarcinoma) Human cancer cell lines A-549 (lung) and THP-1 (leukemia)	Flavonoids, phenol, terpenes, ellagic acid, thymol	Ramya et al., 2017; Sharma and Arora, 2017
Asgandh (*Withania somnifera)*	Whole plant	In vivo In vitro	Lung adenomas (A-549), liver, breast, colon (HCT-15), prostate cancer cell line (PC-3), DU-145, and IMR-32	Withaferin A	Singh et al, 1986; Uma et al., 1992; Prakash et al., 2001; Jayaprakasam et al., 2003; Yadav et al., 2010
Zanjabeel (*Zingiber officinale)*	Rhizome	In vitro	Human cervix carcinoma (HeLa cell line), human breast adenocarcinoma (MDA-MB231)	Zingerone	Katiyar et al., 1996; Vinothkumar et al., 2014; Akimoto, 2015; Ansar et al., 2016

TABLE 3.2 *(Continued)*

Unani drugs	Part used	Nature of study	Type of cancer suppressed	Phytochemical	References
Satawar (*Asparagus racemosus)*	Roots		Non-small-cell lung cancer, breast, colon, kidney	Steroids	Biswas et al., 2018; Mitra et al., 2012
Musli Siyah (Curculigo orchioides)	Roots	In vitro	Human breast cancer cell line (MCF-7)	Saponins	Singh et al., 2008
Filfil Daraz (*Piper longum)*	Fruit	In vivo	Dalton's lymphoma, ehrlich ascites carcinoma	Alkaloid	Sunila and Kuttan, 2004; Sharma et al., 2014
Lehsun (*Allium sativum)*	Bulb	In vivo	Suppresses proliferation of leukemia	Allicin, ajoene	Colic et al., 2002; Ahmed et al., 2001
Asalusoos (Glycyrrhiza glabra)	Root	In vitro	Breast cancer cell line (MCF-7) and HEP-2	Glycyrrhizin	Baltina et al., 2003; Rossi et al., 2003
Darchini (Cinnamomum zeylenicum)	Bark	In vitro	Human hepatoma cancer cells and human cervical tumor	Cinnamic aldehyde	Koppikar et al., 2010; Varalakshmi et al., 2014
Haldi (Curcuma longa)	Rhizome	In vitro	Epidermoid carcinoma cell line (HEp2), suppression of MMP-2 activity	Curcumin	Mitra et al., 2006
Shahm-e-Hanzal (Citrullus colocynthis)	Fruit	In vitro	Liver cancer cell line (HepG2) and breast cancer cell line (MCF7)	Cucurbitales, β-sitosterol, quercetin.	Wasfi et al., 1994; Tannin-Spitz et al., 2007; Ayyad et al., 2012
Methi (*Trigonella foenum-graecum)*	Seeds	In vitro	MCF7, TCP (T-cell lymphoma), FRO (thyroid papillary carcinoma), and brain tumors	Flavonoids, alkaloids, cadence, zinger one, vanillin, and eugenol	Sur et al., 2001; Amin et al., 2005; Hasanzadeh et al., 2010; Alsemari et al., 2014
Balela (*Terminalia bellerica*)		In vitro	Human breast (MCF-7) carcinoma and human lung (A549) carcinoma	Gallic acid, ellagic acid	Nishida et al., 2008

TABLE 3.2 *(Continued)*

Unani drugs	Part used	Nature of study	Type of cancer suppressed	Phytochemical	References
Khajoor (*P. dactylifera*)	Fruit	In vitro	Human breast adenocarcinoma (MCF7), human epithelial colorectal adenocarcinoma (Caco-2), and human melanoma derived cell line (IGR-39)	Polyphenols, flavonoids, folic acid, phenolic, procyanidins	Chakroun et al., 2016; Khan et al., 2016
Afsantin (*Artemisia absinthium* L.)	Aerial parts	In vitro	Breast cancer cell lines—an estrogenic responsive cell line (MCF-7) and an estrogenic-unresponsive cell line (MDA-MB-231).	Artemisinin	Shafi et al., 2012
Gilo (*Tinospora cordifolia*)	Root	In vitro In vivo	Human cervical cancer cell line (HeLa), Ehrlich ascites carcinoma	Tinosporin, columbin, isocolumbin, choloine, palmitine, phenylpropanoids, furan glycosides, norditerpene, diterpene, and phytoecdysones. Tetrahydropalmatine and magnoflorine	Gangan et al., 1997; Jagetia et al., 1998; Jagetia et al., 2006; Sultana et al., 2007
Brahmi (*Centella asiatica*)	Whole plant	In vitro	Dalton's lymphoma ascites, ehrlich ascites carcinoma	Asiaticoside, pectic acid, ascorbic acid, hydrocotyline, vallerine, flavonoids, sterol, stigmasterol, thankunosides	Babu et al., 1995; Sharma and Sharma, 2005; Srivastava and Kumar, 1997
Bhuinamla (*Phyllanthus amarus*)	Fruit	In vivo	Dalton's lymphoma ascites, ehrlich ascites carcinoma	Lignans, flavonoids, and tannins	Rajeshkumar et al., 2002

VEGFR1 (vascular endothelial growth factor receptor-1), VEGFR2, Raf kinase, and PDGFR (platelet derived growth factor). Imatinib acts by inhibiting ab 1 (Abelson proto-oncogene) tyrosine kinase activity, PDGFR, and c-kit. EGFR and HER2 tyrosine kinase activities are inhibited by lapatinib (Sams-Dodd, 2005; Jimeno, 2006).

Plants contain numerous pharmacologically active primary and secondary metabolites like alkaloids, flavonoids, glycosides, terpenes, lignans, saponins, taxanes, vitamins, minerals, gums, and oils that play substantial roles in cancer inhibition. Anticancer efficacy of these bioactive compounds has been studied both in vitro and in vivo. They have complimentary and overlapping mechanism to slow down the carcinogenic process. They act either by inhibiting proteins activated by cancer cells, CDC2, CDK2, and CDK4 kinases signaling pathways, activating DNA repair mechanism (p21, p27, p51, p53 genes and their protein products), inhibiting Bcl-2, cytokines, PI3K, Akt, MAPK/ERK, MMP, TNK, mechanistic target of rapamycin [mTOR]) Bax, Bid, Bak proteins, enzymes (topoisomerase, cyclooxygenase [COX] and COX-2), stimulating the formation of protective enzymes (Caspase-3, 7, 8, 9, 10, 12), inducing antioxidant action (antioxidant enzymes, e.g,. GSH, GST, and GPxn) (Thakore, 2012; Tariq, 2017). A brief mechanism of action of Unani drugs in treatment of cancer has been described in Figure 3.1.

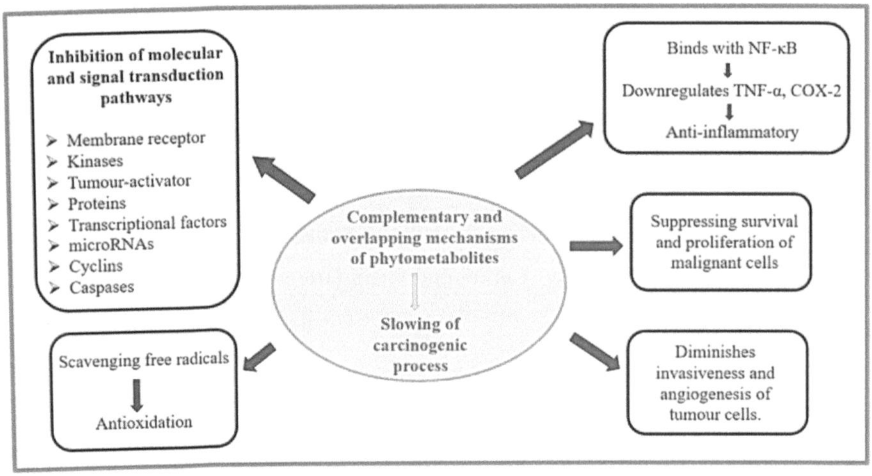

FIGURE 3.1 Mechanism of action of anticancerous plants.

3.5.1 UNANI COMPOUND FORMULATIONS USED IN SARTAN

When there is a mixture of two or more than two drugs and form one drug then this formulation of drugs is called compound formulations. In Unani text, some compound formulations have been given which are used in Sartan these are: *Itrifal-e-Aftimoon, Habb-e-Asgandh, Majoon Najah,Ma ul Jubn, Majoon Ushba, Tiryaq e Faruq,* and *Majoon Baladur.*

Table 3.3 describes those Unani compound formulations which can be used for combating the side effects caused by the chemotherapy and Table 3.4 enlisted some Unani compound formulations that have been studied for various protective activities.

TABLE 3.3 Compound Formulations Used for Combating Side Effects Due to Chemotherapy.

Sr. no	Compound formulations	Side effects of chemotherapy	References
1.	*Jawarish Bisbasa, Hab-e-Tursh Mushtahi, Namak-e-Suleman*	Loss in appetite	NCI, 2015; NFUM, 2006
2.	*Jawarish Mastagi, Hab-e-Ral*	Diarrhoea	NCI, 2015; NFUM, 2006
3.	*Sharbat Bazoori Mautadil*	Oedema	NCI, 2015; NFUM, 2006
4.	*Hab-e-Asgandh, Hab-e-Azraqi*	Nerve problems	NCI, 2015; NFUM, 2006
5.	*Jawarish Anarain, Jawarish Tamarhindi,*	Nausea and vomiting	NCI, 2015; NFU, 2006
6.	*Sharbat Anjbar, Qurs kahruba, Qurs kafoor, Qurs Sartan*	Bleeding and bruising	NCI, 2015; NFUM, 2006
7.	Sharbat Tooth Siyah, Lauq khayarshambar, Lauq Sapistan	Throat problems	NCI, 2015; NFUM, 2006
8.	Majoon Falasfa, kahamira Abresham, Khamira Gauzaban	Memory and concentration problems	NCI, 2015; NFUM, 2006

TABLE 3.4 Compound Formulations with Proven Protective Activities.

S.no	Pharmacological activity	Compound formulations	References
1	Nephro-protective	*Jawarish Zarooni Sada*	Afzal et al., 2004
2	Hepato-protective	*Majoon Dabidulward, Kabideen, Sharbat-e-Deenar, Jigreen*	Shakya et al., 2012; Shakya et al., 2012; Mahim et al., 2015; Najmi et al., 2005
3	Cardio-protective	*Khamira Abresham Hakim Arshad wala*	Goyal et al., 2010
4	Neuro-protective	*Majun Khadar, Majun Baladur*	Yousuf et al., 2011; Yousuf et al., 2007

3.6 CONCLUSION AND FUTURE PERSPECTIVE

Carcinogenesis is a multifactorial disease that is considered to be caused by the dysregulation of numerous physiological and biochemical pathways regulating cell growth, survival, and apoptosis. Considering these facts, the drugs/molecules are of prime importance that are targeting multiple signals which are inclusively contribute to tumor growth or progression. For the prevention and treatment of cancer, numerous traditional medicinal plants are used worldwide in various conventional ways from generations to generations. To fully harness the potential of phytochemicals, a paradigm drug-development strategy is necessary, in which ethnopharmacological expertise is backed up by a wide range of multidisciplinary and integrative approach comprising of biochemistry, medicinal chemistry, pharmacology, molecular, and cellular biology. Additionally, advances in analytical technology and breakthroughs in computational methodologies, along with the development of artificial intelligence network, will lead in finding new phytochemical entities for pharmacological testing. This chapter summarizes the Unani treatment based on the Unani pathophysiology. Unani medicinal plants are having substantial amount of active phytocompounds and they exhibited potential anticancer activities with specific mechanism of action. Most of the investigated phytochemicals in preclinical testing lack their molecular interactions with various signaling molecules. In order to solve concerns with molecular targets and pathways, in-silico technologies such as molecular docking must be used to understand the mechanism, which can then further be validated by means of various in vitro and in vivo models. Furthermore, many traditional plants lack clinical and toxicity studies; hence, there is a requirement of comprehensive studies for the development of clinically approvable novel anticancer drugs.

KEYWORDS

- **anti-cancerous plants**
- **humor**
- **immunomodulation**
- **Sartan**
- **Unani medicine**
- **humor**

REFERENCES

ACS-American Cancer Society. Early History of Cancer [Online] (2014). https://www.cancer.org/ cancer/cancer-basics/history-of-cancer/cancer-causes-theories-throughout-history.html. (accessed Jun 24, 2021).

Afzal, M.; Khan, N. A.; Ghufran, A.; Iqbal, A.; Inamuddin, M. Diuretic and Nephroprotective Effect of Jawarish Zarooni Sada--A Polyherbal Unani Formulation. *J. Ethnopharmacol.* **2004,** *91* (2–3), 219–23.

Ahmed, N.; Laverick, J.; Sammons, J.; Zhang, H.; Maslin, D. J.; Hassan, H. T. Ajoene, a Garlic-Derived Natural Compound, Enhances Chemotherapy-Induced Apoptosis in Human Myeloid Leukaemia CD34-Positive Resistant Cells. *Anticancer Res.* **2001,** *21,* 3519–3529.

Ahmad, R.; Ahmad, N.; Naqvi, A. A.; Shehzad, A.; Al-Ghamdi, M. S. Role of Traditional Islamic and Arabic Plants in Cancer Therapy. *J. Tradit. Complement. Med.* **2016,** *7* (2), 195–204.

Ahmed, N. Z.; Ansari, A. P.; Anwar, N.; Shahid, M. Cancer Perception in Unani Medicine – Conceptual Analysis. *Spatula DD* **2016,** *6* (4), 113–120.

Akimoto, M. Anticancer Effect of Ginger Extract Against Pancreatic Cancer Cells Mainly Through Reactive Oxygen Species-Mediated Autotic Cell Death. *PLoS One* **2015,** *10* (5), e0126605. https://doi.org/10.1371/journal.pone.0126605

Alsemari, A.; Alkhodairy, F.; Aldakan, A.; et al. The Selective Cytotoxic Anti-cancer Properties and Proteomic Analysis of *Trigonella Foenum-graecum. BMC Complement Alternat Med.* **2014,** *14,* 114.

Amin, A.; Alkaabi, A.; Al-Falasi, S.; Daoud, S. A. Chemopreventive Activities of *Trigonella Foenum Graecum* (Fenugreek) Against Breast Cancer. *Cell Biol. Int.* **2005,** 29, 687–694.

Ansar, J. K.; et al. Anticancer and Antioxidant Activity of Ginger Rhizome. *Indian J. Exp. Biol.* **2016,** *54,* 767–773.

Ayyad, S. E. N.; Abdel-Lateff, A.; Alarif, W. M.; Patacchioli, F. R.; Badria, F. A.; Ezmirly, S. T. In Vitro and In Vivo Study of Cucurbitacins-Type Triterpene Glucoside From *Citrullus Colocynthis* Growing in Saudi Arabia Against Hepatocellular Carcinoma. *Environ. Toxicol. Pharmacol.* **2012,** *33,* 245–251.

Babu, T. D.; Kuttan, G.; Padikkala, J. *J. Ethnopharmacol.* **1995,** *48* (1), 53–57.
Baghdadi, I. H. Kitab Al-Mokhtarat Fit Tibb (Urdu Translation); CCRUM, Ministry of Health and Family Welfare, Government of India: New Delhi, 2004; vol 3, pp 90–128.
Baitar, I. Al-Jame al-Mufrada al-Advia Wa al- Aghzia (Urdu Translation); CCRUM: New Delhi, 1999.
Baltina, L. A. Chemical Modification of Glycyrrhizic Acid as a Route to New Bioactive Compounds for Medicine. *Curr. Med. Chem.* **2003,** *10,* 155–171.
Bisset, N. G. *Planta Med.* **1983,** *48,* 225–229.
Biswas, D.; et al. Anticancer Activity of Root Extracts in Non-small Cell Lung Cancer Asparagus Racemosus A549 Cells. *Asian J. Pharmacy Pharmacol.* 2018, *4* (6), 764–770. DOI: org/10.31024/ajpp.2018.4.6.7
Bitar, I. A. AlJame Li-Mofradat al Adwiyah wal Aghthiyah (The Collection of Medical Items and food). Two volumes. Dar Sader Publishing: Beirut (In Arabic), 1874.
Cancer Treatment, Side-effects‖. Cancer National Institute, [Online] 2015. https://www.cancer.gov/about-cancer/treatment/side-effects on June 20, 2021.
Chakroun, M.; Khemakhem, B.; Mabrouk, H. B.; El Abed, H.; Makni, M.; Bouaziz, M.; Drira, N.; Marrakchi, N.; Mejdoub, H. Evaluation of Anti-diabetic and Anti-tumoral Activities of Bioactive Compounds From Phoenix Dactylifera L's Leaf: In Vitro and In Vivo Approach. *Biomed. Pharmacother.* **2016,** *84,* 415–422. DOI: 10.1016/j.biopha.2016.09.062
Chatterjee, D.; Sahu, R. K.; Jha, A. K.; Dwivedi, J. Evaluation of Antitumor Activity of Cuscuta Reflexa Roxb. (Cuscutaceae) Against Ehrlich Ascites Carcinoma in Swiss Albino Mice. *Trop. J. Pharmaceu. Res.* **2011,** *10* (4), 447–454.
Colic, M.; Vucevic, D.; Kilibarda, V.; Radicevic, N.; Savic, M. Modulatory Effects of Garlic Extracts on Proliferation of T-lymphocytes In Vitro Stimulated With Concanavalin A. *Phytomedicine* **2002,** *9,* 117–124.
Cragg, G. M.; Newman, D. J. Medicinal for the Milennia. *Ann. N. Y. Acad. Sci.* **2001,** *953,* 3–25.
Diwanay, S.; Chitre, D.; Patwardhan, B. J. *Ethnopharmacology* **2004**, *90* (1), 49–55.
Ghani. N. *Khazain-ul-Advia*; Idara Kitabul Shifa: New Delhi, 2010.
Goyal, S.; Siddiqui, M. K.; Siddiqui, K. M.; Arora, S.; Mittal, R.; Joshi, S.; Arya, D. S. Cardioprotective Effect of 'Khamira Abresham Hakim Arshad Wala' a Unani Formulation in Isoproterenol-Induced Myocardial Necrosis in Rats. *Exp. Toxicol. Pathol.* **2010,** *62* (1), 61–74.
Gupta, S. C.; Kim, J. H. S.; Prasad, B. B. Regulation of Survival, Proliferation, Invasion, Angiogenesis, and Metastasis of Tumor Cells Through Modulation of Inflammatory Pathways by Nutraceuticals. *Cancer Metastasis Rev.* **2010,** *29,* 405.
Hakeem, M. I. *Bustan ul Muridat*; Idara Taraqi Urdu Publication: Lucknow, India, 1999.
Hasanzadeh, E.; Rezazadeh, S. H.; Shamsa, S. F.; Dolatabadi, R.; Zarringhalam, J. Review on Phytochemistry and Therapeutic Properties of Fenugreek (*Trigonella Foenum-Graceum*). *J. Med. Plants* **2010,** *2* (34), 1–18.
Hussain, et al, Relevance of Traditional Unani (Greco-Arab) System of Medicine in Cancer: An update Chapter 10. In *Anticancer Plants: Clinical Trials and Nanotechnology;* Akhtar, M. S., Swamy, M. K., Eds.; [Online]. https://doi.org/10.1007/978-981-10-8216-0_10
International Agency for Research on Cancer (IARC), World Cancer Factsheet, 2014.
Jagetia, G. C.; Nayak, V.; Vidyasagar, M. S. *Cancer Lett.* **1998,** *127* (1–2), 71–82.

Jagetia, G. C.; Rao, S. K. *Biol. Pharm. Bull.* **2006,** *29* (3), 460–466.

Jayaprakasam, B.; Zhang, Y.; Seeram, N. P.; Nair, M. G. Growth Inhibition of Human Tumor Cell Lines by Withanolides From Withania Somnifera Leaves. *Life Sci.* **2003,** *74*, 125–132.

Jemal, A.; Bray, F.; Melissa, M.; Ferlay, J.; Ward, E.; Forman, D. Global Cancer Statistics. *CA Cancer J. Clin.* **2011,** *61*, 69–90.

Jimeno, A.; Hidalgo, M. Multitargeted Therapy: Can Promiscuity be Praised in an Era of Political Correctness? *Crit. Rev. Oncol. Hematol.* **2006,** *59* (2), 150–158.

Kabeeruddin, M. *Makhzanul Mufradat*; Idara Kitab-Us-Shifa: New Delhi, 2010.

Katiyar, S. K.; Agarwal, R.; Mukhtar, H. Inhibition of Tumor Promotion in SENCAR Mouse Skin by Ethanol Extract of Zingiber Officinale Rhizome. *Cancer Res.* **1996,** *56* (5), 1023–1030.

Khan, A. Avicenna (Ibn Sina): Muslim Physician and Philosopher of the Eleventh Century (Great Muslim Philosophers and Scientists of the Middle Ages). The Rosen Publishing Group: New York, 2006.

Khan, S. A.; Al Kiyumi, A. R.; Al Sheidi, M. S.; Al Khusaibi, T. S.; Al Shehhi, N. M.; Alam, T. In Vitro Inhibitory Effects on α-glucosidase and α-amylase Level and Antioxidant Potential of Seeds of Phoenix Dactylifera L. *Asian Pac. J. Trop. Biomed.* **2016,** *6* (4), 322–329. DOI: 10.1016/j.apjtb.2015.11.008

Koppikar, S. J.; Choudhari, A. S.; Suryavanshi, S. A.; Kumari, S.; Chattopadhyay, S.; Kaul-Ghanekar, R. Aqueous Cinnamon Extract (ACEc) From the Bark of Cinnamomum Cassia Causes Apoptosis in Human Cervical Cancer Cell Line (SiHa) Through Loss of Mitochondrial Membrane Potential. *BMC Cancer* **2010,** *10*, 210.

Krishnamurthi, K. Screening of Natural Products for Anticancer and Antidiabetic Properties. *Cancer* **2007,** *3,* 4.

Lichota, A.; Gwozdzinski, K. Anticancer Ativity of Natural Compounds From Plant and Marine Environment. *Int. J. Mol. Sci.* **2018,** *19*, 1–38.

Mahim, Z.; Abdur, R.; Iqbal, A. Q. Heaptoprotective Activity of a Unani Polyherbal Formulation _Kabideen' in CCl4 Induced Liver Toxicity. *IJABFP* 2015, *6* (1), 8–16.

Maseehi, A. A. I. Q. *Kitabul Umda fil Jarahat*, (Urdu Translation by CCRUM). New Delhi: Ministry of Health and Family Welfare, Govt of India, 1995; vol I & II, pp 169–170, pp 71–75.

Mitra, A.; Chakrabarti, J.; Banerji, A.; Chatterjee, A.; Das, B. *J. Environ. Pathol. Toxicol. Oncol.* **2006,** *25* (4), 679–690.

Mitra, S. K.; Prakash, N. S.; Sundaram, R. Shatavarins (Containing Shatavarin IV) With Anticancer Activity From the Roots of *Asparagus Racemosus. Indian J. Pharmacol.* **2012,** *44* (6), 732–736. DOI: 10.4103/0253-7613.103273

Najmi, J.; Pillai, A. K.; Pal, K. K.; Aqil, M. Free Radical Scavenging and Hepatoprotective Activity of Jigrine Against Galactosamine Induced Hepatopathy in Rats. *Ethnopharmacology* **2005,** *97* (3), 521–525.

National Formulary of Unani Medicne (NFUM). Ministry of Health and Family Welfare, Department of AYUSH, 2006.

Newman, D. J.; Cragg, G. M.; Snader, K. M. Natural Products as Sources of New Drugs Over the Period. *J. Nat. Prod.* **2003,** *66,* 1022–1037.

Nishida, K.; Yamaguchi, O.; Otsu, K. Crosstalk Between Autophagy and Apoptosis in Heart Disease. *Circ. Res.* **2008,** *103*, 343–351.

Park, E. J.; Pezzutto, J. M. Botanicals in Cancer Chemoprevention. *Cancer Metastasis Rev.* **2002,** *21* (3–4), 231–255.

Prakash, J.; Gupta, S. K.; Kochupillai, V.; Singh, N.; Gupta, Y. K.; Joshi, S. Chemotherapy Activity of Withania Somnifera in Experimentally Induced Fibrosarcoma Tumours in Swiss Albino Mice. *Phytother. Res.* **2001,** *15*, 240–244.

Qamari, N. B. M. *Ghana Mina* (Urdu Translation), 1st ed.; CCRUM, Ministry of Health and Family Welfare, Government of India: New Delhi, 2008; pp 508–510.

Rafeequddin, M. Kanzul Advia Mufradat. Aligarh Muslim University Press, 1985.

Rajeshkumar, N. V.; Joy, K. L.; Kuttan, G.; Ramsewak, R. S.; Nair, M. G.; Kuttan, R. *J. Ethnopharmacol.* **2002,** *81* (1), 17–22.

Ramya, N.; Priyadharshini; Prakash, R.; Dhivya, R. Anti Cancer Activity of Trachyspermum Ammi Against MCF7 Cell Lines Mediates by p53 and Bcl-2 mRNA Levels. *J. Phytopharmacol.* **2017,** *6* (2), 78–83.

Razi, A. M. B. Z. *Al Hawi Fit Tib.* (Urdu Translation by CCRUM); CCRUM, Ministry of Health and Family Welfare, Govt. of India; New Delhi, 1997; vol 12, pp 9–24.

Rhazes. *Al Hawy* (The Comprehensive); Dar AlKalam Publishing Beirut (in Arabic), 925.

Rossi, T.; Castelli, M.; Zandomeneghi, G.; Ruberto, A.; Benassi, L.; Magnoni, C. Selectivity of Action of Glycyrrhizin Derivatives on the Growth of MCF-7 and HEP-2 Cells. *Anticancer Res.* **2003,** *23* (5A), 3813–3818.

Rushd, I. *Kitabul Kulliyat*, 1st ed.; (Urdu Translation by CCRUM); Ministry of Health and Family Welfare, Govt. of India, New Delhi, 1980; pp 89–90.

Saad, B.; Azaizeh, H.; Said, O. Tradition and Perspectives of Arab Herbal Medicine: A Review. *Evid. Based Compl. Altern. Med.* **2005,** *2*, 475–479.

Saad, B.; Azaizeh, H.; Said, O. Arab Herbal Medicine. *Bot. Med. Clin. Pract.* **2008,** *4*, 31.

Said, O.; Zaid, H.; Saad, B. Greco-Arab and Islamic Herbal Medicine and Cancer Treatment/Prevention. In *Bioactive Foods and Extracts Cancer Treatment and Prevention*; Watson, R. R., Preedy, R. V. (Eds.); CRC Press, Taylor and Francis: Boca Raton, 2011; pp 49–66.

Samarqandi, A. N. *Moalajat Sharh-e-Asbab* (Urdu Translation by Khuwaja Rizwan); CCRUM, Ministry of Health and Family Welfare, Government of India: New Delhi, 2010; vol 3, pp 369–370.

Sams-Dodd, F. Target-Based Drug Discovery: Is Something Wrong? *Drug Discov. Today* **2005,** *10* (2), 139–147.

Schwartsmann, G.; Ratain, M. J.; Cragg, G. M.; Wong, J. E.; Saijo, N.; Parkinson, D. R.; et al. Anticancer Drug Discovery and Development Throughout the World. *J. Clin. Oncol.* **2002,** *20,* 47S–59S.

Seca, A. M.; Pinto, D. C. Plant Secondary Metabolites as Anticancer Agents: Successes in Clinical Trials and Therapeutic Application. *Int. J. Mol. Sci.* **2018,** *19* (263), 1–22.

Shafi, G.; Hasan, T. N.; Syed, N. A.; Al-Hazzani, A. A.; Alshatwi, A. A. Artemisia Sbsinthium (AA): A Novel Potential Complementary and Alternative Medicine for Breast Cancer. *Mol. Biol. Rep.* **2012,** *39* (7), 7373–7379.

Shakya, A. K.; Sharma, N.; Saxena, M.; Shrivastava, S.; Shukla, S. Evaluation of the Antioxidant and Hepatoprotective Effect of Majoon-e-Dabeed-ul-Ward Against Carbon Tetrachloride Induced Liver Injury. *Exp. Toxicol. Pathol.* **2012,** *64* (7–8), 767–773.

Shakya, A. K.; Saxena, M.; Sharma, N.; Shrivastava, S.; Shukla, S. Hepatoprotective Efficacy of Sharbat-e-Deenar Against Carbon Tetrachloride-Induced Liver Damage. *J. Environ. Pathol. Toxicol. Oncol.* **2012,** *31* (2), 131–141.

Shamsi, Y.; Khan, A. A.; Alam, T.; Jabeen, A. Management of Cancer With Munzij and Mus'hil Therapy: A Regimen of Ilaj Bit Tadbeer (Regimenal Therapy) in Unani System of Medicine. *Int. J. Curr. Rev. Res.* **2016,** *8,* 4–9.

Sharma, E.; Arora, B. S. Phytochemical Investigation of Seeds of Trachyspermum Ammi Linn. by GC-MS. *J. Chem. Environ. Sci. Appl.* **2017,** *3* (2), 91–100. DOI: https://doi.org/10.15415/jce.2017.32007

Sharma, R.; Sharma, J. *Phytother. Res.* **2005,** *19* (7), 605–611.

Sharma, A. H.; et al. Cell Cycle Inhibitory Activity of Piper Longum Against A549 Cell Line and its Protective Effect Against Metal-Induced Toxicity in Rats. *Indian J. Biochem. Biophys.* **2014,** *51,* 358–364.

Sina, I. *Al-Qanoon Fit Tibb* (Urdu Translation by Gulam Husain Kanturi); Nigarishat Miyan Chambers: Lahore, 1992; vol 4, pp 175–176.

Singh, N.; Singh, S. P.; Nath, R. Prevention of Urethane-Induced Lung Adenomas by Withania Somnifera (L.) Dunal in Albino Mice. *Int. J. Crude Drug Res.* **1986,** *24,* 90–100.

Singh, R.; et al. Antimicrobial and Antitumor Activity of the Fractionated Extracts of Kalimusli. *Int. J. Green Pharm.* **2008,** *2* (1), 34–36.

Srivastava, R.; Kumar, S. *Ind. J. Med. Arom. Plants* **1997,** *19,* 1049–1056.

Srivastava, S. K.; Rai, V.; Srivastava, M.; Ra, A. K.; wat, S.; Mehrotra, S. Estimation of Heavy Metals in Different Berberis Species and its Market Samples. *Environ. Monit. Assess* **2006,** *116,* 315–320.

Sultana, N.; Lee, N. H. *Phytother. Res.* **2007,** *21* (12), 1171–1176.

Sun, Y.; Xun, K.; Wang, Y.; Chen, X. A Systematic Review of the Anticancer Properties of Berberine, A Natural Product From Chinese Herbs. *Anticancer Drugs* **2009,** *20,* 757–769.

Sunila, E. S.; Kuttan, G. Immunomodulatory and Antitumor Activity of Piper Longum Linn. and Piperine. *J. Ethnopharmacol.* **2004,** *90,* 339–346. DOI: 10.1016/j.jep.2003.10.016

Sur, P.; Das, M.; Gomes, A.; et al. *Trigonella Foenum Graecum* (Fenugreek) Seed Extract as an Antineoplastic Agent. *Phytother. Res.* **2001,** *15,* 257–259.

Tabri, A. A. M. Molejate Buqratiyah, (Urdu Translation by CCRUM). Ministry of Health and Family Welfare, Govt of India: New Delhi, 1995; *II,* 244–248.

Tabri, R. *Firdousul Hikmat*; Idarae Kitabushifa: New Delhi, 2010.

Tannin-Spitz, T.; Grossman, S.; Dovrat, S.; Gottlieb, H. E.; Bergman, M. Growth Inhibitory Activity of Cucurbitacin Glucosides Isolated From *Citrullus Colocynthis* on Human Breast Cancer Cells. *Biochem. Pharmacol.* **2007,** *73,* 56–67.

Tariq, A.; Sadia, S.; Pan, K.; Ullah, I.; Mussarat, S.; Sun, F.; et al. A Systematic Review on Ethnomedicines of Anti-Cancer Plants. *Phytother. Res.* **2017,** *31,* 202–264.

Thakore, P.; Mani, R. K.; Kavitha, S. J. A Brief Review of Plants Having Anti-Cancer Property. *Int. J. Pharm. Res. Dev.* **2012,** *3,* 129–136.

Thomas, J. In *Medicinal and Aromatic Plants Research in India.* UNDP Proceeding of Training Course on Industrial Exploitation of Indigenous Medicinal and Aromatic Plants, Beijing, China, 1997; pp 17–27.

Uma Devi, P.; Sharada, A. C.; Solomon, F. E.; Kamath, M. S. In Vivo Growth Inhibitory Effects of Withania Somnifera (Ashwagandha) on a Transplantable Mouse Tumor, Sarcoma180. *Cancer Lett.* **1992,** *30,* 169–172.

Varalakshmi, B.; Anand, V.; Karpagam, T.; Suguna, B. J.; Manikandan, R. In Vitro Antimicrobial and Anticancer Activity of Cinnamomum Zeylanicum Linn Bark Extracts. *Int. J. Pharm. Pharm. Sci.* **2014,** *6,* Suppl 1, 12–18.

Vinothkumar, R.; Sudha, M.; Nalini, N. Chemopreventive Effect of Zingerone Against Colon Carcinogenesis Induced by 1,2-dimethylhydrazine in Rats. *Eur. J. Cancer Prev.* **2014,** *23* (5), 361–371.

Vogelstein, B.; Kinzler, K. W. Cancer Genes and the Pathways They Control. *Nat. Med.* **2004,** *10* (8), 789–799.

Wasfi, I. A. Some Pharmacological Studies on *Citrullus Colocynthis. J. Herbs Spices Med. Plants* **1994,** *2* (2), 65–79.

Yadav, B, A.; Bajaj, A.; Saxena, M.; Saxena, A. K. In Vitro Anticancer Activity of the Root, Stem and Leaves of Withania Somnifera Against Various Human Cancer Cell Lines. *Indian J. Pharm. Sci.* **2010,** *72* (5), 659–663.

Yousuf, S.; Atif, F.; Ahmad, M.; Ishrat, T.; Khan, B.; Islam, F. Neuroprotection Offered by Majun Khadar, a Traditional Unani Medicine, During Cerebral Ischemic Damage in Rats. *Evid. Based Complement. Alternat. Med.* **2011,** 754025.

Yousuf, S.; Atif, F.; Hoda, N.; Ahmad, M.; Saleem, S.; Ishrat, T.; Khan, M. B.; Ahmad, A. S.; Islam, F. Oral Supplementation of Majun Baladar Ameliorates Antioxidant Enzyme Activities in Cerebral Ischaemic Damage. *Basic Clin. Pharmacol. Toxicol.* **2007**, *101* (4), 246–253.

Zaid, H.; Silbermann, M.; Ben-Arye, E.; Saad, B. Greco-Arab and Islamic Herbal-Derived Anticancer Modalities: From Tradition to Molecular Mechanisms. *Evid. Based Complement. Alternat. Med.* **2012,** *2012,* 1–14.

Zohar, A. M. A. M. I. *Kitabul Taiseer,* 1st ed.; Urdu Translation by CCRUM; Ministry of Health and Family Welfare, Govt. of India: New Delhi, 1986; p 217.

CHAPTER 4

Exploration of Anticancer Medicinal Plants of the Northern Hemisphere

YOUNIS AHMAD HAJAM,[1] AISHWARYA SHARMA,[2] and RAJESH KUMAR[3]

[1]*Department of Life Sciences and Allied Health Sciences, Sant Baba Bhag Singh University, Jalandhar, Punjab, India*

[2]*Department of Biosciences, Division Zoology, Career Point University, Hamirpur, Himachal Pradesh, India*

[3]*Department of Biosciences, Himachal Pradesh University, Shimla, Himachal Pradesh, India*

ABSTRACT

Since earlier times of human history, many plants have been known, identified, studied, and used for various medicinal purposes and can be regarded as the basis of modern medicine. Kingdom Plantae has an essential metabolism which has a capacity to develop a various type of compounds on large scale, which can be utilized by various industries like pharmaceutical in order to obtain and produce a new variety of innovative medicines. The continuous search for antitumor and anticancer agents from plant sources is an essential way to figure out various ways for safe and effective treatment for much health-related problems. According to the ethnobotanical historical sources, various uses and wide applications of medicinal plants have led to more attention. Many natural products having various significant chemical structures are isolated as anticancer agents. Certain side effects occur due to chemotherapy, whereas natural therapies like utilization of plant-derived products in cancer treatment do not cause such adverse effects. Thus, protection of medicinal plants by

Plant-Derived Anticancer Drugs in the OMICS Era: Biosynthesis, Functions, and Applications. Deepu Pandita, Anu Pandita (Eds.)

import and export monitoring trade is highly symbolic and the best way for conservation of medicinal plants is plant cultivation.

4.1 INTRODUCTION

Cancer is acting as an aggressive killer in the world. Clinically, the novel synthetic chemotherapeutic agents are not working so well in order to meet the expectations and instead of their consideration costs about 17 million deaths occur due to cancer per year (Thun et al., 2010). In spite of decades in medical research and advancements, problems like cancer still remain as a big huddle in healthcare system (Yabroff et al., 2011). Globally, cancer is known to be the major mortality as well as morbidity cause. Moreover, apart from cardiovascular diseases, cancer has become the second most leading consequence of death among communicable diseases (Sener et al., 2005). Incidence as well as mortality of cancer is more in countries like New Zealand and Australia if compared with other parts of the world (Parkin, 2004). The cases of deaths occurring because of cancer are supposed to elevate from 7.1 million at 2002 to 11.5 million in 2030 across the globe (Mathers and Loncar, 2006).

India is known as a leading country for having scientific literature highlighting cancer based on phytochemical, ethnomedicinal, and pharmacological aspects. Moreover, a large part of the Himalayan region comes beneath Indian Territory constituting a strong and effective traditional system (Mathur and Joshi, 2013). Cancer is regarded as a primordial disease which is evident from record of fossil bones and mummies found in Egypt (Mackay et al., 2006). According to studies, after cardiovascular diseases, cancer is regarded as the highest cause for death (Park et al., 2008). About 50% of anticancer drugs employed these days are obtained by naturally occurring products or are isolated as either semisynthetic or synthetic compounds, out of which plants act as essential sources (Newman and Cragg, 2012).

The 6500-year-old text from Rigveda has an emphasis on the use of Himalayan plants for various medicinal uses (Malla and Shakya, 1984). Himalaya serves to be the planet's largest biodiversity zone accounting for plant resource diversity (Kala and Mathur, 2002). Every year, thousands of deaths due to cancer are reported in various Himalayan countries such as India, Nepal, and Pakistan (Akhtar, 2007; Bhatia et al., 2011). Identification as well as evaluation of effective anticancer plants along with their mechanisms and uses may be beneficial for the novel drug development which will then be employed for treatment of cancer (Krishnaswamy, 2008). About 10 million new cases are diagnosed every year with occurrence of approximately 6 million deaths all over the world (Hanif et al., 2009; Ismail et al., 2012). By 2030, WHO projected about 11 million deaths (WHO, 2007).

Approximately about more than 10,000 medicinal plants reported from the Himalayas are known to support primary health care as well as livelihoods of about 600 million people of the area (Shengji, 2001). Indigenous aspect of knowledge applied for the formation of different ethnomedicines is essential for the treatment of cancer (Gautam, 2011). Medicinal plants have contributed a lot to the discovery of anticancer drugs like camptothecine, podophyllotoxon, paclitaxel, and taxol (Oberlies and Kroll, 2004; Singh et al., 2013). The International Agency for Research on Cancer has estimated the chances of prevalence and mortality with regard to the disease. About 14.1 million cases of cancer were reported and then they further resulted in about 8.2 million of deaths along with 32.6 million patients suffering with diseases like cancer as per 2012 census of 184 countries worldwide (WHO, 2016). Medicinal plants form an essential constituent of health care for population as they are greatly used in terms of traditional and modern medicines (Luseba et al., 2010). An important income source is being provided to rural as well as urban people as a trade value for global trade whose estimation is accounted to be 32.6 billion per year (Brinckmann, 2016). Apart from accessibility and productivity, climate change affects the phytochemical content of the existing populations which potentially affects the pharmaceutical properties (Gairola et al., 2010). Despite the considerable development cost, novel synthetic chemotherapeutic agents who are in use were unavailable in fulfilling expectations (Coseri, 2009). Thus, a need for developing new, effective, and affordable anticancer drugs arises. Over past 30 years, natural products have been receiving much attention for having a great efficiency as a cancer therapeutic cum preventive agent (Newman, 2008). Plant kingdom acts as the most significant source as about 60% of drugs employed in treatment of cancer are extracted by the naturally occurring sources (Gordaliza et al., 2007).

4.2 TOXICITY DUE TO CHEMOTHERAPEUTIC TREATMENT

Consistent discovery and development have given rise to the collection of various chemotherapeutic agents although treatments involving such drugs not even devoid of their self-intrinsic problems. As a result of chemotherapeutic treatment, many toxicities are produced like 5-fluorouracil which also behaves like a vasoplastic and may cause myelotoxicity and cardiotoxicity (Macdonald, 1999). Cardiac toxicity (Rexroth and Scotland, 1994), toxicity of renal system (Manil et al., 1995), as well as myelotoxicity (Andreux et al., 1994) may be caused by doxorubin, whereas bleomycin causes pulmonary toxicity (Golding et al., 1982) along with cutaneous toxicity (Klaus et al., 1973). A cyclophosphamide helps in treatment of many malignant conditions and may cause bladder toxicity and may be in the form of immunosuppression, alopecia, hemorrhagic cystitis, and cardiotoxicity (Kanekal and Kehrer, 1991).

Medicinal plants serve to have a common alternative for treatment of cancer among different countries and more than 300 plants are being identified to exhibit anticancer properties worldwide. Data reflect that product derived from plants has 10–40% incidence for cancer treatment at global level, reporting about 50% of patients from Asia (Cassileth and Deng, 2004), whereas estimation of anticancer herbal product cost is approximately about 5 billion dollars per year (Jong et al., 2006).

4.3 PLANTS AS SOURCE OF DRUGS

The natural compounds obtained from plant source have an essential role in pharmacological activities, and Taxol, Vina alkaloids, camptothecine, and podophyllotoxins along with their semisynthetic derivatives are examples of such cooperation (Malik et al., 2014). Compounds having therapeutic properties in plants were identified by scientists and are thus used to treat various diseases (Shankari and Gurunathan, 201). As per the World Health Organization, curcumin can be taken into consideration in order to study the decreased rates of cancers like colorectal, lung, and prostate in India and is under clinical trials in order to study its safety and effectiveness (Dahmke et al., 2014). The anticancer action of the green tea from *Camellia sinensis* along with its main constituent like an epigallocatechin-3-gallate with regard to various tumor cell-related models has been proven, although more studies are still required for proving their role as anticancer drugs (Rahmani et al., 2015).

4.4 DEMANDS FOR MEDICINAL PLANTS

The successful trials have been made in the drug development originating from plants with regard to the clinical development. Some species are investigated and selected by various developing countries like Africa or Asia practicing herbal therapies with their enormous use in the cancer treatment (Ochwang et al., 2014). It was estimated by the World Health Organization during 2007 that the trade based on plant-derived drugs contributed about US$100 billion approximately, and by 2050, it is expected to reach US$5 trillion. Factors like deforestation, population growth along with rapid urbanization are contributing to an issue of protecting medicinal plants which is need of an hour as many medicinal plants having high value are being threatened and are on the verge of extinction due to over-exploitation (Parveen et al., 2013).

4.5 PLANT METABOLITES EXTRACTED FROM THE NATURAL SOURCES

For about 60,000 years approximately, plants have been used as medicines having ability of cocktail production by secondary metabolites accounting for a broad and wide range of pharmacological properties exhibiting anticancer activity (Kuttan et al., 1997). Phenolic compounds such as flavonoids account to be the most promising plant-derived secondary metabolites which are useful in treating cancer (Asensi et al., 2011; Wahl et al., 2011). All the extracts which have been reported so far would be able to show replication in their anticancer effects in larger scale tests and that may be essential in making them compatible for various strategies employed during treatment of cancer (Fritz et al., 2013; Ioannidis, 2005).

Tubulin depolymerization is inhibited by paclitaxel which stabilizes the microtubule cytoskeleton and block mitosis in a manner depending upon concentration (Wani and Horwitz, 2014). Various other molecular anticancer agents are found in plants naturally like genistein, lycopene, and resveratrol which are under further clinical trials (Bosviel et al., 2012;

King-Batoon et al., 2008). Several pregnane glycosides as well as alkaloids are some other examples of plant-obtained metabolites which show anticancer activity in vitro and serve to inhibit breast growth and prostate cancer lines (Jagadeesh et al., 2007). Nonpsychoactive cannabinoids have also been reported to show antitumor activities (McAllister et al., 2015) and likewise such activities are being reported for increasing number of secondary plant metabolites (Schnekenburger et al., 2014).

TABLE 4.1 Some Anticancer Medicinal Plants of Northern Hemisphere.

S. no.	*Botanical name*	*Common name*	*Plant part used*
1.	*Tinospora cordifolia*	Miers	*Stem, root*
2.	*Curcuma longa*	Turmeric	Rhizome
3.	*Ziziphus nummularia*	*Jujube*	*Root, stem, bark, seed, and flower*
4.	*Cedrus deodara*	Deodar	Resins, bark
5.	*Centella asiatica*	*Pennywort*	*Whole plant, especially leaves*
6.	*Andrographis paniculata*	Creat	Roots, leaves
7.	*Phyllanthus amarus*	Gale of wind	*Whole plant*
8.	*Mappia foetida amruta*	Amruta	*Whole plant*
	Taxus baccata	English yew	Pollen, needles, root, stem, bark, and wood
9.	*Podophyllum peltatum*	Indian May Apple	Rhizomes
10.	*Taraxacum officinale*	Common dandelion root	Root

4.5.1 *TINOSPORA CORDIFOLIA (WILD) MIERS)*

Botanical name: *Tinospora cordifolia*
Common name: Miers
It is also known as guduchi, giloya, heartleaf moonseed plant
Plant part used: Stem, roots

It is a smooth, bulky, deciduous shrub devoid of bristles. *Tinospora cordifolia* is among the noncontroversial and largely used herbs in Ayurveda medicine. It belongs to Menispermaceae family. It is also known as amrita because of its ability of imparting vitality and longevity. Stem of this plant is beneficial in treating debility, fever, jaundice, dyspepsia, jaundice, anemia, vomiting, piles, and certain skin diseases (Srivastava et al., 2003). Its roots have curative properties useful as antidote for snakebite (Wang

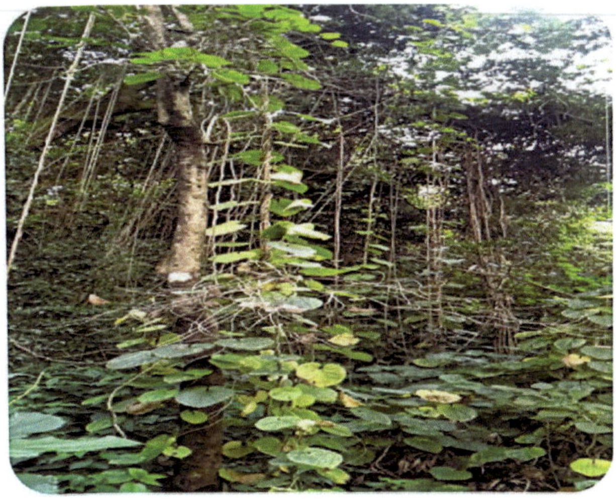

FIGURE 4.1 *Tinospora cordifolia.*

et al., 1991). Apart from this, it also has some beneficial properties in the modern medicine as it is immunomodulatory and adaptogenic along with essential anti-inflammatory, anti-arthritic as well as antioxidant properties (Chitre et al., 2004). Roots of this plant contain various alkaloids such as choline, tinosporin, isocolumbin, columbin, palmatine tetrahydropalmatine, and magnoflorine (Qazi et al., 2008). *T. cordifolia* helps in killing HeLa cells in vitro and this indicates that it can act as an anticancer agent and thus its extract shows an increase in tumor-free survival capacity which is dose dependent along with highest survivors (Vidyasagar et al., 1998). Leaves of *Tinospora* are protein-rich which accounts for 11.2% and also constitutes of calcium as well as phosphorus. Diterpene compounds are active adaptogenic constituents which include tinosporic acid, tinosporone, cordifolisides, yellow alkaloid, giloin, and berberine along with certain polysaccharides like arabinogalactan polysaccharides (Winston et al., 2007).

4.5.1.1 ANTICANCER ACTIVITY IN T. CORDIFOLIA

Response surface methodology is used to extract alkaloid palmatine from *T. cordifolia* species which then indicates anticancer efficiency in dimethylbenz anthracene (DMBA)-inducing skin cancer with reference to animal models like mice. Before 24 h of cyclophosphamide (50 mg/kg) administration, a single dose of *Tinospora* extract that is 200, 400, and

600 mg/kg dry weight, respectively, helps in preventing the formation of micronucleus in bone marrow of mice (Ali and Dixit, 2013). An increase in the life span along with a decrease in size of tumor with comparison to the control was studied at a dose of 750 mg/kg body weight C57 BI mice were administrated with 50% of *T. cordifolia* methanolic extract consecutively for 30 days (Verma et al., 2011). It was also found in a study that antibrain cancer potential accounts for 50% ethanolic *T. cordifolia* extract along with the use of C6 glioma cells (Mishra and Kaur, 2013). Cell proliferation was reduced by TCE in dose-dependent manner, whereas it helped in inducing differentiation in C6 glioma cells. Then, it was reported that all the extracts taken were much active in response to KB as well as CHOK-1 cells, while palmatine was known to be much responsive against the KB and HT-29; yangambin against the KB cells whereas tinocordiside against the KB and CHOK-1 (Bala et al., 2015). There were two molecules marked as hexane as well as methanol fractions and were represented as T1 and T2. *T. cordifolia* plant showed that in case of MCF-7 cells, T1 treatment suppresses the process of proliferation and invasion, thereby increasing E-cadherin transcription while the migration of MCF-7 cells is mainly regulated by T1 as compared with T2 (Shilpa et al., 2015).

TABLE 4.2 Various Chemical Constituents of *T. cordifolia.*

Sr. no.	Chemical	Plant part	Active compound
1	Sesquiterpenoid	Stem	Tinocordifolin
2	Glycosides	Stem	Euranoid diterpene glucoside, 18-norclerodane glucoside cordioside, cordifolioside A, cordiofolioside B, cordifoliside C, cordifoliside D, cordifolisides E palmatosides C, palmatosides F
3	Steroids	Aerial partStem	B-sitosterol, δ-sitosterol, 20 β-hydroxy ecdysones
			Ecdysterone, makisterone A, giloinosterol
4	Diterpenoids lactones	Whole plant	Euranolactone, clerodane derivatives, tinosporon, tinosporides, jateorine, columbin
5	Alkaloids	Stem as well as root	Palmatine choline berberine, tembetarine, magnoflorine, tinosporin, tetrahydropalmatine, isocolumbin, palmatine magnoflorine
6	Aliphatic compound	Whole plant	Heptacosanol, octacosanol

4.5.2 CURCUMA LONGA

Botanical name: *Curcuma longa*
Common name: Turmeric
It is also known as haridra and haldi.
Plant part used: Rhizome.

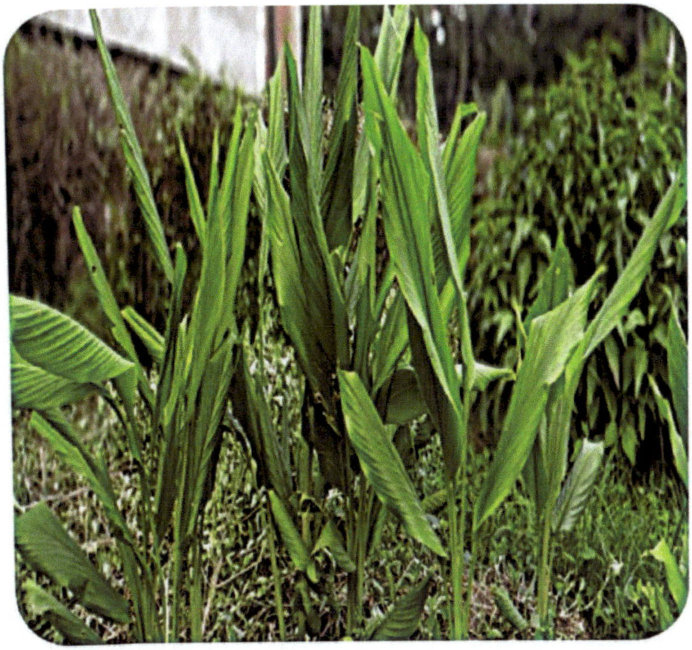

FIGURE 4.2 *Curcuma longa.*

It has an ability of proliferation inhibition in a large variety of tumor cells which accounts for its anticancer potential (Aggrawal and Kumar, 2015). This antiproliferative potential can be related to property of downregulating the expression of various genes like NF-kappa B, activator protein 1, or AP-1, lysyl oxidase (LOX), cycloxygenase 2 (COX2), nitric oxide synthase (NOS), epidermal growth receptor 1 (EGR-1), matrix metallopeptidase 9 (MMP-9) as well as tumor necrosis factor (Shen et al., 2002). It also causes inhibition of the action of c-Jun kinase present at N-terminal as well as inhibits kinase and serine proteins. Turmeric causes reduction in expression of surface adhesion molecules, chemokines, cyclins, and growth receptors such as EGFR and HER2 (Aggrawal and Kumar, 2015). Turmeric also helps in inhibition of tumor cell invasion along with metastasis process occurring in vitro as it reduces MMP-2 action and also inhibits cell invasion of HEp2 (Chakrabati et al., 2006). Various studies show that apoptosis is induced by curcumin. It also leads to proliferation inhibition and interrupt progression of cell cycle (Chen and Huang, 1998). A rapid decrease in membrane potential of mitochondria is caused due to curcumin, release of cytochrome *c*, caspases 3 and 9 activation along with anti-apoptotic protein downregulation and inhibition of apoptosis protein leading to apoptosis occurring in vitro (Goswami et al., 2004; Kumar et al., 2004). Multiple molecular targets along with enzymes, proteins, transcription factors, cytokines, and cell cycles are revealed as experimental evidence (Sharma et al., 2005; Shishodia et al., 2005).

4.5.2.1 ANTICANCER ACTIVITY

A polyphenol (diferuloylmethane) curcumin is derived from *Curcuma longa* plant called turmeric whose constituents are much active. Out of all such constituents, curcumin is the most active as found in research. In raw turmeric, it is present between 0.3% and 5.4% and it is nontoxic comprising numerous therapeutic properties (Cikrikci et al., 2008). Anticancer pigment known as curcumin is exhibited by *C. longa* that can cause inhibition of cancer growth under in-vivo as well as in-vitro conditions (Sharma et al., 2006). Activity of proliferation of cells is suppressed by it in different cancer cell lines and is also known to cause tumor inhibition. G1/S arrest along with induction of apoptosis is also seen as an effect of curcumin apart from mitotic block found in various cell lines of tumor (Shishodia et al., 2005; Sa and Das, 2008). It shows effect on various biological pathways which are involved in activities like oncogenic expression, mutagenesis, apoptosis, metastasis, tumorigensis, and regulation of cell cycle. It also acts as radiotherapy enhancer as it leads to cancer cell arrest during phase G2/M in the cell cycle, where various cells show increased susceptibility toward various cytotoxic effects caused because of radiotherapy (Wilken et al., 2011).

4.5.3 *ZIZIPHUS NUMMULARIA*

Botanical name: *Ziziphus nummularia*
Common name: *Jujube.*
It is also known as bhukamtaka, harbor, and wild jujube.
Plant part used: *root, stem, bark, seed, and flower.*

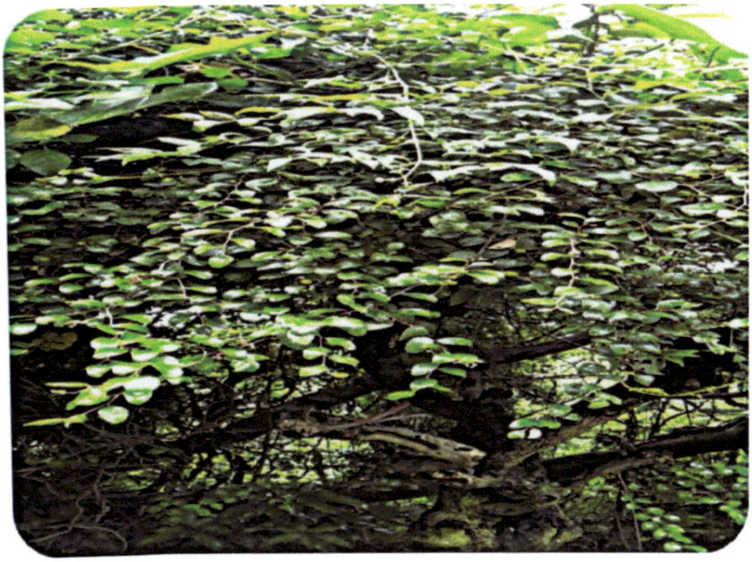

FIGURE 4.3 *Ziziphus nummularia.*

It is a shrub or can be called a thorny bush having purplish stems with velvet-like prickles present in pairs.

It is found in the countries like India, Afghanistan, Pakistan, Iraq, Iran, Egypt, and Israel. Within the bark and stem of this plant, some chemicals are present like betulin and betulinic acid which exhibit antitumor properties (Urban et al., 2005). Cytotoxicity is generated by glycosides of betulinic acid so that cancer cell lines are much sensitive as compared to the normally occurring cells (Legault et al., 2006). Betulinic acid is a pentacyclic triterpenoid that occurs naturally and marks cytotoxicity in response to different cell lines with regard to tumor (Eiznhamer et al., 2004). Betulinic acids have an ability to cause destruction of cancer cells which are even much resistant toward some other chemotherapeutic agents. It is also known for inducing apoptosis process through the production of ROS, inhibiting topoisomerase-I, activating mitogen protein kinase cascade, inhibiting angiogenesis, modulating progrowth transcriptional activators along with aminopeptidase-N activity (Eiznhamer, et al., 2004). The effect as a result of apoptosis of anticancer drugs targeting various cell lines of tumor is potentiated by betulinic acid, which includes *p53* mutant cells, along with primary tumor cells, and not by fibroblast cells of humans, which indicates specificity of tumor to some extent (Simone et al., 2005).

4.5.3.1 ANTICANCER ACTIVITY

In *Z. nummularia*, medicinal properties are present in tremendous amount which can be confirmed by the presence of secondary metabolites having unique and wide number of therapeutic properties. This plant constitutes 16 glycosides and flavonoids along with 64 glycosides as well as 14 terpenoids.

4.5.3.2 PHYTOCHEMISTRY (Z. NUMMULARIA)

TABLE 4.3 Presence of Various Alkaloids, Flavonoids, Saponins, Triterpenoids, and Fatty Acids Has Been Marked with Regard to the Phytochemistry of *Z. nummularia.*

Phytochemicals		Reference
Alkaloids	Nummularine-T, a 13-membered formylcyclopeptide alkaloid extracted from the bark of Z. nummularia	Singh and Pandey (1995)
Cyclopeptide alkaloids	Two peptide alkaloids, namely, nummularine-M as well as nummularine-N, are extracted by the *Z. nummularine*	Pandey et al. (1984)
Glycosides and saponin	Zizynummin is extracted by the dry leaves of the *Ziziphus*	Sharma et al. (1983)
Glycosides	25Spirostane (25S-3 alpha-hydroxy-5 alpha-spirostane-2,12-dione)	Srivastava et al. (1984)

4.5.4 CEDRUS DEODARA

Botanical name: *Cedrus deodara*

Name "Deodar" is derived from Sanskrit name "devdar" which means "timber of the god."

Common name: Deodar.

It is also known as Himalayan cedar, Devdar.

Plant part used: Resins, bark.

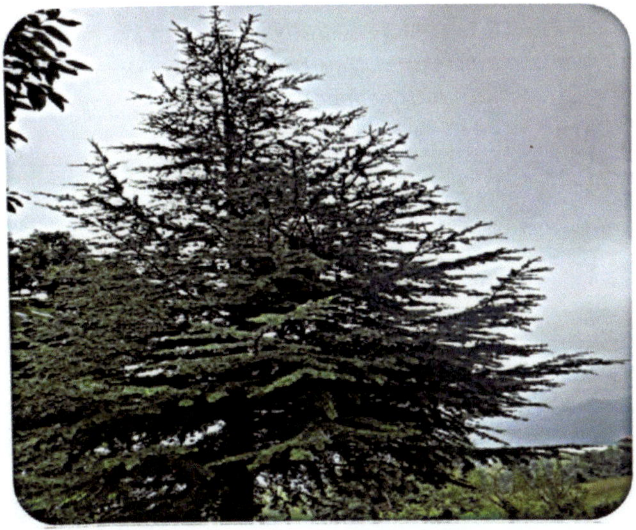

FIGURE 4.4 *Cedrus deodara.*

It is found in countries like Afghanistan, Pakistan, India, Nepal, and Tibet. Its bark is used in the treatment of fevers, rheumatoid arthritis, ulcers, diarrhea, dysentery, and cancer as a remedy (Kirtikar et al., 1918). Oil is extracted from Cedarwood and it has various applications as it exhibits anti-inflammatory, antidiabetic as well as antiulcer properties and acts as an expectorant, arthritis pain reliever, and catarrhal in respiratory tract (Desai et al., 2008). Resins have anti-obesity properties which are effective in cleaning the respiratory tract by reducing cough and cold. Insecticidal as well as antifungal properties are also exhibited by the *Cedrus* oil. Stem wood leads to production of lignin composition which exhibits cytotoxicity in cancer cell lines of humans (Jaswant et al., 2006). Some studies show that the lignin mixture mediates early formation of NO which leads to activation of caspases, generation of peroxides along with depolarization of mitochondria which is ultimately the reason of mitochondrial-dependent as well as independent apoptotic pathways that result in destroying leukemia cells (Shashi et al., 2006).

4.5.5 CENTELLA ASIATICA

Botanical name: *Centella asiatica*
Common name: *Pennywort, leafspade*
It is also known as mandukaparni, brahmamanduki.
Plant part used: *Whole plant especially leaves.*

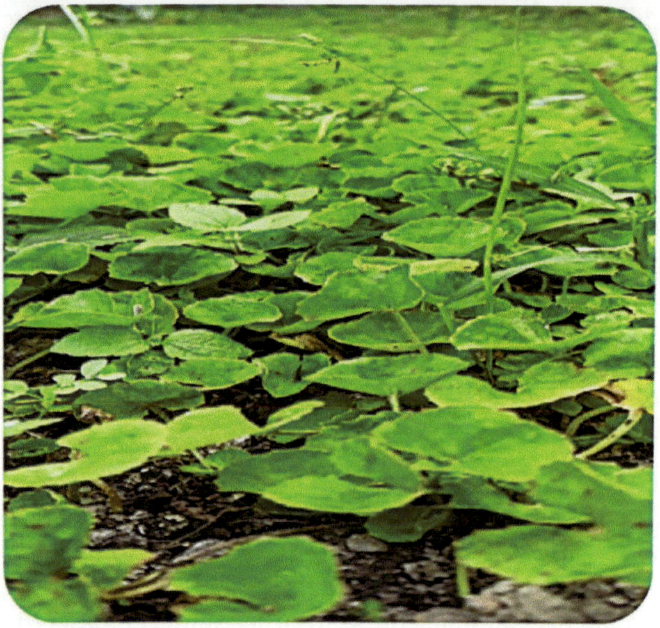

FIGURE 4.5 *Centella asiatica*

It is found in various countries like Australia, Malaysia, India, New Guinea, Iran, India, and Pacific Islands. Transformed cell lines proliferation along with the Ehrlich tumor cells ascites along with Dalton's lymphoma tumor cells ascites are inhibited by partially purified *C. asiatica* dose fractions (Kuttan et al., 1995). It is also known to suppress proliferation of fibroblast cells present in mouse lungs. Studies also show that the development of solid and as cite tumors was slowed and span of life in case of tumor-bearing mice was increased through the oral administration of *C. asiatica* extract and this mechanism which shows emphasis on the antitumor activity exhibited by *C. asiastica* and was recommended to cause a direct inhibition in synthesis of DNA (Babu, 1995). Number of compounds like hydrocotyline, vallerine, asiaticoside, sterol, thankunosides, stigmasterol, flavonoids, and ascorbic acid are present in *C. asiatica* extract (Sharma and Sharma, 2005). Anti-elastase activity is exhibited by this plant and thus it acts like a free radical scavenger. It decreases the ATPase, Mg^{+2} ATPase, Na^{+}, and K^{+} ATPase level and leads to an increase in the Ca^{+} ATPase level and such processes then help in defending the tissue against the reaction of peroxidation, showing protection from cell damage and highlighting its anticancer property (Singh et al., 2008).

4.5.6 *ANDROGRAPHIS PANICULATA*

Botanical name: *Andrographis paniculata*
Common name: Creat
It is also called as bhunimba, kalmegha, kiryat, king of bitters, and chiretta.
Plant part used: Roots and the leaves.

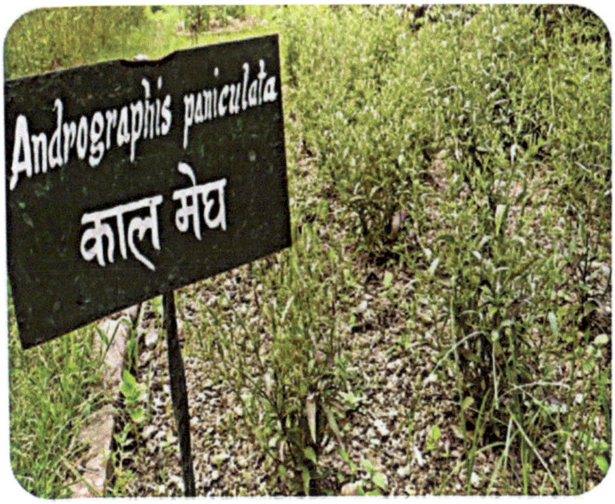

FIGURE 4.6 *Andrographis paniculata.*

It is found in various countries like India and Sri Lanka. Extract of *A. paniculata* constitutes of flavonoids, diterpenes, and stigmasterols. It is identified as diterpene lactone because of its structure which seems ring-like. It also has colorless crystalline structure with bitter taste (Taylor et al., 1992). It has an ability to activate both antigen-specific as well as nonspecific immune response; thus, it is also regarded as potent-stimulator. It acts as chemoprotective agent and is much effective against many infectious as well as oncogenic agents (Saxena et al., 1993).

Cytotoxic activity is observed in response to different cancer cell verities (Tewari et al., 2010). Examples of such cells where andrographolide has cytotoxic activity are p388 lymphocytic leukemia cells, KB human epidermoid cancer cells, and HCT-116 colon cancer cells along with MCF-7 cancer cells (Surbur et al., 2007). It causes growth inhibition in cancer cells of colon and further enhances development along with peripheral blood lymphocyte divisions exerting differentiate effects upon myeloid leukemia M1 cell line present in mouse (Kuroyangi et al., 1994). In immune-competent Swiss albino mice, in-vivo results showed that andrographolide leads to inhibition of proliferative cancer cell devoid of any toxicity symbols even at increased doses (Nirmal et al., 2016).

4.5.7 PHYLLANTHUS AMARUS

Botanical name: *Phyllanthus amarus*
Common name: Gale of wind
It is also known as bhumyamalaki and jaramla.
Plant part used: Whole plant including leaves, roots, and shoots.

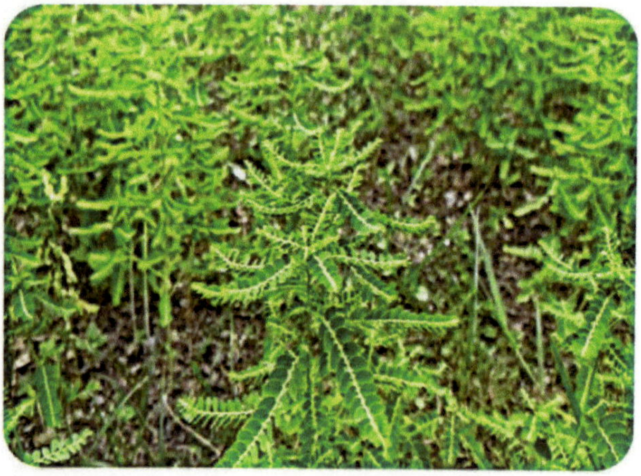

FIGURE 4.7 *Phyllanthus amarus*

It can be found in tropical Asia, especially in the warmer regions of country like India. Various constituents like lignans, flavonoids, and tannins are present in *P. amarus*. *Its* extract is known to exert antitumor effects while its oral administration leads to an increase in the life span and reduce the size of tumor in mice having Dalton's lymphoma ascites and Erlich ascites carcinoma. This plant has property to cause metabolic inhibition of carcinogenic compounds, inducing the arrest of cell cycle and interference in DNA repair process (Joy et al., 2002). *P. amarus* extract shows DNA polymerase inhibition in hepatitis B virus and it also causes downregulation of hepatitis B virus, mRNA transcription along with translation (Gupta et al., 1996). It has been shown to cause inhibition of aniline hydroxylase, a P-450 enzyme that contributes to a reason for carcinogen activation and its extract also inhibits cdc 25 tyrosine phosphate activity which accounts for the key enzyme employed in the regulation of cell cycle (Kuttan et al., 2000). It has an anti-angiogenic effect on mice having Lewis lung carcinoma and is known to interrupt vascular endothelial cell migration (Yang et al., 2006).

4.5.8 MAPPIA FOETIDA

Botanical name: *Mappia foetida amruta*
Common name: Amruta, Kalgur, Narkya whole plant
Plant part used: Whole plant

It is found in tropical countries and has acquired attention at international level. Active and effective constituent of its tree wood is camptothecine in which a potent chemotherapy drug is employed for leukemia treatment (Wall and Wani, 1996). Moreover, endophytic funguses that grow on such plants also produce substances like camptothecine (Verma et al., 2005). Camptothecines serve to have broad spectrum of antitumor activities. They also exhibit antineoplastic activity which leads to inhibitory action upon nuclear enzyme like DNA topoisomerase and topo-1 (Potmesil, 1994). Various clinical trials have been done in order to access anticancer action of camptothecine along with their analogs and such trails have revealed wide range of actions against leukemia, lymphoma, and epithelial tumors (Rowinsky et al., 1993).

4.5.9 TAXUS

It is a genus of 12 species that are distributed across the northern hemisphere, among which about four species are present in North America in Europe, and others are native to Southeast Asia.

Botanical name: *Taxus baccata*
Common name: English yew
Plant part used: Pollen, needles, root, stem, bark, and wood.

Taxus was taken into consideration by various research institute such as Triangle Research Institute, NC, USA. A novel anticancer molecule diterpene amide commonly known as "taxol" was extracted from bark(Wani et al., 1971; Edgington, 1991). *Taxus* constitutes various compounds including taxane derivatives, flavonoids, and polysaccharides. An oxygen-rich diterpene known as taxol is of great significance as it can be employed in inhibition of cancer cell growth.

Taxus species show slow growth with 1.5–2 years of seed dormancy (Steinfeld, 1992). Taxol shows significant action of malignant melanoma treatment, lung cancer, and other kinds of tumors (Wickremesinhe and Arteca, 1993). It is a diterpene alkaloid which has been derived from *Taxus* species having a high market value which is approximately about more than $1 billion each year (Malik et al., 2011). Taxol stabilizes microtubules and inhibits the process of depolymerization into tubulin that then stops the cell cycle at G2/M phase causing the death of cells (Schiff et al., 1979; Horwitz, 1994). Yew trees related to *Taxus* are common and distributed in the Northern hemisphere and are classified into eight species on the basis of their geographical location (Cope, 1998; Gupta, 2015).

Plant culture is regarded as most relevant and efficient way for sustainable production of the taxol along with concerned taxoids at industrial level (Exposito et al., 2009). Since 1990, the taxol's biotechnological production had been started through cell culture obtained from the *Taxus* (Fett-Neto et al., 1992; Wicremesinhe and Arteca, 1993). Successfully, it has been isolated from other *Taxus* species including various plant parts like pollen, needles, bark, root, stem, and wood (Wani et al., 1971; Vidensek et al., 1990; Witherup et al., 1990; Fett-Neto et al., 1992). Extraction procedures show that about 7000 kg bark is required in order to produce 1 kg taxol (Cragg et al., 1993).

4.5.10 *PODOPHYLLUM*

Botanical name: *Podophyllum peltatum*
Common name: Indian May apple
Plant part used: Rhizomes

It is found in Indian Himalayas, Bhutan, Pakistan, Afghanistan, Nepal, China, and Taiwan. *Podophyllum* in India has been distributed among the restricted regions of the Himalayan zone at an altitude ranging from the 2000 to 4000 m.a.s.l. (Bhadula et al., 1996). It is an herbaceous as well as rhizomatous species with much medicinal importance which was announced to be in danger of getting extinct by CITES in 1989 (Foster, 1993). Its rhizomes are used for extraction of podophyllotoxin lignin which then produces semi-synthetic byproducts, teniposide, and etoposide that are used for cancer treatment (Bruneton, 2009). Since 1966, routes for the podophyllotoxin synthesis have been improved (Gensler and Gatsonis, 1966), although this is still not viable commercially because of its complicated and complex structure; thus, there is a need for podophyllotoxin production as along with that derived anticancer drugs have also known to stimulate exploration of another source of plant (Gordaliza et al., 2004; Malik et al., 2014).

4.5.11 *TARAXACUM OFFICINALE*

Botanical name: *Taraxacum officinale*
Common name: Common dandelion root
Plant part used; Root

It is quite popular for its medicinal properties existing in various cultures and is employed for treating diseases like anemia, hepatitis, cirrhosis, cancer, and inflammation. It has also been used in Jordan folk medicine for male infertility treatment (Tahtamouni et al., 2016). An effective antimicrobial as well as anticancer drugs having cheap cum eco-friendly nature can be developed by dandelion-mediated synthesis of nanoparticles as stated in a study (Saratale et al., 2018) and some recent in-vitro studies also show that anticancer potential for an aqueous dandelion root extract constitutes of cancer cell-killing effect on colon cancer cell models (Bahrambeygi et al., 2014). In-vitro apoptosis activity can be induced in hepatocellular carcinoma cells of humans (Yoon et al., 2016). It has a potential that leads to induction of apoptosis and autophagy in case of human pancreatic cells causing no specific effect on the noncancerous cells (Venezuela et al., 2021). It contains taraxerol, saponins, taraxasterol, sesquiterpenes, flavonoids as well as phenolic compounds which are known to have anticancer property (Ivanov et al., 2018).

4.6 PLANTS ACTING AS AN EXPRESSION SYSTEM

Tropical rainforests as well as coral reefs are well known to harbor molecule plethora which are undiscovered along with similar or greater efficiency as anticancer reagents, although modes of action are still unknown (Mukherjee et al., 2001; Pereira et al., 2018). This perspective is endowed with much huge damage as well as destruction of forests and reefs in relation to extinction of various species (van Oppen et al., 2017). Many plant species are employed as expression systems for the recombinant therapeutic proteins in addition to native protein production along with anticancer activity (Spiegel et al., 2016). Plants used for the formulation of recombinant therapeutic proteins and these proteins are important for the treatment of diseases (Buyel, 2015; Fischer et al., 2013). Plants are beneficial in context with biopharmaceutical manufacturing as they are capable of producing various complex proteins along with the significant post-translational modifications having low-cost upstream production inheriting safety on the basis of human pathogen inability to cause replication in the plants giving rise to the potential for smooth as well as flexible production accounting at a larger scale (Buyel et al., 2017). Some natural compounds obtained from plant source show an essential part in the activities related to pharmacology and Taxol, Vina alkaloids, camptothecine, and podophyllotoxins along with their semi-synthetic derivatives are examples of such cooperation (Malik et al., 2014).

4.7 NANOPARTICLES ACTING AS CARRIERS IN ANTICANCER AGENTS RELATED TO PLANT VIRUSES

Nanoparticles acting as carriers in the site-specific delivery of anticancer agents have gained much interest since many years (van der Meel et al., 2017). These particles are proteinaceous and biodegradable in nature. With only about 104 formulations of polymers in the field of the clinical trials in comparison to 2800 trials for mAbs, it can be stated that success as inapplicable approval of anticancer nanoparticles is still inadequate (Venditto and Szoka, 2013). Size of nanoparticles may have hindered the success rate by reducing tumor penetration efficiency, or even due to some uncertainties regarding biocompatibility as well as biodegradability of nanoparticles in vivo, potentially causing their accumulation inside the body with long-term side effects which are still unknown (Lammers et al., 2012). Study shows that particles of Cowpea mosaic virus with different lengths deprived of cargo anticancer drugs lead to a spectacular collapse in case of solid tumors within 3 days, when directly administrated into the tumors (Lizotte et al., 2016). Based on native research, plant virus nanoparticles like Potato virus X or Cowpea mosaic virus are used for presenting HER2 epitopes as an anticancer vaccine (Shukla et al., 2017) and for delivery of compounds constituting small molecules targeting toward specific cells which leads to the reduction in side effects related with chemotherapy (Le et al., 2017).

4.8 ENVIRONMENTAL CONDITIONS AFFECTING MEDICINAL PLANTS

Environmental conditions are being altered at some areas which create unideal and unsurvival conditions for species inhabiting them, although suitable range for species is specified and medicinal plants then narrow and move substantially as per changes in the climate. The risk, due to which species will not be able to migrate, increases because of habitat fragmentation (Pompe et al., 2008). Phenological change leads to disruption in relationship between pollinators and other commensal organisms (Kharouba et al., 2018). Factors like smoking tobacco, alcohol consumption, and infections caused due to the *Helicobacter pylori*, hepatitis B and C, and environmental pollutants leading to genetic mutations (Futreal et al., 2004; Park et al., 2008). An additional threat of unsustainable harvesting pressures is exhibited by medicinal plants of high value (Cho et al., 2014). There is a wide demand for the medicinal plants including illegal harvesting which has become a serious problem leading to decline in species abundance as well as average stature (McGraw, 2001; Case et al., 2007). Complete extinction of valued species occurs due to factors like commercial harvest and destruction of habitat including decline in size as well as abundance (Kiehn, 2007), for example, snow lotus (*Saussurea laniceps* Hand. Mazz), goldenseal (*Hydrastis canadensis*), *and silphium* (*Ferula* species) (Law and Salick, 2005; Albercht and McCarthy, 2006; Brinckmann et al., 2020). More than 10,000 Himalayan medicinal plants are known to support primary healthcare as well as livelihoods of about 600 million people of the area (Shengji, 2001). Indigenous knowledge is essential in the preparation of different ethnomedicines for treating cancer-like disease (Gautam, 2011). Medicinal plants have contributed much into the discovery of anticancer-related drugs like camptothecine, podophyllotoxon, paclitaxel, and taxol (Oberlies and Kroll, 2004; Singh et al., 2013). Conservationists have recognized the unsustainability of herbaceous root harvesting and have regarded related medicinal plants to be under a higher threat (Verma et al., 2007; Maroyi, 2011). Secondary metabolite production like polyphenols, alkaloids, and terpenes has been reported for anticancer properties on the basis physiological adaptations in biochemical profile of plant tissues (Bhatia et al., 2011).

4.9 SUMMARY

Only chemotherapy is the most preferred way for cancer treatment in spite of many side effects. Thus, the idea of using natural as well as harmless ways like ethnoplants exhibiting anticancerous properties is of significant importance in relation to health as well as biodiversity exploration. Study states that there is huge variety of discovered and undiscovered anticancerous plants in the northern hemisphere. More research and exploration with this regard would be highly beneficial to pharmaceutical industries which would contribute toward the increase in economy and improvement in health-related sector. Access to medicinal plants creates resilience which focuses on the decline due to the increase in environmental extremes and economic losses as a result of climate change. Thus, actions by local and national governments and ethnobotanical communities are of great significance in helping the people as well as communities who are dependent upon medicinal plants for income, medicine, or healthcare. Such actions will lead to promotion of medicinal plant cultivation in order to maintain access for local people along with preservation of traditional knowledge and values preserving their sustainable use. Ex-situ seed banking as well as assisted migration can be beneficial for preventing extinction of useful species at the global level.

KEYWORDS

- **anticancer**
- **medicinal plants**
- **Northern Hemisphere**
- **phytochemicals**
- **therapy**
- **mechanism**

REFERENCES

Aggrawal, B. B.; Kumar, A.; Phatric, A. C. Anticancer Potential of Curcumin. *Anticancer Res*. **2003,** *23*, 366–378.

Albrecht, M. A.; McCarthy, B. C. Comparative Analysis of Goldenseal (Hydrastis Canadensis L.) Population Re-growth Following Human Harvest: Implications for Conservation. *Am. Midl. Nat.* **2006,** *156*, 229–236.

Ali, H.; Dixit, S. Extraction Optimization of Tinospora Cordifolia and Assessment of the Anticancer Activity of its Alkaloid Palmatine. *Sci. World J.* **2013,** *28,* 376216.

Amin, A.; Gali-Muhtasib, H.; Ocker, M.; Schneider-Stock, R. Overview of Major Classes of Plant-Derived Anticancer Drugs. *Int. J. Biomed. Sci. IJBS*, **2009,** *5*, 1.

Applequist, W. L.; Brinckmann, J. A.; Cunningham, A. B.; Hart, R. E.; Heinrich, M.; Katerere, D. R.; Van Andel, T. Scientists' Warning on Climate Change and Medicinal Plants. *Planta Med.* **2020,** *86*, 10–18.

Asensi, M.; Ortega, A.; Mena, S.; Feddi, F.; Estrela, J. M. Natural Polyphenols in Cancer Therapy. *Crit. Rev. Clin. Lab. Sci.* **2011,** *48*, 197–216.

Babu, T. D.; Kuttan, G.; Padikkala, J. Cytotoxic and Anti-Tumour Properties of Certain Taxa of Umbelliferae With Special Reference to Centella asiatica (L.) Urban. *J. Ethnopharmacol.* **1995,** *48*, 53–57.

Bahrambeygi, Y.; Ahmadi, R.; Joshagani, R. Anticancer Effect of Taraxacum officinale Flower Extract on Cervical Cancer Cells. *Med. Plant*. **2014,** *3*, 908–915.

Bala, M.; Pratap, K.; Verma, P. K.; Singh, B.; Padwad, Y. Validation of Ethnomedicinal Potential of Tinospora Cordifolia for Anticancer and Immunomodulatory Activities and Quantification of Bioactive Molecules by HPTLC. *J. Ethnopharmacol.* **2015,** *175*, 131–137.

Bhatia, A., Arora, S., Singh, B., Kaur, G., Nagpal, A. Anticancer Potential of Himalayan Plant. *Phytochem. Rev.* **2011,** *10,* 309–329.

Bosviel, R.; Durif, J.; Guo, J.; Mebrek, M.; Kwiatkowski, F.; Bignon, Y. J.; Bernard-Gallon, D. J. BRCA2 Promoter Hypermethylation in Sporadic Breast Cancer. *OMICS* **2012,** *16,* 707–710.

Brinckmann, J. A. Sustainable Sourcing: Markets for Certified Chinese Medicinal and Aromatic Plants. International Trade Centre: Geneva, **2016;** vol *22*.

Buyel, J. F.; Twyman, R. M.; Fischer, R. Very-Large-Scale Production of Antibodies in Plants: The Biologization of Manufacturing. *Biotechnol. Adv.* **2017,** *35*, 458–465.

Case, M. A.; Flinn, K. M.; Jancaitis, J.; Alley, A.; Paxton, A. Declining Abundance of American Ginseng (Panax Quinquefolius L.) Documented by Herbarium Specimens. *Biol. Conserv.* **2007,** *134*, 22–30.

Cassileth, B. R.; Deng, G. Complementary and Alternative Therapies for Cancer. *Oncologist* **2004,** *9*, 80–89.

Cencic, R.; Robert, F.; Pelletier, J. Identifying Small Molecule Inhibitors of Eukaryotic Translation Initiation. *Methods Enzymol.* **2007,** *431*, 269–302.

Che, E.; Gao, Y.; Wan, L.; Zhang, Y.; Han, N.; Bai, J.; Li, J.; Sha, Z.; Wang, S. Paclitaxel/Gelatin Coated Magnetic Mesoporous Silica Nanoparticles: Preparation and Antitumor Efficacy in Vivo. *Microporous Mesoporous Mater.* **2015,** *204*, 226–234.

Chen, H. W.; Huang, H. C. Effect of Curcumin on Cell Cycle Progression and Apoptosis in Vascular Smooth Muscle Cells. *Br. J. Pharmacol.* **1998,** *124*, 1029–1040.

Cho, Y. J.; Son, H. J.; Kim, K. S. A 14-Week Randomized, Placebo-Controlled, Double-Blind Clinical Trial to Evaluate the efficacy and Safety of Ginseng Polysaccharide (Y-75). *J. Transl. Med.* **2014,** *12*, 1–7.

Cikrikci, S.; Mozioglu, E.; Yilmaz, H. Biological Activity of Curcuminoids Isolated From Curcuma longa. *Rec. Nat. Prod.* **2008,** *2*, 19.

Cohen, I. S.; Mosher, M. B.; O'Keefe, E. J.; Klaus, S. N.; De Conti, R. C. Cutaneous Toxicity of Bleomycin Therapy. *Arch. Dermatol.* **1973,** *107*, 553–555.

Cope, C. Diagnosis and Treatment of Postoperative Chyle Leakage via Percutaneous Transabdominal Catheterization of the Cisterna Chyli: A Preliminary Study. *J. Vasc. Interv. Radiol.* **1998,** *9*, 727–734.

Cornblatt, B. S.; Ye, L.; Dinkova-Kostova, A. T.; Erb, M.; Fahey, J. W.; Singh, N. K.; Chen, M. S. A.; Stierer, T.; Garrett-Mayer, E.; Argani, P.; Davidson, N. E. Preclinical and Clinical Evaluation of Sulforaphane for Chemoprevention in the Breast. *Carcinogenesis* **2007,** *28*, 1485–1490.

Coseri, S. Natural Products and Their Analogues as Efficient Anticancer Drugs. *Mini Rev. Med. Chem.* **2009,** *9*, 560–571.

Cragg, G. M.; Newman, D. J. Plants as a Source of Anti-Cancer Agents. *J. Ethnopharmacol.* **2005,** *100*, 72–79.

Dahmke, I. N.; Boettcher, S. P.; Groh, M.; Mahlknecht, U. Cooking Enhances Curcumin Anti-Cancerogenic Activity Through Pyrolytic Formation of "Deketene Curcumin. *Food Chem.* **2014,** *151*, 514–519.

Desai, A. G.; Qazi, G. N.; Ganju, R. K.; El-Tamer, M.; Singh, J.; Saxena, A. K.; Bedi, Y. S.; Taneja, S. C.; Bhat, H. K. Medicinal Plants and Cancer Chemoprevention. *Curr. Drug Metabol.* **2008,** *9*, 581–591.

Diwanay, S.; Chitre, D.; Patwardhan, B. Immunoprotection by Botanical Drugs in Cancer Chemotherapy. *J. Ethnopharmacol.* **2004,** *90*, 49–55.

Eiznhamer, D. A.; Xu, Z. Q. Betulinic Acid: A Promising Anticancer Candidate. *IDrug* **2004,** *7*, 359–373.

Expósito, O.; Bonfill, M.; Moyano, E.; Onrubia, M.; Mirjalili, M. H.; Cusido, R. M.; Palazon, J. Biotechnological Production of Taxol and Related Taxoids: Current State and Prospects. *Anti-Cancer Agents Med. Chem.* **2009,** *9*, 109–121.

Fett-Neto, A. G.; DiCosmo, F.; Reynolds, W. F.; Sakata, K. Cell Culture of Taxus as a Source of the Antineoplastic Drug Taxol and Related Taxanes. *Biotechnology* **1992,** *10*, 1572–1575.

Fischer, A.; Rosen, A. C.; Ensslin, C. J.; Wu, S.; Lacouture, M. E. Pruritus to Anticancer Agents Targeting the EGFR, BRAF, and CTLA-4. *Dermatol. Ther.* **2013,** *26*, 135–148.

Fraiser, L. H.; Kanekal, S.; Kehrer, J. P. Cyclophosphamide Toxicity. *Drugs* **1991,** *42*, 781–795.

Fritz, H.; Seely, D.; Kennedy, D. A.; Fernandes, R.; Cooley, K.; Fergusson, D. Green Tea and Lung Cancer: A Systematic Review. *Integr. Cancer Ther.* **2013,** *12*, 7–24.

Fulda, S.; Debatin, K. M. Sensitization for Anticancer Drug-Induced Apoptosis by Betulinic Acid. *Neoplasia* **2005,** *7*, 162–170.

Gairola, S.; Shariff, N. M.; Bhatt, A. Influence of Climate Change on Production of Secondary Chemicals in High Altitude Medicinal Plants: Issues Needs Immediate Attention. *J. Med. Plants Res.* **2010,** *4*, 1825–1829.

Gauthier, C.; Legault, J.; Lebrun, M.; Dufour, P.; Pichette, A. Glycosidation of Lupane-Type Triterpenoids as Potent In Vitro Cytotoxic Agents. *Bioorg. Med. Chem.* **2006,** *14*, 6713–6725.

Gensler, W. J.; Gatsonis, C. D. Synthesis of Podophyllotoxin1, 2. *J. Org. Chem.* **1966,** *31*, 4004–4008.

Gibaud, S.; Andreux, J. P.; Weingarten, C.; Renard, M.; Couvreur, P. Increased Bone Marrow Toxicity of Doxorubicin Bound to Nanoparticles. *Eur. J. Cancer*. **1994,** *30*, 820–826.

Golding, R. P.; van Zanten, T. E. G.; Vermorken, J. B. Bleomycin Pleuropneumonitis. *Br. J. Radiol.* **1982,** *55*, 672–674.

Gordaliza, M. Natural Products as Leads to Anticancer Drugs. *Clin. Transl. Oncol.* **2007,** *9*, 767–776.

Gordaliza, M.; Garcıa, P. A.; Del Corral, J. M.; Castro, M. A.; Gómez-Zurita, M. A. Podophyllotoxin: Distribution, Sources, Applications and New Cytotoxic Derivatives. *Toxicon* **2004,** *44*, 441–459.

Greenwell, M.; Rahman, P. K. S. M. Medicinal Plants: Their use in Anticancer Treatment. *Int. J. Pharmaceut. Sci. Res.* **2015,** *6*, 4103.

Gupta, A. P.; Pandotra, P.; Kushwaha, M.; Khan, S.; Sharma, R.; Gupta, S. Alkaloids: A Source of Anticancer Agents From Nature. *Stud. Nat. Prod. Chem.* **2015,** *46,* 341–445. Elsevier.

Hakim, I. A.; Harris, R. B.; Brown, S.; Chow, H. S.; Wiseman, S.; Agarwal, S.; Talbot, W. Effect of Increased Tea Consumption on Oxidative DNA Damage Among Smokers: A Randomized Controlled Study. *J. Nutri.* **2003,** *133*, 3303S–3309S.

Heiss, E.; Herhaus, C.; Klimo, K.; Bartsch, H.; Gerhäuser, C. Nuclear Factor κB is a Molecular Target for Sulforaphane-Mediated Anti-Inflammatory Mechanisms. *J. Biol. Chem.* **2001,** *276*, 32008–32015.

Henary, M.; Narayana, L.; Ahad, S.; Gundala, S. R.; Mukkavilli, R.; Sharma, V.; Owens, E. A.; Yadav, Y.; Nagaraju, M.; Hamelberg, D.; Tandon, V. Novel Third-Generation

Water-Soluble Noscapine Analogs as Superior Microtubule-Interfering Agents With Enhanced Antiproliferative Activity. *Biochem. Pharmacol.* **2014,** *92*, 192–205.
Horwitz, S. B. Taxol (Paclitaxel): Mechanisms of Action. *Ann. Oncol.* **1994,** *5*, S3–S6.
Huang, S. T.; Yang, R. C.; Lee, P. N.; Yang, S. H.; Liao, S. K.; Chen, T. Y.; Pang, J. H. S. Anti-Tumor and Anti-Angiogenic Effects of Phyllanthus urinaria in Mice Bearing Lewis Lung Carcinoma. *Int. Immunopharmacol.* **2006,** *6*, 870–879.
Ioannidis, J. P. Contradicted and Initially Stronger Effects in Highly Cited Clinical Research. *JAMA*. **2005,** *294*, 218–228.
Ivanov, I.; Petkova, N.; Tumbarski, J.; Dincheva, I.; Badjakov, I.; Denev, P.; Pavlov, A. GC-MS Characterization of n-hexane Soluble Fraction From Dandelion (Taraxacum officinale Weber ex FH Wigg.) Aerial Parts and its Antioxidant and Antimicrobial Properties. *Z. Naturforsch.* **2018,** *73*, 41–47.
Jada, S. R.; Subur, G. S.; Matthews, C.; Hamzah, A. S.; Lajis, N. H.; Saad, M. S.; Stevens, M. F.; Stanslas, J. Semisynthesis and In Vitro Anticancer Activities of Andrographolide Analogues. *Phytochemistry* **2007,** *68*, 904–912.
Jagadeesh, S.; Sinha, S.; Pal, B. C.; Bhattacharya, S.; Banerjee, P. P. Mahanine Reverses an Epigenetically Silenced Tumor Suppressor Gene RASSF1A in Human Prostate Cancer Cells. *Biochem. Biophys. Res. Commun.* **2007,** *362*, 212–217.
Jagetia, G. C.; Nayak, V.; Vidyasagar, M. S. Evaluation of the Antineoplastic Activity of Guduchi (Tinospora Cordifolia) in Cultured HeLa Cells. *Cancer Lett.* 1998, *127*, 71–82.
Jagetia, G. C.; Rao, S. K. Evaluation of the Antineoplastic Activity of Guduchi (Tinospora Cordifolia) in Ehrlich Ascites Carcinoma Bearing Mice. *Biol. Pharmaceut. Bull.* **2006,** *29*, 460–466.
Jana, N. R.; Dikshit, P.; Goswami, A.; Nukina, N. Inhibition of Proteasomal Function by Curcumin Induces Apoptosis Through Mitochondrial Pathway. *J. Biol. Chem.* **2004,** *279*, 11680–11685.
Jordan, M. A.; Kamath, K.; Manna, T.; Okouneva, T.; Miller, H. P.; Davis, C.; Littlefield, B. A.; Wilson, L. The Primary Antimitotic Mechanism of Action of the Synthetic Halichondrin E7389 is Suppression of Microtubule Growth. *Mol. Cancer Therapeut.* **2005,** *4*, 1086–1095.
Jose, J. K.; Kuttan, G.; George, J.; Kuttan, R. Antimutagenic and Anticarcinogenic Activity of Emblica Officinalis Gaertn. *J. Clin. Biochem. Nutr.* **1997,** *22*, 171–176.
Jyoti, K.; Kaur, K.; Pandey, R. S.; Jain, U. K.; Chandra, R.; Madan, J. Inhalable Nanostructured Lipid Particles of 9-Bromo-Noscapine, a Tubulin-Binding Cytotoxic Agent: In Vitro and In Vivo Studies. *J. Colloid Interface Sci.* **2015,** *445*, 219–230.
Kala, C. P.; Mathur, V. B. Patterns of Plant Species Distribution in the Trans-Himalayan Region of Ladakh, India. *J. Veg. Sci.* **2002,** *13*, 751–754.
Kaplan, I. W. Condylomata Acuminate. *New Orleans Med. Surg. J.* 1942, *94*, 388–390.
Katerere, D. R.; Luseba, D. Eds.; *Ethnoveterinary Botanical Medicine: Herbal Medicines for Animal Health*; CRC Press, 2010.
Kharouba, H. M.; Ehrlén, J.; Gelman, A.; Bolmgren, K.; Allen, J. M.; Travers, S. E.; Wolkovich, E. M. Global Shifts in the Phenological Synchrony of Species Interactions Over Recent Decades. *Proc. Natl. Acad. Sci.* **2018,** *115*, 5211–5216.
Kiehn, M. Silphion Revisited. *Med. Plant Conserv.* 2007, *13*, 4–8.
King-Batoon, A.; Leszczynska, J. M.; Klein, C. B. Modulation of Gene Methylation by Genistein or Lycopene in Breast Cancer Cells. *Environ. Mol. Mutagen.* **2008,** *49*, 36–45.

Kirtikar, K. R.; Basu, B. D. Indian Medicinal Plants. *Indian Med. Plants.* 1918.

Kuttan, R.; Bhanumathy, P.; Nirmala, K.; George, M. C. Potential Anticancer Activity of Turmeric (Curcuma Longa). *Cancer Lett.* **1985,** *29*, 197–202.

Lammers, T.; Kiessling, F.; Hennink, W. E.; Storm, G. Drug Targeting to Tumors: Principles, Pitfalls and (Pre-) Clinical Progress. *J. Control. Release* **2012,** *161*, 175–187.

Law, W.; Salick, J. Human-Induced Dwarfing of Himalayan Snow Lotus, Saussurealaniceps (Asteraceae). *Proc. Natl. Acad. Sci.* **2005,** *102*, 10218–10220.

Le Grazie, M.; Biagini, M. R.; Tarocchi, M.; Polvani, S.; Galli, A. Chemotherapy for Hepatocellular Carcinoma: The present and the Future. *World J. Hepatol.* 2017, *9*, 907.

Lee, C. D.; Ott, M.; Thyagarajan, S. P.; Shafritz, D. A.; Burk, R. D.; Gupta, S. Phyllanthus amarus Down-Regulates Hepatitis B Virus mRNA Transcription and Replication. *Eur. J. Clin. Investig.* **1996,** *26*, 1069–1076.

Lizotte, P. H.; Wen, A. M.; Sheen, M. R.; Fields, J.; Rojanasopondist, P.; Steinmetz, N. F.; Fiering, S. In Situ Vaccination With Cowpea Mosaic Virus Nanoparticles Suppresses Metastatic Cancer. *Nat. Nanotechnol.* **2016,** *11*, 295–303.

Macdonald, J. S. Toxicity of 5-Fluorouracil. *Oncology* **1999,** *13*, 33–34.

Malik, S.; Cusidó, R. M.; Mirjalili, M. H.; Moyano, E.; Palazón, J.; Bonfill, M. Production of the Anticancer Drug Taxol in Taxus baccata Suspension Cultures: A Review. *Process Biochem.* **2011,** *46*, 23–34.

Malik, M.; Wysokiński, R.; Zierkiewicz, W.; Helios, K.; Michalska, D. Raman and Infrared Spectroscopy, DFT Calculations, and Vibrational Assignment of the Anticancer Agent Picoplatin: Performance of Long-Range Corrected/Hybrid Functionals for a Platinum (II) Complex. *J. Phys. Chem. A*, **2014,** *118*, 6922–6934.

Manil, L.; Mahieu, P.; Couvreur, P. Acute Renal Toxicity of Doxorubicin (Adriamycin)-Loaded Cyanoacrylate Nanoparticles. *Pharmaceut. Res.* **1995,** *12*, 85–87.

Mariotto, A. B.; Robin Yabroff, K.; Shao, Y.; Feuer, E. J.; Brown, M. L. Projections of the Cost of Cancer Care in the United States: 2010–2020. *J. Natl. Cancer Inst.* **2011,** *103*, 117–128.

Mathers, C. D.; Loncar, D. Projections of Global Mortality and Burden of Disease From 2002 to 2030. *PLoS Med.* **2006,** *3*, 442.

Mathur, A.; Joshi, H. Ethnobotanical Studies of the Tarai Region of Kumaun, Uttarakhand, India. *Ethnobot. Res. Appl.* **2013,** *11*, 174–203.

Matsuda, T.; Kuroyanagi, M.; Sugiyama, S.; Umehara, K.; Ueno, A.; Nishi, K. Cell Differentiation-Inducing Diterpenes From Andrographis paniculata Nees. *Chem. Pharmaceut. Bull.* **1994,** *42*, 1216–1225.

McGraw, J. B. Evidence for Decline in Stature of American Ginseng Plants From Herbarium Specimens. *Biol. Conserv.* **2001,** *98*, 25–32.

Mehta, K.; Pantazis, P.; McQueen, T.; Aggarwal, B. B. Antiproliferative Effect of Curcumin (Diferuloylmethane) Against Human Breast Tumor Cell Lines. *Anticancer Drugs* **1997,** *8*, 470–481.

Mishra, R.; Kaur, G. Aqueous Ethanolic Extract of Tinospora Cordifolia as a Potential Candidate for Differentiation Based Therapy of Glioblastomas. *PLoS One* **2013,** *8*, 78764.

Mitra, A.; Chakrabarti, J.; Banerji, A.; Chatterjee, A.; Das, B. R. Curcumin, A Potential Inhibitor of MMP-2 in Human Laryngeal Squamous Carcinoma Cells HEp2. *J. Environ. Pathol. Toxicol. Oncol.* **2006,** *25*.

Mukherjee, A. K.; Basu, S.; Sarkar, N.; Ghosh, A. C. Advances in Cancer Therapy With Plant Based Natural Products. *Curr. Med. Chem.* 2001, *8*, 1467–1486.

Newcomb, E. W. Flavopiridol: Pleiotropic Biological Effects Enhance its Anti-Cancer Activity. *Anticancer Drugs* 2004, *15*, 411–419.

Newman, D. J. Natural Products as Leads to Potential Drugs: An Old Process or the New Hope for Drug Discovery? *J. Med. Chem.* 2008, *51*, 2589–2599.

Newman, D. J.; Cragg, G. M. Natural Products as Sources of New Drugs Over the 30 Years From 1981 to 2010. *J. Nat. Prod.* 2012, *75*, 311–335.

Niranjan, A.; Tewari, S. K.; Lehri, A. Biological Activities of Kalmegh (Andrographis PaniculataNees), 2010.

Ochwang'I, D. O.; Kimwele, C. N.; Oduma, J. A.; Gathumbi, P. K.; Mbaria, J. M.; Kiama, S. G. Medicinal Plants Used in Treatment and Management of Cancer in Kakamega County Kenya *J. Ethnopharmacol.* 2014, *151,* 1040–1055.

Pandey, V. B.; Singh, J. P.; Seth, K. K.; Shah, A. H.; Eckhardt, G. Cyclopeptide Alkaloids From Zizyphus Nummularia. *Phytochemistry* 1984, *23*, 2118–2120.

Park, E. J.; Pezzuto, J. M. Botanicals in Cancer Chemoprevention. *Cancer Metastasis Rev.* 2002, *21*, 231–255.

Parkin, D. M. International Variation. *Oncogene* 2004, *23*, 6329–6340.

Parveen, S.; Jan, U.; Kamili, A. Importance of Himalayan Medicinal Plants and Their Conservation Strategies. *Aust. J. Herb. Med.* 2013, *25*, 63–67.

Pereira, I.; Sousa, F.; Kennedy, P.; Sarmento, B. Carcinoembryonic Antigen-Targeted Nanoparticles Potentiate the Delivery of Anticancer Drugs to Colorectal Cancer Cells. *Int. J. Pharmaceut.* 2018, *549*, 397–403.

Pledgie-Tracy, A.; Sobolewski, M. D.; Davidson, N. E. Sulforaphane Induces Cell Type–Specific Apoptosis in Human Breast Cancer Cell Lines. *Mol. Cancer Therapeut.* 2007, *6*, 1013–1021.

Pompe, S.; Hanspach, J.; Badeck, F.; Klotz, S.; Thuiller, W.; Kühn, I. Climate and Land Use Change Impacts on Plant Distributions in Germany. *Biol. Lett.* 2008, *4*, 564–567.

Potmesil, M. Camptothecins: From Bench Research to Hospital Wards. *Cancer Res.* 1994, *54*, 1431–1439.

Puri, A.; Saxena, R.; Saxena, R. P.; Saxena, K. C.; Srivastava, V.; Tandon, J. S. Immunostimulant Agents From Andrographis Paniculata. *J. Nat. Prod.* 1993, *56*, 995–999.

Puri, S. C.; Verma, V.; Amna, T.; Qazi, G. N.; Spiteller, M. An Endophytic Fungus From Nothapodytes foetida that Produces Camptothecin. *J. Nat. Prod.* 2005, *68*, 1717–1719.

Rahmani, A. H.; Allemailem, K. S.; Aly, S. M.; Khan, M. A. Implications of Green Tea and its Constituents in the Prevention of Cancer Via the Modulation of Cell Signalling Pathway. *BioMed Res. Int.* 2015.

Rahul V.; Hotam S. C.; Agrawal R. C. Evaluation of Ant Carcinogenic and Ant Mutagenic Effect of Tinospora Cordifolia in Experimental Animals. *J. Chem. Pharm. Res.* 2011, *3*, 877–881.

Rajeshkumar, N. V.; Joy, K. L.; Kuttan, G.; Ramsewak, R. S.; Nair, M. G.; Kuttan, R. Antitumour and Anticarcinogenic Activity of Phyllanthus amarus Extract. *J. Ethnopharmacol.* 2002, *81*, 17–22.

Rajeshkumar, N. V.; Kuttan, R. Phyllanthus amarus Extract Administration Increases the Life Span of Rats With Hepatocellular Carcinoma. *J. Ethnopharmacol.* **2000,** *73*, 215–219.

Rashmi, R.; Kumar, S.; Karunagaran, D. Ectopic Expression of Bcl-XL or Ku70 Protects Human Colon Cancer Cells (SW480) Against Curcumin-Induced Apoptosis While Their Down-Regulation Potentiates it. *Carcinogenesis* **2004,** *25*, 1867–1877.

Raza, H.; John, A. Green Tea Polyphenol Epigallocatechin-3-Gallate Differentially Modulates Oxidative Stress in PC12 Cell Compartments. *Toxicol. App. Pharmacol.* **2005,** *207*, 212–220.

Rexroth, G.; Scotland, V. J. M. K. Cardiac Toxicity of 5-Fluorouracil. *Med. Klin.* **1994,** *89*, 680–688.

Sa, G.; Das, T. Anti Cancer Effects of Curcumin: Cycle of Life and Death. *Cell Div.* **2008,** *3*, 1–14.

Sahu, R. P.; Batra, S.; Srivastava, S. K. Activation of ATM/Chk1 by Curcumin Causes Cell Cycle Arrest and Apoptosis in Human Pancreatic Cancer Cells. *Br. J. Cancer*. **2009,** *100*, 1425–1433.

Saratale, R. G.; Benelli, G.; Kumar, G.; Kim, D. S.; Saratale, G. D. Bio-Fabrication of Silver Nanoparticles Using the Leaf Extract of an Ancient Herbal Medicine, Dandelion (Taraxacum officinale), Evaluation of Their Antioxidant, Anticancer Potential, and Antimicrobial Activity Against Phytopathogens. *Environ. Sci. Pollut. Res.* **2018,** *25*, 10392–10406.

Sarek, J.; Kvasnica, M.; Urban, M.; Klinot, J.; Hajduch, M. Correlation of Cytotoxic Activity of Betulinines and Their Hydroxy Analogues. *Bioorg. Med. Chem. Lett.* **2005,** *15*, 4196–4200.

Schiff, P. B.; Fant, J.; Horwitz, S. B. Promotion of Microtubule Assembly in Vitro by Taxol. *Nature* **1979,** *277*, 665–667.

Schnekenburger, M.; Dicato, M.; Diederich, M. Plant-Derived Epigenetic Modulators for Cancer Treatment and Prevention. *Biotechnol. Adv.* **2014,** *32*, 1123–1132.

Sener, G.; Kapucu, C.; Cetinel, S.; Cikler, E.; Ayanoğlu-Dülger, G. Gastroprotective Effect of Leukotriene Receptor Blocker Montelukast in Alendronat-Induced Lesions of the Rat Gastric Mucosa. *Prostaglandins Leukot. Essent. Fatty Acids*. **2005,** *72*, 1–11.

Shah, U.; Shah, R.; Acharya, S.; Acharya, N. Novel Anticancer Agents From Plant Sources. *Chin. J. Nat. Med.* **2013,** *11*, 16–23.

Shankari, V.; Gurunathan, S. Drug Discovery: An Appraisal. *Int. J. Pharm. Sci.* **2015,** *7*, 59–66.

Shao, Z. M.; Shen, Z. Z.; Liu, C. H.; Sartippour, M. R.; Go, V. L.; Heber, D.; Nguyen, M. Curcumin Exerts Multiple Suppressive Effects on Human Breast Carcinoma Cells. *Int. J. Cancer*. **2002,** *98*, 234–240.

Sharma, R. A.; Gescher, A. J.; Steward, W. P. Curcumin: The Story so Far. *Eur. J. Cancer* **2005,** *41*, 1955–1968.

Sharma, S.; Kulkarni, S. K.; Agrewala, J. N.; Chopra, K. Curcumin Attenuates Thermal Hyperalgesia in a Diabetic Mouse Model of Neuropathic Pain. *Eur. J. Pharmacol.* **2006,** *536*, 256–261.

Sharma, S.C.; Kumar, R. Zizynummin, a dammarane saponin from zizyphus nummularia. *Phytochem.* **1983,** *22*, 1469–1471.

Sharma, R.; Sharma, J. Modification of Gamma Ray Induced Changes in the Mouse Hepatocytes by Centella Asiatica Extract: In Vivo Studies. *Phytother. Res.* **2005,** *19*, 605–611.

Shashi, B.; Jaswant, S.; Madhusudana, R. J.; Kumar, S. A.; Nabi, Q. G. A Novel Lignan Composition from Cedrus deodara Induces Apoptosis and Early Nitric Oxide Generation in Human Leukemia Molt-4 and HL-60 Cells. *Nitric Oxide* **2006,** *14*, 72–88.

Shilpa, P.; Balaraju, Y.; Salimath, B. P. Antimetastatic Activity of Tinospora Cordifolia Involves Inhibition of Cell Migration and Invasion Regulated By Twist and Snail Genes. *Int. J. Pharm. Biol. Sci.* **2015,** *10*, 44–49.

Shishodia, S.; Amin, H. M.; Lai, R.; Aggarwal, B. B. Curcumin (Diferuloylmethane) Inhibits Constitutive NF-kappaB Activation, Induces G1/S Arrest, Suppresses Proliferation, and Induces Apoptosis in Mantle Cell Lymphoma. *Biochem. Pharmacol.* **2005,** *70*, 700–713.

Shishodia, S.; Sethi, G.; Aggarwal, B. B. Curcumin: Getting Back to the Roots. *Ann. N. Y. Acad. Sci.* **2005,** *1056*, 206–217.

Singh, B.; Pandey, V. B. An N-formyl Cyclopeptide Alkaloid From Zizyphus Nummularia Bark. *Phytochemistry* **1995,** *38*, 271–273.

Singh, S. S.; Pandey, S. C.; Srivastava, S.; Gupta, V. S.; Patro, B.; Ghosh, A. C. Chemistry and Medicinal Properties of Tinospora Cordifolia (Guduchi), 2003.

Siripong, P.; Kongkathip, B.; Preechanukool, K.; Picha, P.; Tunsuwan, K.; Taylor, W. C. Cytotoxic Diterpenoid Constituents From Andrographis PaniculataNees Leaves. *J. Sci. Soc. Thailand* **1992,** *18*, 187–194.

Slichenmyer, W. J.; Rowinsky, E. K.; Donehower, R. C.; Kaufmann, S. H. The Current Status of Camptothecin Analogues as Antitumor Agents. *JNCI: J. Natl. Cancer Inst. Monogr.* **1993,** *85*, 271–291.

Srivastava, S.K. Nummularogenin, a new spirostane from Zizyphus nummularia. *J. Nat. Prod.* **1984,** *47*, 781–783.

Tahtamouni, L. H.; Al-Khateeb, R. A.; Abdellatif, R. N.; Al-Mazaydeh, Z. A.; Yasin, S. R.; Al-Gharabli, S.; Elkarmi, A. Z. Anti-spermatogenic Activities of Taraxacum officinale Whole Plant and Leaves Aqueous Extracts. In *Veterinary Research Forum*; Faculty of Veterinary Medicine, Urmia University: Urmia, Iran, **2016;** vol 7, p 89.

Tariq, A.; Mussarat, S.; Adnan, M. Review on Ethnomedicinal, Phytochemical and Pharmacological Evidence of Himalayan Anticancer Plants. *J. Ethnopharmacol.* **2015,** *164*, 96–119.

Tascilar, M.; de Jong, F. A.; Verweij, J.; Mathijssen, R. H. Complementary and Alternative Medicine During Cancer Treatment: Beyond Innocence. *Oncologist* **2006,** *11*, 732–741.

Thun, M. J.; DeLancey, J. O.; Center, M. M.; Jemal, A.; Ward, E. M. The Global Burden of Cancer: Priorities for Prevention. *Carcinogenesis* **2010,** *31*, 100–110.

Tiwari, D.; Sah, A. N.; Bawari, S.; Bussmann, R. W. Ethnobotanical Investigations on Plants Used in Folk Medicine by Native People of Kumaun Himalayan Region of India. *Ethnobot. Res. Appl.* **2020,** *20*, 1–35.

van der Meel, R.; Lammers, T.; Hennink, W. E. Cancer Nanomedicines: Oversold or Underappreciated? *Expert Opin. Drug Deliv.* **2017,** *14*, 1–5.

Van Oppen, M. J.; Gates, R. D.; Blackall, L. L.; Cantin, N.; Chakravarti, L. J.; Chan, W. Y.; Cormick, C.; Crean, A.; Damjanovic, K.; Epstein, H.; Harrison, P. L. Shifting Paradigms in Restoration of the World's Coral Reefs. *Glob. Change Boil.* **2017,** *23*, 3437–3448.

Venditto, V. J.; Szoka Jr, F. C. Cancer Nanomedicines: So Many Papers and So Few Drugs! *Adv. Drug Delivery Rev.* **2013,** *65*, 80–88.

Venezuela, R. F.; Mosmann, J. P.; Mugas, M. L.; Kiguen, A. X.; Montoya, S. C. N.; Konigheim, B. S.; Cuffini, C. G. Dandelion Root Extract Affects the Proliferation, Survival and Migration of Cervical Cancer Cell Lines, 2021.

Vikhe, S.; Nirmal, S.; Siddheshwar, S. Protagonist Role of Herbal Medicament in Malignant Chemokinesis, 2016.

Wahl, O.; Oswald, M.; Tretzel, L.; Herres, E.; Arend, J.; Efferth, T. Inhibition of Tumor Angiogenesis by Antibodies, Synthetic Small Molecules and Natural Products. *Curr. Med. Chem.* **2011,** *18*, 3136–3155.

Wani, M, C.; Horwitz, S. B. Nature as a Remarkable Chemist: A Personal Story of the Discovery and Development of Taxol. *Anticancer Drugs* 2014, *25,* 482–487.

Wall, M. E.; Wani, M. C. Discovery to Clinica. *Ann. N.Y. Acad. Sci.* 1996, *803*, 1–12.

Wicremesinhe, E. R. M.; Arteca, R. N. Taxus callus Cultures: Initiation, Growth Optimization, Characterization and Taxol Production. *Plant Cell Tissue Organ Cult.* **1993,** *35,* 181–193.

Wild, C. P.; Stewart, B. W. Eds.; *World Cancer Rep.* World Health Organization: Geneva, Switzerland, **2014;** pp 482–494.

Wilken, R.; Veena, M. S.; Wang, M. B.; Srivatsan, E. S. Curcumin: A Review of Anti-Cancer Properties and Therapeutic Activity in Head and Neck Squamous Cell Carcinoma. *Mol. Cancer*. **2011,** *10*, 1–19.

Winston, D.; Maimes, S. Adaptogens : Herbs for Strength, Stamina and Stress Relief, Healing Arts Press, 2007.

World Health Organization and International Agency for Research on Cancer; Globocan, 2016.

Yoon, J. Y.; Cho, H. S.; Lee, J. J.; Lee, H. J.; Jun, S. Y.; Lee, J. H.; Song, H. H.; Choi, S.; Saloura, V.; Park, C. G.; Kim, C. H. Novel TRAIL Sensitizer Taraxacum officinale FH Wigg Enhances TRAIL-Induced Apoptosis in Huh7 Cells. *Mol. Carcinog.* **2016,** *55*, 387–396.

Zhao, T.; Wang, X.; Rimando, A. M.; Che, C. T. Folkloric Medicinal Plants: Tinospora Sagittata var. Cravaniana and Mahonia Bealei. *Planta Med.* **1991,** *57*, 505–505.

CHAPTER 5

Genetic Engineering of Plants for Enhanced Anticancer Potential

BUSHRA HAFEEZ KIANI

Department of Biological Sciences (Female Campus), International Islamic University, Islamabad, Pakistan

ABSTRACT

Secondary plant metabolites were first utilized for pharmaceutical use as herbal medicines. These metabolites can be used for curing cancer as they have cell division-inhibiting properties. Recombinant DNA technology and gene-altering platforms like CRISPR/Cas9 have recently enabled plants to produce cancer-targeting medicines. Enhanced resistance to diseases, insects, and herbicides, as well as increased yield and concentration of active ingredients, can be achieved in medicinal plants through recombinant DNA technology. These engineering technologies have facilitated increased production of active substances and heterologous expression of recombinant proteins like antibodies, vaccine candidates, and lectins for pharmaceutical use. Plant-derived anticancer agents in nature and the application of genetic engineering to increase selectivity minimize side effects, and the potential of these agents to revolutionize medical systems are discussed in this chapter.

5.1 INTRODUCTION

Numerous Kingdom Plantae species have potential medical applications. Antitumor, anti-inflammation, antioxidants, antiseptics, and lowering

Plant-Derived Anticancer Drugs in the OMICS Era: Biosynthesis, Functions, and Applications.
Deepu Pandita, Anu Pandita (Eds.)

blood glucose are some of those properties that are present in plants due to secondary metabolites. Ferulic acid, paclitaxel, betulinic acid, chlorogenic acid, and vinblastine are some of the probable metabolites for medical applications as they possess remedial and health-promoting qualities. Presently, the call for naturally occurring active compounds that have preventative and restorative effects has increased to prevent death from cancer, diabetes, cardiovascular disease, or respiratory disease (Zaynab et al., 2018). Secondary metabolites make up the majority of phytochemicals utilized for this purpose. These compounds are produced either constitutively or through different stimuli responses from different primary metabolites in plant cells and have varying structures and functions. Protection of plants from ultraviolet light (Kohler et al., 2017; Takshak and Agrawal, 2019), various pathogens (Bednarek et al., 2008), and herbivores (Huber et al., 2016; Huang et al., 2019), providing distinct scents and colors for effective pollination and distribution of seeds, are some of the important roles of these compounds. They are also essential signaling and regulating molecules for major metabolic processes.

Cancer is affecting humans all over the world which is why there is a continuous need for new therapies to stop this deadly disease. Scientists are now shifting their attention toward naturally derived agents for cancer treatment as they are comparatively less toxic than treatments like chemotherapy that are in use today. Secondary metabolites with anticancer abilities are synthesized by plants in nature and have initiated the development of new pharmaceutical medicines. New technologies are being further developed for cancer treatment after producing staple drugs by these compounds (Howe and Jander, 2008).

Traditional breeding procedures were used by conventional plant breeders to cultivate plants with desired characteristics in the past. Traditional breeding procedures, on the other hand, can only be utilized in closely related species that may crossbreed. Furthermore, traditional breeding cannot be used to get characteristics that are not present in the gene pool of the target plants. With recent developments in recombinant DNA technology, it is now feasible to transfer desired traits from another species or even kingdom into a host plant, resulting in genetically modified plants with a variety of desirable characteristics (Hammond-Kosack and Jones, 2000).

Genetically modified plants have altered genomes either by the addition of a transgene or by removing damaged DNA with the help of recombinant

DNA technology (Jhansi and Usha, 2013). The gene added to the target plant could be from a different species or even different kingdoms. For example, the tobacco plant was the first plant that was transgenically modified by the addition of the *nptII* bacterial antibiotic resistance gene (Framond et al., 1983). Since then, a wide range of genetically modified plants with vital agronomic characteristics such as resistance to pests and water scarcity have been developed in dicots and monocots that are receptive to genetic engineering, owing to recent advances in plant molecular biology, and recombinant DNA technology. The primary motivation for developing genetically modified plants is to create crops with optimal characteristics, high production, and excellent quality. Apart from agricultural importance, plants can act as a vehicle in pharmaceutical protein production (Lai et al., 2015).

New recombinant DNA techniques aim at administering the release of compounds to increase the anticancer ability of plant-derived drugs and look into new methods for administration. This chapter will be covering the use of genetic engineering to increase the production of anticancer drugs using medicinal plants and their properties that make them a valuable source for anticancer treatments.

5.2 FORMULATION OF ANTICANCER PRODUCTS

Despite the obstacles faced in the production of personalized medication are ignored, the challenges for producing high-quality anticancer medicines that can satisfy today's expectations are enormous (Siddiqui and Rajkumar, 2012). Because of their complicated structure, low reaction yields, and high costs, synthesizing small-molecule drugs and proteins by chemical means is not preferred.

Using prokaryotes as an expression system is usually not favorable for mAbs and some therapeutic proteins as prokaryotes do not have post-translational modifications such as N-linked glycosylation, which is required for the effective working of therapeutic proteins and the inefficient bond formation such as disulfide bonding, which is necessary for true protein folding. Reduced yield and high production cost have to be incurred if there is an inefficient formation of disulfide bonds that makes protein insoluble, resulting in the accumulation of inclusion bodies. These inclusion bodies have to be solubilized and refolded again in the lab

(Eiberle and Jungbauer, 2010). Expression systems like Chinese hamster ovary (CHO) cells, which are based on mammalian cells, are not ideal for producing small anticancer agents. This is because anticancer agents are deliberately created to be fatal for mammalian cells; an example of this is through impairing the cell cycle. Not only this, even less hazardous chemicals can be difficult to produce in mammalian expression systems since their economics rely on high yield, which is dependent on high cell division and optimal cell growth.

5.2.1 ANTICANCER PLANT-DERIVED DRUGS

Drugs derived from plants hold an important place in treating cancer as they are sourced naturally. They can be eaten as part of a patient's diet (Cornblatt et al., 2007; Amin et al., 2009) and as they are obtained from plants, so they are more bearable and safer than normal human cells (Unnati et al., 2013). But cyanogenic glycosides, lectins, saponins, lignans, lectins, and some taxanes are some of the exceptions (Phillipson, 1999; Unnati et al., 2013). These drugs derived from plants can be clinically tested for future therapeutic development if they are selective, meaning they are toxic to cancer cells and not normal cells. DNA damage preventive drugs or antioxidants, mitotic disruptors, methyltransferase inhibitors, and histone deacetylases inhibitors are the four classes of plant-derived drugs (Amin et al., 2009).

Histone deacetylase inhibitors include compounds like sulforaphane, isoflavones, isothiocyanates, and pomiferin. The activity of cancer-causing proteins is inhibited by these inhibitors. Sulforaphane, for example, has been found to block key targets in breast cancer growth. Histone deacetylase inhibition by sulforaphane therapy in breast cancer cell lines caused a decrease in the expression of estrogen receptors, epidermal growth factor receptor, and human epidermal growth factor receptor 2 (Pledgie-Tracy et al., 2007). Histone deacetylase inhibitors activate genes that are repressed by epigenetics and are involved in chromatin acetylation in cancer cells, which then go through programmed cell death. Chemotherapeutic susceptibility of malignant tumors in humans can be improved by plant-derived compounds as they block histone deacetylase enzymes (Pledgie-Tracy et al., 2007; Amin et al., 2009).

Vincristine, vinblastine, vinflunine, vindesine, and vinorelbine are products of *Vinca* alkaloids. These products bind to β-tubulin and disrupt the microtubule dynamics. Taxanes like paclitaxel and its counterpart docetaxel also inhibit microtubule dynamics. These substances inhibit the transition of the cell cycle from metaphase to anaphase, resulting in no cell division and programmed cell death. Paclitaxel reduces cell division by stabilizing or polymerizing the microtubules of cancer cells (Amos and Lowe, 1999; Jordan and Wilson, 2004; Khazir et al., 2014). Paclitaxel is one of the first drugs that were found to be effective against cancer cells while vincristine and vinblastine were among the first isolated drugs (Khazir et al., 2014).

Plant extracts containing a combination of medicines produced from *Podophyllum* lignans, *Vinca* alkaloids, *Camptotheca* alkaloids, and *Taxus* diterpenes not only increase the anticancer activity but also have an impact on therapeutic effectiveness (Khazir et al., 2014; Solowey et al., 2014). Solowely et al. (2014) studied the effects of the extracts from *Urtica membranaceae*, *Artemesia monosperma*, and *Origanum dayi Post* on cancer cells extracted from the cancerous breast, lung, colon, and prostate tissues. A combination of plant extracts with anticancer agents showed specificity, as they did not affect normal lymphocytes and fibroblasts and only killed cancerous cells. This makes plant extracts superior to chemically synthesized therapeutic drugs. Apoptosis caused by plant extracts is characterized by elevated levels of cells in the sub-G1 phase where cells have low genetic content and condensed chromatin. Moreover, after extract treatment, an increase in caspase 3 activation was reported which is one of the basic stages in programmed cell death (Solowey et al., 2014). Clinical trials are being considered for anticancer extracts that exclusively target cancerous cells, and have the ability to kill and halt cancer cells from growing (Fig. 5.1A, 5.1B, 5.1C, 5.1D).

Plants are eukaryotic cells with mechanisms for protein folding and post-translational alterations that are also present in mammal cells. Since plant cell activities differ, they have the advantage of producing molecules that are otherwise lethal to animal cells. Another advantage of plant cells is that recombinant DNA technology can be used to increase the production, scalability, and sustainability of anticancer agents.

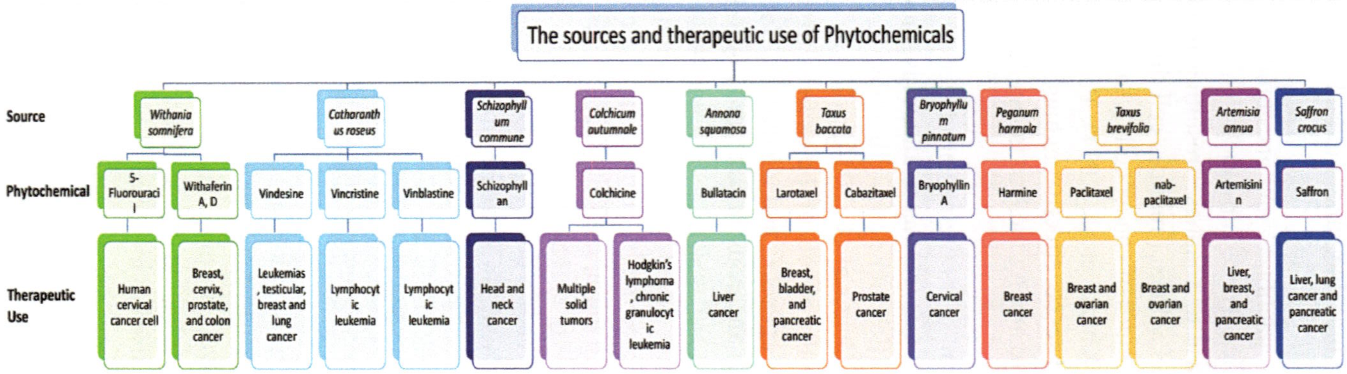

FIGURE 5.1A Known phytochemicals, their source, and therapeutic use.

Source: Adapted with permission from Buyel, 2018. © 2018 Elsevier.

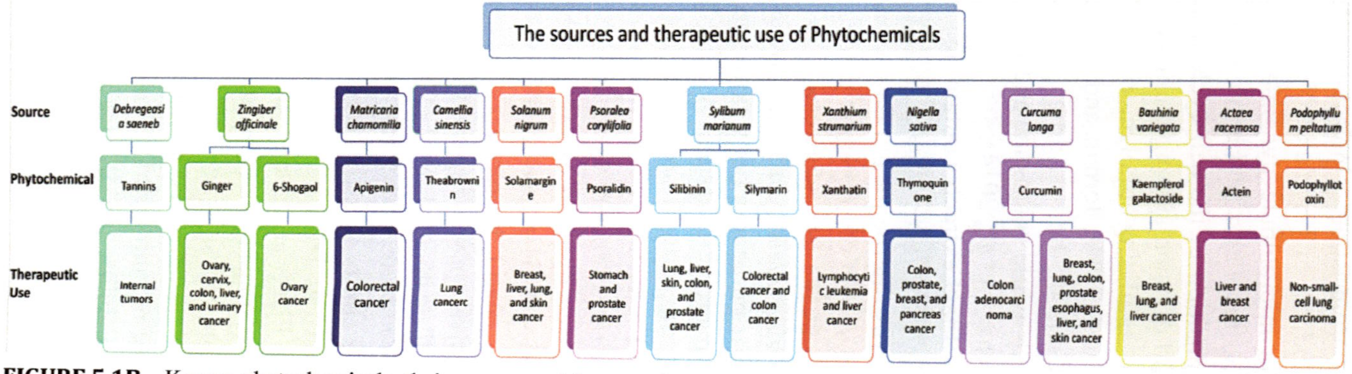

FIGURE 5.1B Known phytochemicals, their source, and therapeutic use.

Source: Adapted with permission from Buyel, 2018. © 2018 Elsevier.

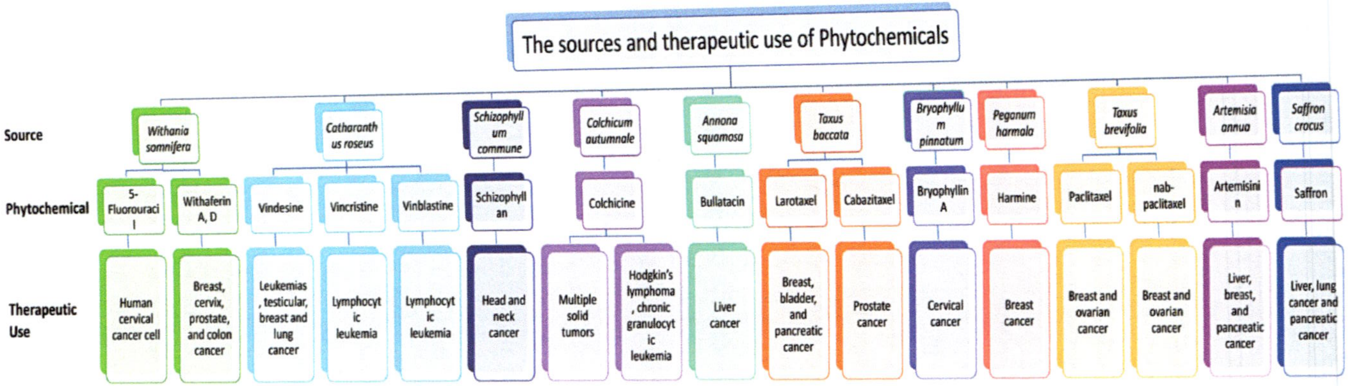

FIGURE 5.1C Known phytochemicals, their source, and therapeutic use.

Source: Adapted with permission from Buyel, 2018. © 2018 Elsevier.

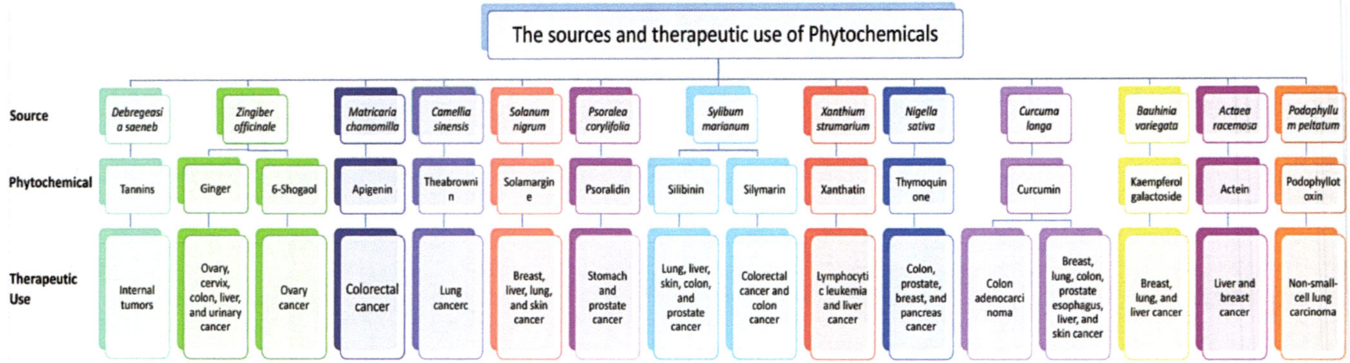

FIGURE 5.1D Known phytochemicals, their source, and therapeutic use.

Source: Adapted with permission from Buyel, 2018. © 2018 Elsevier.

5.3 ANTICANCER PRODUCTS DEVELOPED FROM PLANT SECONDARY METABOLITES

5.3.1 NATURAL SOURCES OF PLANT METABOLITES HAVING ANTICANCER PROPERTIES

For at least 60,000 years, plants have been utilized for medicinal purposes (Fabricant and Farnsworth, 2001) which demonstrates their capacity to generate a wide range of secondary metabolites having wide pharmaceutical applications including the treatment of cancer (Kuttan et al., 1997; Zarkovic et al., 1998). The most effective secondary metabolites derived from plants that are anticancer are phenolic compounds like flavonoids (Asensi et al., 2011; Wahl et al., 2011). In the past, drugs produced by plants were taken through the mouth either by consuming plant tissues or by making raw extracts, both of which are beneficial as both of the previously mentioned techniques are cost-effective and simple.

Moreover, it is safe and painless to consume and there is no use of a syringe or need for any invasive method. There is an extensive increase in publications describing the anticancer effect of extracts obtained from plants. A significant increase in publications has been observed since the beginning of the 21st century with 531 review articles and 4753 hits with the term "plant extract anticancer" when searching on July 1, 2019, at http://www.ncbi.nlm.nih.gov/pubmed (Fig. 5.2). It is impossible to provide an outline of all the plant agents that can potentially serve as cancer treatment and their working principle and effectiveness. Moreover, it is improbable that all the plant extracts discovered until now will show anticancer properties when tests would be replicated on a larger scale, which is compulsory for developing strategies for a cure against cancer (Fritz et al., 2013; Ioannidis, 2005; Nuzzo, 2014). In case plant extracts are effective against cancer (Kwon et al., 2016), it can still not be used at a commercial level until it is tested for its effectiveness and safety. It is a possibility that these raw mixtures may contain undesirable compounds and it would be difficult to control the relative concentrations of active pharmaceutical ingredients (APIs) and other components. The crude extract obtained from *Papaver somniferum* seeds, for example, includes sanguinarine which is an alkaloid processing antitumor properties (Selvi et al., 2009); however, it is an addictive opioid that causes hallucinations.

APIs consisting of anticancer properties are extracted from flora and tested at certain concentrations to avoid harmful effects. Taxane paclitaxel is an important anticancer plant metabolite synthesized in nature (Camidge, 2001; Wani and Horwitz, 2014). In 1992, the US Food and Drug Administration authorized taxane paclitaxel to be used on humans. Ovarian, breast, and pancreatic cancers are some of the cancers treated by paclitaxel (Committee for Medicinal Products for Human Use (CHMP), 2015a; Wani and Horwitz, 2014) similarly if gemcitabine is combined with paclitaxel, it is reported that median survival time is increased by less than 25% for pancreatic cancer patients in comparison to just gemcitabine treatment (Von Hoff et al., 2013). Depolymerization of tubulin is inhibited by paclitaxel that stabilizes microtubule cytoskeleton and stops mitosis in a dose-dependent manner (Wani and Horwitz, 2014).

Some of the tiny anticancer agent molecules that occur naturally in plants and are being clinically tested for their efficiency against oral and breast cancer include genistein, lycopene, and resveratrol (Bosviel et al., 2012; King-Batoon et al., 2008; Schnekenburger et al., 2014; Zlotogorski et al., 2013). Many pregnane glycosides such as desmiflavaside D and alkaloids like mahanine are some of the plant-derived metabolites that were found to stop the growth of prostate and breast tumors, sequentially (Jagadeesh et al., 2007; Raees et al., 2016). According to McAllister et al. (2015), nonpsychoactive cannabinoids possess cancer-fighting properties and many other plant metabolites have been seen to exhibit such properties (Schnekenburger et al., 2014).

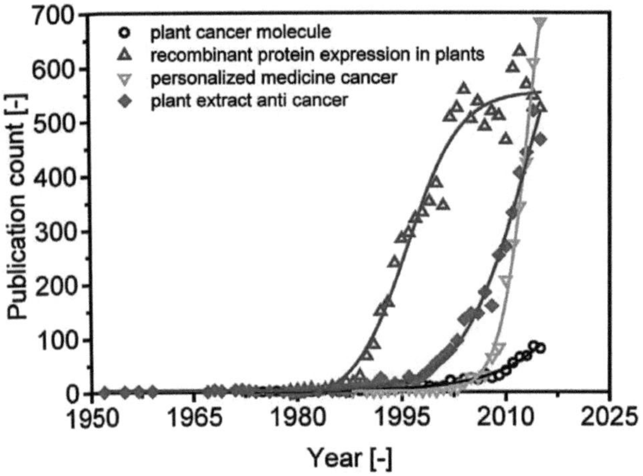

FIGURE 5.2 Publication history for four search queries related to anticancer compounds derived from or produced in plants. The most relevant query is shown as green diamonds indicating the production of anticancer compounds in plants (adapted from Buyel, 2018).

Ecologically varied areas like tropical rainforests and coral reefs are believed to be the habitat of many unexplored compounds that could be more efficiently serve as a similar purpose or have undiscovered mechanisms as anticancer agents (Mukherjee et al., 2001; Pereira et al., 2012). The devastation and harm being done to tropical rainforests and coral reefs, which is also linked with the loss of many species, dims this outlook (Van Oppen et al., 2017). This condition is gaining severe momentum as species that produce probable cancer-fighting compounds are being harvested for medicinal purposes driving them toward extinction. This scenario happened to be with Pacific yew, which was the only foundation of paclitaxel at the time (Wani and Horwitz, 2014). Frequently increased amounts of plant biofuel are needed to meet market demands. Paclitaxel, for example, is required in high doses ~3 g for liters on a single patient (Small and Catling, 1999) but local plants produce them in less amount (Kelsey and Vance, 1992) and the recovery rate of these chemicals could be as less as 0.004% after extraction (Wani and Horwitz, 2014). As a result, the plant's natural ability to produce these cancer-fighting agents is often inadequate to fulfill market needs. In certain situations, this restriction can be overcome by using therapeutic plants for increasing plant tissue cultures (AbouZid, 2014; Hussain et al., 2012; Yue et al., 2016).

5.4 GENETIC ENGINEERING OF PLANTS FOR PRODUCING ANTICANCER AGENTS

5.4.1 PRODUCTION OF ANTICANCER AGENTS IN GENETICALLY ENGINEERED PLANTS

Genetic engineering can be used to extend the preexisting plant metabolome or introduce new metabolic pathways that can be used to mass-produce anticancer agents in plants such as Pacific yew that are not suitable for cultivating. This would eliminate the manufacturing restrictions for anticancer reagents and prevent the temporary consumption of plant species in the ecosystem (Farre et al., 2014; Staniek et al., 2013; Wilson and Roberts, 2012). High growth rates, low generation times, high biomass production, and adaptability for biomass processing are all characteristics that impart compatibility (Verpoorte et al., 2002). Paclitaxel extraction by Pacific yew trees, for example, will need a huge cultivation area and up to 200 years for enough trees to develop (Wani and Horwitz, 2014). The trees have to be stripped of bark and cut for paclitaxel extraction; hence, the trees are killed during the process. As the trees are huge with rigid bark, expensive large-scale equipment is required. Productivity rate with respect to the area would remain low even if cultivation and infrastructure are ideal. Suppose a century-old yew tree contains ~3 kg of bark that can provide 0.14 g^{-1} kg^{-1} of paclitaxel (Small and Catling, 1999) but these trees require approximately 30 m^2 area for growing, hence the productivity rate will only be 0.14 mg a^{-1} m^{-2}. *Nicotiana tabacum*, on the other hand, generates biomass at a rate of 10 kg a^{-1} m^{-2} (Stoger et al., 2002). Although tobacco gives 10% in yew trees through transgenic modification, the productivity rate will still be 140 mg a^{-1} m^{-2} and hence a thousand-fold more compared to natural sources. External variables such as lighting conditions might also boost secondary metabolite synthesis (Buyel et al., 2015a).

Plant cell cultures can also be used to synthesize small anticancer agent molecules (Korkina and Kostyuk, 2012; Rischer et al., 2013; Tabata, 2004) at the rate of almost 1000 L or more (Georgiev and Weber, 2014). The equipment needed for fermentation and sterilized handling is costly requirement for upstream manufacturing. Cell cultures can still be beneficial since they can be derived from the original species or near relatives and their useful intrinsic metabolic capabilities can be intensified by adding elicitors or through genetic modification to enhance yield. Phyton Biotech (Delta BC, Canada) used such a method to generate GMP-compliant paclitaxel on a 75,000-L scale by the use of *Taxus* sp. cells to produce the APIs for Bristol-Myers Squibb (New York, USA) (Zhong, 2002). The annual sale of the product was US$1.592 billion in 2000 and has been in the market since 1992 (Exposito et al., 2009). Many strategies have since then been developed for increasing the 75,000-L yield of paclitaxel titers in the course of the cultivation process, such as using methyl jasmonate elicitor (Cusido et al., 2014). The research on other anticancer agents has been facilitated by this, for example, shikonin which is formed in *Lithospermum erythrorhizon* and berberine that is formed in *Coptis japonica* cells (Fujita, 2007).

5.4.2 GENETICALLY MODIFIED CROPS AND THE POTENTIAL MASS PRODUCTION OF ANTICANCER AGENTS

Genetically modified crops can be grown as multicellular individual organisms as opposed to microbes and other higher eukaryotic cell cultures.

In order to fulfill market demands, tons of recombinant proteins can be produced through transgenic plants as sterile cultivation environment and use of antibiotics is not needed for the upstream manufacturing and medicinal plants could be cultivated on a similar cultivating level as other plants (Buyel et al., 2017; Fischer and Schillberg, 2006). In 2015, 179.7 million hectares of transgenic plants were cultivated which is a 100-fold increase from 1996 (James, 2015). One more benefit of genetically modified crops is that they comparatively have a much more stable gene integration that is transferred through mammal cells or microorganisms (Baneyx and Mujacic, 2004; Gerngross, 2004; Hellwig et al., 2004; Wurm, 2004). The latter guarantees a proper and secure gene transfer providing a generation with ideal and functioning seed banks (Fischer et al., 2012). In order to create transgenic lines, transformation is done through *Agrobacterium tumefaciens* or particle bombardment (a physical method to transfer target genes in the host) before regenerating into crops (Lorence and Verpoorte, 2004; Newell, 2000; Rivera et al., 2012). The first transformants go through three to eight breeding cycles to produce plants that are homozygous and genetically modified. Depending on the genetic construct and plant species, this process of transformation and breeding can take up to 8–24 months, which is in correspondence with the cell line development of the CHO (Fan et al., 2017; Sack et al., 2015). Preparing seed banks for mass production may require more time (Twyman et al., 2003); CRISPR/Cas9 or other genome-editing tools can lower the period (Bortesi and Fischer, 2015; Puchta and Fauser, 2014) but genetically modified plants may be unfit for the immediate needs like individualized cancer treatments that are indispensable for patients. Transgenic plants, on the other hand, offer a superior mass production method for proteins needed for conventional treatments in a sizeable proportion of cancer patients, such as anticancer vaccinations or rituximab which is a recombinant monoclonal antibody (mAb) (Buyel et al., 2017).

The major issue in producing anticancer vaccines and antibodies by plant source is that plant glycans that are attached to the proteins differ structurally from those synthesized in humans, meaning that the APIs that are injected can potentially elicit an immune response. The same restrictions are applied to CHO-derived recombinant mAbs, although the amount of data available is many times more, lowering the uncertainty level. Despite the fact that human serum contains antibodies against plant glycans, no harmful effects for plant recombinant proteins have been seen so far in humans (Bardor et al., 2003; Chargelegue et al., 2000; Koprivova et al., 2004). Plant-produced glycans can also be beneficial in some instances, for example, modifying the effector activities of some mAbs that are plant-based because the Fc region is linked to carbohydrates. These glycans can also benefit to simplify production if the glycan antenna does not need to be cut off for product uptake, as it is for glucocerebrosidase enzyme (Grabowski et al., 2014). Plants could thus be viewed as a possible source of "biobetters" as well as an alternate manufacturing method. Plants can be modified if the need for human-type glycosylation is required in treatment by removing residues that are present in plants but absent in mammals like core α1,3-fucose, and β1,2-xylose and adding human genes that code for proteins needed to produce terminal sialic acids, glycans core 1,6-fucose, and 1,4-galactose, which are multi-antennary in nature (Bakker et al., 2006; Strasser, 2013, 2016; Strasser et al., 2008). Recombinant proteins that have true mammalian glycans can now be produced by these glyco-modified plants.

5.4.3 RECOMBINANT PROTEIN PRODUCTS

5.4.3.1 MONOCLONAL ANTIBODIES

mAbs are extremely selective and effective anticancer APIs (Chiarella, 2011; Gaughan, 2015; Scott et al., 2012). A gross total of about 10 t of mAbs were produced in 2013, with a US$75 billion market value (Ecker et al., 2015). According to 10% annual growth rate estimates (Research, 2013), before 2025, this industry will surpass US$ 200 billion (Research, 2013). Rituximab and etanercept had an annual demand of one-ton bulk API (Kelley, 2007) but this demand will likely increase since then as these agents would be supplied to nations that have a lack of resources for expensive cancer treatments. Suppose every second patient amongst the new 14.1 million cancer patients reported annually (Pritzkuleit et al., 2010; Rottenberg et al., 2010) needs a typical dose of 10 g protein in mAb therapy per person (Chames et al., 2009). The need for cancer-treating mAbs would go up to 70.5 t annum^{-1}. This estimate excludes the possibility of increased cancer cases in the future because of shifting demographics and improved cancer diagnostics, as well as the possibility of increased per-patient mAbs dose due to higher survival rates.

The production of MABs at a large scale is difficult to achieve if only utilizing traditional expression systems, although mAb titers of 5–10 g^{-1} L^{-1} are normally attainable now (Li et al., 2010; Shukla and Thommes, 2010). Even extremely large-scale fermenters with capacities of 10,000–25,000 L would be too expensive (Kelley, 2007; Li et al., 2010) and will generate about 5.0 t of mAb each year only, if the 12-day batch length is assumed (Kelley, 2007). This would therefore satisfy less than 10% of the expected demand. Moreover, single-use technologies are not preferred for large-scale productions as disposable fermenters have a capacity of about 2000 L, necessitating the utilization of several manufacturing trains. Even with the greater initial expenses, a stainless-steel fixed fermenter will overall be less priced in this case (Eibl et al., 2010; Shukla and Gottschalk, 2013).

Plants, on the other hand, come with their single-use built-in bioreactors, and the price difference between different production sizes is irrelevant as the number of plants can be scaled up as needed, and the required greenhouses or land is the primary cost element. Instead of open-field cultivation if vertical farming units (VFUs) are used (Buyel et al., 2017; Holtz et al., 2015). The biomass yield of some of the crops can be increased, for example, tobacco biomass can be increased from 10,000 t a^{-1} km^{-2} (Stoger et al., 2002) to 91,000 t a^{-1} km^{-2} by using VFUs. When antibody expression levels of 2 g^{-1} kg^{-1} are combined with these biomass yields (Zischewski et al., 2015) and a standard mAb recovery of 70% by purifying transgenic plants (Ma et al., 2015), ~0.555 km^{-2} of VFU area is enough to generate 70 t of purified mAb (Buyel et al., 2017).

Improved containment and highly regulated growth conditions are some of the extra advantages that can be practiced better in VFUs in comparison with open-land crops or greenhouse spaces, which can be beneficial for good manufacturing practice GMP (Fischer et al., 2012), along with the prospect of complete automation in the handling process even in GMP-compliant conditions (Wirz et al., 2012). A bioreactor of volume greater than 350,000 L would be needed in order to get the same yield through the fermentation process. It will also be a huge capital risk due to contamination and other repeated batch failures (Lolas, 2013). A loss of US$ 19–32 million would be incurred per failed batch if the CHO media is priced at $US 55–90 L^{-1}. There is a more comprehensive explanation of the advantages of plants for mass-producing mAbs elsewhere (Buyel et al., 2017). After considering these upstream benefits, downstream processes, and scale-up factors would be comparable to expression systems based on cell cultures (Ma et al., 2015; The CMC Biotech Working Group, 2009), such as constant production and preference of single-use technology (Angarita et al., 2015; Baur et al., 2015; Klutz et al., 2015).

The knowledge gained for mass production in the food manufacturing industry can be of use for plant-based systems (Goody, 1997). In conclusion, using plant-based expression systems might unlock the full potential of mAbs as medicines for a wide population of people suffering from cancer in both developed and developing nations.

5.4.3.2 LECTINS

Lectins can also be developed as a drug candidate against cancer. Viscumin, for example, is currently in clinical trials and is produced in compliance with the GMP by using the expression system of *Escherichia coli* (Schoffski et al., 2004; Zwierzina et al., 2011). Nonetheless, a low recovery rate of ~5% was recorded because of re-solubilization and refolding of the inclusion bodies formed by both A and B polypeptide chains that were constructed by two distinct strains of the bacterial species (Eiberle and Jungbauer, 2010). Moreover, glycosylation was absent, which might affect the stability and efficacy of the product (Li et al., 2012). The expression system for other plant lectins is *Pichia pastoris* yeast and these lectins are expressed at a rate of 6–20 mg^{-1} L^{-1} (Lannoo et al., 2007; Oliveira et al., 2008) but the yeast-synthesized glycoproteins generally have a lower concentration of complex glycans than mannose (Strasser, 2016). Viscumin expression is not generally a better option in mammal cells as a high concentration of lectin would have harmful effects on them (Endo et al., 1988). Since lectins are naturally produced plant metabolites, and the heterologous expression of lectins is not usually harmful to plants, these types of issues are generally resolved by using plants as expression systems. The development of a plant-based expression system that has ~5 mg^{-1} kg^{-1} yield has been started by the Fraunhofer Institute for Molecular Biology and Applied Ecology IME. This is similar to the 1.5 mg^{-1} mL^{-1} yield obtained after refolding with *Escherichia coli* as an expression system but this does not need re-solubilization or refolding of viscumin (Fuqua et al., 2015).

The production of heterodimeric viscumin from one gene and the monomeric precursor has been processed in the same manner as in the original host, reducing the complexities of the process by eliminating the need for distinct A and B chain synthesis and purification procedures. Separating viscumin from intricate plant matrix is not difficult as the affinity resin lactosyl-sepharose and purifying proteins from plant extracts through affinity chromatography purification do not appear to be hindered by the higher released amounts of host cell proteins in comparison with products secreted by CHO cells into the fermentation broth, as recently demonstrated for a mAb (Ma et al., 2015). Moreover, plants can manufacture a lectin called griffithsin, which has the power to stop the transmission of HIV (O'Keefe et al., 2009; Vamvaka et al., 2016).

5.4.3.3 ANTICANCER VACCINES

The most economical and least incision-dependent method for preventing or treating cancer is vaccines. In comparison with the anticancer agents described above, anticancer vaccines are limited to cancers that are caused by biotic factors like viruses. According to studies, one microgram dose of one or more antigens could be enough to activate a permanent defense against certain types of cancer. Several doses or booster shots could be required after some years (Ouattara and Laurens, 2015).

Vaccinations are subjected to greater critical examination regulators than chemotherapeutic agents since vaccines are generally administered in healthy people, and the ratio of risk to benefit does not bear intense negative effects which may be more tolerable by cancer sufferers in their later stages who have no other options (Kwok, 2011). As subunit vaccines only possess antigenic components like surface proteins of pathogens, they cannot cause virulence or replicate in patients, making them the preferable choice for vaccines (Baxter, 2007). These small proteins stimulate a weaker immune response as compared to vaccines that are more complicated and relatively larger (Bachmann and Jennings, 2010). Immunologic adjuvants like alum are used to increase the immune response and hence increase protection, but virus-like particles possess greater immunogenicity. Virus-like particles are made up of normal viral structural proteins but no nucleic acid content, therefore cannot reproduce or cause illness (Wang and Roden, 2013). Microorganisms could be used for manufacturing structural proteins, but as previously discussed; problems such as the production of high-mannose glycans in yeast and the absence of posttranslational modifications in bacteria are why higher eukaryotes are preferred. Mammal cells generate properly altered subunits but have a higher possibility of exposure to adventitious or endogenous viruses, which may lead to discarding the batches or evacuating the facilities completely (Bethencourt, 2009). Virus filtering is an essential element of all productions based on mammalian cell cultures to ensure that no intact or contagious viruses end up in the final therapeutic agent.

Since VLPs are generally the same size as live virus particles, this provides a distinct problem during the manufacturing process. Virus filtering is not required as the propagation of human-trophic viruses is not sustained by the plants (Commandeur and Twyman, 2005). Several VLPs, including those based on human papillomavirus, have therefore been effectively generated in plants (Commandeur and Twyman, 2005). Subunit vaccines can also be produced in plants, for example, the fusion protein with an altered form of human papillomavirus E7 protein (Buyel et al., 2012). This vaccine contender was not only as effective as the Cervarix and Gardasil vaccines available in the market for preventing cervical cancer but can also be used in the form of a preventive vaccine to hinder cervical cancer growth in people who already have the human papillomavirus (Massa et al., 2007; Venuti et al., 2009). Vaccines for other diseases like malaria have been produced through plants (Spiegel et al., 2015).

5.4.3.4 TRANSIENT EXPRESSION SYSTEMS AS POTENTIAL TARGETS FOR INDIVIDUALIZED CANCER TREATMENTS

Genetically modified plants are the most ideal expression platform for individualized treatments since antibodies, lectins, vaccinations, and VLPs described above are delivered to a large number of patients (or high-risk persons for vaccines). Nonetheless, mAbs can be used as individualized medicines and target the specific characteristics of cancer cells in individuals (Duffy, 2015). Comparatively, the market need for individualized treatments is in a lower grams range than general treatments which are in kg or tonne scale (Kelley, 2007). Individualized treatments, on the other hand, are only limited by the number of diagnosed cancer patients, whereas just a small amount of mAbs will need to be created by the tonne. This means that, in order to achieve reasonable turnaround times, the regulatory approval process for individualized medications will have to deviate from standard methods (Schork, 2015). The typical methods which are based on cell cultures or genetically modified plants as expression systems are not preferable as they need much time for development and time is a crucial aspect of cancer therapy. In comparison to these lengthy developmental processes, transient expression in plants is much more suitable as we can obtain results after receiving the DNA sequence that codes for the individualized antibody within weeks (Rosenberg et al., 2013; Shoji et al., 2012).

Infecting plants with replicating viruses that contain genes for a recombinant protein that results in systematic infection, allows for transient expression. Tobacco plants infected with modified *Tobacco mosaic virus* produce individualized antibodies that have been tested on non-Hodgkin's lymphoma patients and similar experiments have been carried out on a variety of viruses and plants (McCormick et al., 1999). Infiltrating wild-type plants like *Nicotiana benthamiana* with bioengineered *Agrobacterium tumefaciens* with resident plasmids containing transfer DNA with an appropriate transgene that is frequently used in binary vector strategy, can also result in transient expression (Glick et al., 2010). T-DNA is transferred to the cytoplasm of the plant cell and eventually the nucleus via type IV secretion system, where it is retained transiently as an episome, enabling foreign gene expression (Valentine, 2003). Viral-based and bacterial infiltration systems have also been coupled, resulting in the delivery of a partial viral genome by bacterial cells that have localized instead of systemic proliferation (Gleba et al., 2014). Although concentrations of recombinant protein increase after many weeks and then decrease (Buyel et al., 2013a), transient gene expression often provides greater yield in the near term than transgenic plants. Plants periodically carry several copies of episomal vectors in their cells, permitting the accumulation of large amounts of proteins. One disadvantage is that previous transient expression experiments showed notable differences in product yield in every batch (O'Neill et al., 2008), which has raised concerns regarding process repeatability by regulators (Fischer et al., 2012). Improved process parameters such as tight regulation of incubation time and temperature can help to solve this problem (Buyel and Fischer, 2012, 2013; Buyel et al., 2013a; Larsen and Curtis, 2008). VFUs can help with process control, as previously highlighted, and in fact, transient expression technologies are used in the majority of the mass-production factories that have been recently developed (Holtz et al., 2015; Wirz et al., 2012). This approach has been used in various situations like manufacturing emergency drugs, for example, to combat a widespread influenza outbreak (Shoji et al., 2012; Stoger et al., 2014) and has also received widespread government support, particularly in the United States (Paul et al., 2013). As a result, recombinant expression of pharmaceutically useful proteins combines the rapidity and versatility needed to quickly deliver appropriate quantities of anticancer drugs as individualized medicines.

5.5 SUMMARY

Cancer diagnoses are projected to grow as a result of demographic trends in developed countries and improved widely available diagnostics. Anticancer agents will be in high demand as more people have access to health care in developing nations. However, biotechnological processes involving mammalian cell cultures and microbes have high manufacturing costs, impediments, and side effects which will make it difficult to meet high market demands. Anticancer agents such as viscumin and paclitaxel produced in plants have the potential to meet the market demands. Recent advancements in bioprocess design, biotechnology, and plant molecular farming can further enhance these cancer-fighting compounds. For example, transient expression systems can be utilized to produce personalized medicines more efficiently or genetically modified plants can be used to mass-produce APIs.

KEYWORDS

- **anticancer drugs**
- **CRISPR/Cas9**
- **genetic engineering**
- **herbal medicines**

REFERENCES

AbouZid, S. Yield Improvement Strategies for the Production of Secondary Metabolites in Plant Tissue Culture: Silymarin From *Silybum marianum* Tissue Culture. *Nat. Prod. Res.* **2004,** *28* (23), 2102–2110.

Amin, A.; Gali-Muhtasib, H.; Ocker, M.; Schneider-Stock, R. Overview of Major Classes of Plant-Derived Anticancer Drugs. *Int. J. Biomed. Sci.* **2009,** *5* (1), 1–11.

Amos, L. A.; Löwe, J. How Taxol® Stabilises Microtubule Structure. *Chem. Biol.* **1999,** *6* (3), 65–69.

Angarita, M.; Muller-Spath, T.; Baur, D.; Lievrouw, R.; Lissens, G.; Morbidelli, M. Twin-Column CaptureSMB: A Novel Cyclic Process for Protein A Affinity Chromatography. *J. Chromatogr. A* **2015,** *1389,* 85–95.

Asensi, M.; Ortega, A.; Mena, S.; Feddi, F.; Estrela, J. M. Critical Reviews in Clinical Laboratory Sciences. *Crit. Rev. Clin. Lab. Sci.* **2011,** *48* (5–6), 197–216.

Ashraf, M. A. Phytochemicals as Potential Anticancer Drugs: Time to Ponder Nature's Bounty. *BioMed. Res. Int.* [Online] 2020. https://doi.org/10.1155/2020/8602879.

Bachmann, M. F.; Jennings, G. T. Vaccine Delivery: A Matter of Size, Geometry, Kinetics and Molecular Patterns. *Nat. Rev. Immunol.* **2010,** *10* (11), 787–796.

Bakker, H.; Rouwendal, G. J. A.; Karnoup, A. S.; Florack, D. E. A.; Stoopen, G. M.; Helsper, J. P. F. G.; Van Ree, R.; Van Die, I.; Bosch, D. An Antibody Produced in Tobacco Expressing a Hybrid Beta-1,4-galactosyltransferase is Essentially Devoid of Plant Carbohydrate Epitopes. *Proc. Natl. Acad. Sci. USA* **2006,** *103* (20), 7577–7582.

Baneyx, F.; Mujacic, M. Recombinant Protein Folding and Misfolding in *Escherichia Coli. Nat. Biotechnol.* **2004,** *22* (11), 1399–1408.

Bardor, M.; Faveeuw, C.; Fitchette, A. C.; Gilbert, D.; Galas, L.; Trottein, F.; Faye, L.; Lerouge, P. Immunoreactivity in Mammals of Two Typical Plant Glyco-Epitopes, Core Alpha(1,3)-fucose and Core Xylose. *Glycobiology* **2003,** *13* (6), 427–434.

Baur, D.; Angarita, M.; Muller-Spath, T.; Morbidelli, M. Pareto-optimal Design of the Twin-Column CaptureSMB Process Improves Capacity Utilization and Productivity in Protein A Affinity Capture. *Biotechnology* **2015,** *11* (1), 135–145.

Baxter, D. Active and Passive Immunity, Vaccine Types, Excipients and Licensing. *Occup. Med. Oxford* **2007,** *57* (8), 552–556.

Bednarek, P.; Schulze-Lefert, P. In *Role of Plant Secondary Metabolites at the Host-Pathogen Interface*. Molecular Aspects of Plant Disease Resistance 2018; Parker, J., Ed.; Wiley-Blackwell: Hoboken, NJ, USA, 2008**;** vol 34, pp. 220–260.

Bethencourt, V. Virus Stalls Genzyme Plant. *Nat. Biotechnol.* **2009,** *27* (8), 681.

Bortesi, L.; Fischer, R. The CRISPR/Cas9 System for Plant Genome Editing and Beyond. *Biotechnol. Adv.* **2015,** *33* (1), 41–52.

Bosviel, R.; Dumollard, E.; Dechelotte, P.; Bignon, Y. J.; Bernard-Gallon, D. Can Soy Phytoestrogens Decrease DNA Methylation in BRCA1 and BRCA2 on Cosuppressor Genes in Breast Cancer? *OMICS* **2012,** *16* (5), 235–244.

Buyel, J. F. Plants as Sources of Natural and Recombinant Anti-Cancer Agents. *Biotechnol. Adv.* **2018,** *36* (2), 506–520. DOI: 10.1016/j.biotechadv.2018.02.002. Epub 2018 Feb 3. PMID: 29408560.

Buyel, J. F.; Buyel, J. J.; Haase, C.; Fischer, R. The Impact of Pseudomonas Syringae Type III Effectors on Transient Protein Expression in Tobacco. *Plant Biol.* **2015a,** *17* (2), 484–492.

Buyel, J. F.; Fischer, R. Predictive Models for Transient Protein Expression in Tobacco (Nicotiana Tabacum L.) can Optimize Process Time, Yield, and Downstream Costs. *Biotechnol. Bioeng.* **2012,** *109* (10), 2575–2588.

Buyel, J. F.; Fischer, R. Processing Heterogeneous Biomass: Overcoming the Hurdles in Model Building. *Bioengineered* **2013,** *4* (1), 21–24.

Buyel, J. F.; Kaever, T.; Buyel, J. J.; Fischer, R. Predictive Models for the Accumulation of a Fluorescent Marker Protein in Tobacco Leaves According to the Promoter/ 5'UTR Combination. *Biotechnol. Bioeng.* **2013a,** *110* (2), 471–482.

Buyel, J. F.; Twyman, R. M.; Fischer, R. Very-Large-Scale Production of Antibodies in Plants: The Biologization of Manufacturing. *Biotechnol. Adv.* **2017,** *35* (4), 458–465.

Camidge, R. The Story of Taxol: Nature and Politics in the Pursuit of an Anti-Cancer Drug. *Br. Med. J.* **2001,** *323* (7304), 115.

Chames, P.; Van Regenmortel, M.; Weiss, E.; Baty, D. Therapeutic Antibodies: Successes, Limitations and Hopes for the Future. *Br. J. Pharmacol.* **2009,** *157* (2), 220–233.

Chargelegue, D.; Vine, N. D.; Van Dolleweerd, C. J.; Drake, P. M. W.; Ma, J. K. C. A Murine Monoclonal Antibody Produced in Transgenic Plants With Plant-Specific Glycans is not Immunogenic in Mice. *Transgenic. Res.* **2000,** *9* (3), 187–194.

Chiarella, P. Production, Novel Assay Development and Clinical Applications of Monoclonal Antibodies. *Recent Pat. Anti-Canc.* **2011,** *6* (2), 258–267.

Commandeur, U.; Twyman, R. M. Biosafety Aspects of Molecular Farming in Plants. In *Molecular Farming;* Fischer, R., Schillberg, S. (Eds.); Wiley-VCH Verlag GmbH & Co. KGaA: Hoboken, USA, 2005; 251–266.

Cornblatt, B. S.; Ye, L.; Dinkova-Kostova, A. T.; Erb, M.; Fahey, J. W.; Singh, K.; Chen, M. A.; Stierer, T.; Garrett-Mayer, E.; Argani, P.; Davidson, N. E.; Talalay, P.; Kensler, T.W.; Visvanathan, K. Preclinical and Clinical Evaluation of Sulforaphane for Chemoprevention in the Breast. *Carcinogenesis* **2007**, *28* (7), 1485–1490.

Cusido, R. M.; Onrubia, M.; Sabater-Jara, A. B.; Moyano, E.; Bonfill, M.; Goossens, A.; Angeles Pedreno, M. Palazon, J. A Rational Approach to Improving the Biotechnological Production of Taxanes in Plant Cell Cultures of Taxus Spp. *Biotechnol. Adv.* **2014,** *32* (6), 1157–1167.

Duffy, M. J. Personalized Treatment for Patients With Colorectal Cancer: Role of Biomarkers. *Biomark. Med.* **2015,** *9* (4), 337–347.

Ecker, D. M.; Jones, S. D.; Levine, H. L. The Therapeutic Monoclonal Antibody Market. *MAbs* **2015,** 7 (1), 9–14.

Eiberle, M. K.; Jungbauer, A. Technical Refolding of Proteins: Do We Have Freedom to Operate? *Biotechnol. J.* **2010,** *5* (6), 547–559.

Eibl, R.; Kaiser, S.; Lombriser, R.; Eibl, D. Disposable Bioreactors: The Current State of-the-Art and Recommended Applications in Biotechnology. *Appl. Microbiol. Biotechnol.* **2010,** *86* (1), 41–49.

Endo, Y.; Tsurugi, K.; Franz, H. The Site of Action of the A-chain of Mistletoe Lectin I on Eukaryotic Ribosomes. The RNA N-glycosidase activity of the protein. *FEBS Lett.* **1988,** *231* (2), 378–380.

Exposito, O.; Bonfill, M.; Moyano, E.; Onrubia, M.; Mirjalili, M. H.; Cusido, R. M.; Palazon, J. Biotechnological Production of Taxol and Related Taxoids: Current State and Prospects. *Anticancer Agents Med. Chem.* **2009,** *9* (1), 109–121.

Fabricant, D. S.; Farnsworth, N. R. The Value of Plants Used in Traditional Medicine for Drug Discovery. *Environ. Health Perspect.* **2001,** *109*, 69–75.

Fan, L.; Rizzi, G.; Bierilo, K.; Tian, J.; Yee, J. C.; Russell, R.; Das, T. K. Comparative Study of Therapeutic Antibody Candidates Derived From Mini-Pool and Clonal Cell Lines. *Biotechnol. Prog.* **2017,** *33* (6), 1456–1462.

Farre, G.; Blancquaert, D.; Capell, T.; Van Der Straeten, D.; Christou, P.; Zhu, C. Engineering Complex Metabolic Pathways in Plants. *Annu. Rev. Plant Biol.* **2014,** *65,* 187–223.

Fischer, R.; Schillberg, S. Molecular Farming: Plant-made Pharmaceuticals and Technical Proteins. Plant Cell Cultures for the Production of Recombinant Proteins. *Nat. Biotechnol.* **2006,** *22* (11), 1415–1422.

Fischer, R.; Schillberg, S.; Hellwig, S.; Twyman, R. M.; Drossard, J. GMP Issues for Recombinant Plant-Derived Pharmaceutical Proteins. *Biotechnol. Adv.* **2012**, *30* (2), 434–439.

Framond, A. J.; Bevan, M. W.; Barton, K. A.; Flavell, R.; Chilton, M. D. Mini-Ti Plasmid and a Chimeric Gene Construct: New Approaches to Plant Gene Vector Construction. In *Advances in Gene Technology: Molecular Genetics of Plants and Animals,* 20th ed.; Downey K, Voellmy RW, Ahmad F, (Ed.); Miami Winter Symp, Elsevier: Florida, 1983; pp. 159–170.

Fritz, H.; Seely, D.; Kennedy, D. A.; Fernandes, R.; Cooley, K.; Fergusson, D. Green Tea and Lung Cancer: A Systematic Review. *Integr. Cancer Ther.* **2013,** *12* (1), 7–24.

Fujita, Y. Industrial Production of Shikonin and Berberine. In *Ciba Foundation Symposium 137 - Applications of Plant Cell and Tissue Culture*; Bock, G., Marsh, J. (Eds.); John Wiley & Sons, Ltd.: Hoboken 2007; pp. 228–238.

Fuqua, J. L.; Hamorsky, K.; Khalsa, G.; Matoba, N.; Palmer, K. E. Bulk Production of the Antiviral Lectin Griffithsin. *Plant Biotechnol. J.* **2015,** *13* (8), 1160–1168.

Gaughan, C. L. The Present State of the Art in Expression, Production and Characterization of Monoclonal Antibodies. *Mol. Divers.* **2015,** *20* (1), 255–270.

Georgiev, M. I.; Weber, J. Bioreactors for Plant Cells: Hardware Configuration and Internal Environment Optimization as Tools for Wider Commercialization. *Biotechnol. Lett.* **2014,** *36* (7), 1359–1367.

Gerngross, T. U. Advances in the Production of Human Therapeutic Proteins in Yeasts and Filamentous Fungi. *Nat. Biotechnol.* **2004,** *22* (11), 1409–1414.

Gleba, Y. Y.; Tuse, D.; Giritch, A. Plant Viral Vectors for Delivery by Agrobacterium. *Curr. Top. Microbiol. Immunol.* **2014,** *375,* 155–192.

Glick, B. R.; Patten, J. P. J.; Li, C. *Molecular Biotechnology: Principles and Applications of Recombinant DNA* 2010, 4th ed.; John Wiley & Sons: Hoboken.

Goody, J. Industrial food. Towards the development of a world cuisine. In: Counihan, C., van Esterik, P. (Eds.), Food and Culture. Routledge, London **1997**, pp. 338–356.

Grabowski, G.A.; Golembo, M.; Shaaltiel, Y. Taliglucerase alfa: an enzyme replacement therapy using plant cell expression technology. Mol. Genet. Metab **2014**, 112 (1), 1–8.

Hammond-Kosack, K.; Jones J.D. Responses to plant pathogens. Biochemistry and Molecular Biology of Plants. Jan **2000**, 1(1):1102-1156

Holtz, B. R.; Berquist, B. R.; Bennett, L. D.; Kommineni, V. J.; Munigunti, R. K.; White, E. L.; Wilkerson, D. C.; Wong, K. Y.; Ly, L. H.; Marcel, S. Commercial-Scale Biotherapeutics Manufacturing Facility for Plant-made Pharmaceuticals. *Plant Biotechnol. J.* **2015,** *13* (8), 1180–1190.

Howe, G. A; Jander, G. Plant Immunity to Insect Herbivores. *Ann. Rev. Plant Biol.* **2008,** *59* (1), 41–66.

Huang, W.; Gfeller, V.; Erb, M. Root Volatiles in Plant–Plant Interactions II: Root Volatiles Alter Root Chemistry and Plant–Herbivore Interactions of Neighbouring Plants. *Plant Cell Environ.* **2019,** *42*, 1964–1973.

Huber, M.; Epping, J.; Schulze Gronover, C.; Fricke, J.; Aziz, Z.; Brillatz, T.; Swyers, M.; Köllner, T. G.; Vogel, H.; Hammerbacher, A.; et al. A Latex Metabolite Benefits Plant Fitness Under Root Herbivore Attack. *PLoS Biol.* **2016,** *14,* 1–27.

Ioannidis, J. P. A. Why Most Published Research Findings are False. *Plos Med.* **2005,** *2* (8), 696–701.

Jagadeesh, S.; Sinha, S.; Pal, B. C.; Bhattacharya, S.; Banerjee, P. P. Mahanine Reverses an Epigenetically Silenced Tumor Suppressor Gene RASSF1A in Human Prostate Cancer Cells. *Biochem. Biophys. Res. Commun.* **2007,** *362* (1), 212–217.

James, C. *Global Status of Commercialized Biotech/GM Crops*; International Service for the Acquisition of Agri-biotech Applications, Ithaca, 2015; pp 20.

Jhansi, R. S; Usha R. Transgenic Plants: Types, Benefits, Public Concerns and Future. *J. Pharm. Res.* **2013**, *6* (8), 879–883. Transgenic Plants: Gene Constructs, Vector and Transformation Method. http://dx.doi.org/10.5772/intechopen.7936955

Jordan, M. A.; Wilson, L. Microtubules as a Target for Anticancer Drugs. *Nat. Rev. Cancer* **2004,** *4,* 253–266.

Kelley, B. Very Large Scale Monoclonal Antibody Purification: The Case for Conventional Unit Operations. *Biotechnol. Prog.* **2007,** *23* (5), 995–1008.

Khazir, J.; Mir, B. A.; Pilcher, L.; Riley, D. L. Role of Plants in Anticancer Drug Discovery. *Phytochem. Lett.* **2014,** *7*, 173–181.

King-Batoon, A.; Leszczynska, J. M.; Klein, C. B. Modulation of Gene Methylation by Genistein or Lycopene in Breast Cancer Cells. *Environ. Mol. Mutag.* **2008,** *49* (1), 36–45.

Klutz, S.; Magnus, J.; Lobedann, M.; Schwan, P.; Maiser, B.; Niklas, J.; Temming, M.; Schembecker, G. Developing the Biofacility of the Future Based on Continuous Processing and Single-Use Technology. *J. Biotechnol.* **2015,** *213,* 120–130.

Köhler, H.; Contreras, R. A.; Pizarro, M.; Cortés-Antíquera, R.; Zúñiga, G. E. Antioxidant Responses Induced by UVB Radiation in Deschampsia Antarctica Desv. *Front. Plant Sci.* **2017,** *8,* 1–10.

Koprivova, A.; Stemmer, C.; Altmann, F.; Hoffmann, A.; Kopriva, S.; Gorr, G.; Reski, R.; Decker, E. L. Targeted Knockouts of Physcomitrella Lacking Plantspecific Immunogenic N-glycans. *Plant Biotechnol. J.* **2004,** *2* (6), 517–523.

Korkina, L.; Kostyuk, V. Biotechnologically Produced Secondary Plant Metabolites for Cancer Treatment and Prevention. *Curr. Pharm. Biotechnol.* **2012,** *13* (1), 265–275.

Kuttan, G.; Menon, L. G.; Antony, S.; Kuttan, R. Anticarcinogenic and Antimetastatic Activity of Iscador. *Anti-Cancer Drugs* **1997,** (Suppl. 1), 1a5–16.

Kwok, R. The Real Issues in Vaccine Safety. *Nature* **2011,** *473* (7348), 436–438.

Kwon, S. B.; Kim, M. J.; Yang, J. M.; Lee, H. P.; Hong, J. T.; Jeong, H. S.; Kim, E. S.; Yoon, D. Y. Cudrania Tricuspidata Stem Extract Induces Apoptosis Via the Extrinsic Pathway in SiHa Cervical Cancer Cells. *PloS One* **2016,** *11* (3), e0150235.

Lai, K. S.; Yusoff, K.; Mahmood, M. Heterologous Expression of Hemagglutinin-Neuraminidase Protein From Newcastle Disease Virus Strain AF2240 in *Centella Asiatica. Acta Biol. Crac.Ser. Bot.* **2015,** *24* (1), 142–147

Lannoo, N.; Vervecken, W.; Proost, P.; Rouge, P.; Van Damme, E. J. Expression of the Nucleocytoplasmic Tobacco Lectin in the Yeast Pichia Pastoris. *Protein Expr. Purif.* **2007,** *53* (2), 275–282.

Larsen, J. S.; Curtis, W. R. Reducing Batch-to-Batch Variability of Agrobacterium Mediated Transient Protein Expression in Plant Tissue Culture. In AIChE (Ed.); The **2008** Annual Meeting; AIChE: Philadelphia, PA.

Li, C. H.; Narhi, L. O.; Wen, J.; Dimitrova, M.; Wen, Z. Q.; Li, J.; Pollastrini, J.; Nguyen, X.; Tsuruda, T.; Jiang, Y. J. Effect of pH, Temperature, and Salt on the Stability of Escherichia Coli- and Chinese Hamster Ovary Cell-Derived IgG1 Fc. *Biochemistry* **2012,** *51* (50), 10056–10065.

Li, F.; Vijayasankaran, N.; Shen, A.; Kiss, R.; Amanullah, A. Cell Culture Processes for Monoclonal Antibody Production. *MAbs* **2010,** *2* (5), 466–479.

Lolas, A. Microbial Control Strategies in Bioprocessing Falling Short of Assuring Product Quality and Satisfying Regulatory Expectations, American Pharmaceutical Review 2013**,** Compare Networks, Fishers.

Lorence, A.; Verpoorte, R. Gene Transfer and Expression in Plants. *Methods Mol. Biol.* **2004,** *267,* 329–350.

Ma, J. K.; Drossard, J.; Lewis, D.; Altmann, F.; Boyle, J.; Christou, P.; Cole, T.; Dale, P.; Van Dolleweerd, C. J.; Isitt, V.; Katinger, D.; Lobedan, M.; Mertens, H.; Paul, M. J.; Rademacher, T.; Sack, M.; Hundleby, P. A.; Stiegler, G.; Stoger, E.; Twyman, R. M.; Vcelar, B.; Fischer, R. Regulatory Approval and a First-in-Human Phase I Clinical Trial of a Monoclonal Antibody Produced in Transgenic Tobacco Plants. *Plant Biotechnol. J.* **2015,** *13* (8), 1106–1120.

Massa, S.; Franconi, R.; Brandi, R.; Muller, A.; Mett, V.; Yusibov, V.; Venuti, A. Anti-cancer Activity of Plant-Produced HPV16 E7 Vaccine. *Vaccine* **2007,** *25* (16), 3018–3021.

McAllister, S. D.; Soroceanu, L.; Desprez, P. Y. The Antitumor Activity of Plant-Derived Non-Psychoactive Cannabinoids. *J. Neuroimmune Pharm.* **2015,** *10* (2), 255–267.

McCormick, A. A.; Kumagai, M. H.; Hanley, K.; Turpen, T. H.; Hakim, I.; Grill, L. K.; Tuse, D.; Levy, S.; Levy, R. Rapid Production of Specific Vaccines for Lymphoma by Expression of the Tumor-Derived Single-Chain Fv Epitopes in Tobacco Plants. *Proc. Natl. Acad. Sci. USA* **1999,** *96* (2), 703–708.

Mukherjee, A. K.; Basu, S.; Sarkar, N.; Ghosh, A. C. Advances in Cancer Therapy With Plant Based Natural Products. *Curr. Med. Chem.* **2001,** *8* (12), 1467–1486.

Newell, C. A. Plant Transformation Technology - Developments and Applications. *Mol. Biotechnol.* **2000,** *16* (1), 53–65.

Nuzzo, R. Scientific Method: Statistical Errors. *Nature* **2014,** *506* (7487), 150–152.

O'Keefe, B. R.; Vojdani, F.; Buffa, V.; Shattock, R. J.; Montefiori, D. C.; Bakke, J.; Mirsalis, J.; d'Andrea, A. L.; Hume, S. D.; Bratcher, B.; Saucedo, C. J.; McMahon, J. B.; Pogue, G. P.; Palmer, K. E. Scaleable Manufacture of HIV-1 Entry Inhibitor Griffithsin and Validation of its Safety and Efficacy as a Topical Microbicide Component. *Proc. Natl. Acad. Sci. USA* **2009,** *106* (15), 6099–6104.

Oliveira, C.; Felix, W.; Moreira, R. A.; Teixeira, J. A.; Domingues, L. Expression of Frutalin, an Alpha-D-Galactose-Binding Jacalin-Related Lectin, in the Yeast Pichia Pastoris. *Protein Expr. Purif.* **2008,** *60* (2), 188–193.

O'Neill, K. M.; Larsen, J. S.; Curtis, W. R. Scale-up of Agrobacterium-Mediated Transient Protein Expression in Bioreactor-Grown Nicotiana Glutinosa Plant Cell Suspension Culture. *Biotechnol. Prog.* **2008,** *24* (2), 372–376.

Ouattara, A.; Laurens, M. B. Vaccines Against Malaria. *Clin. Infect. Dis.* **2015,** *60* (6), 930–936.

Paul, M. J.; Teh, A. Y. H.; Twyman, R. M.; Ma, J. K. C. Target Product Selection – Where can Molecular Pharming Make the Difference? *Curr. Pharm. Des.* **2013,** *19* (31), 5478–5485.

Pereira, D. M.; Valentao, P.; Correia-da-Silva, G.; Teixeira, N.; Andrade, P. B. Plant Secondary Metabolites in Cancer Chemotherapy: Where Are We? *Curr. Pharm. Biotechnol.* **2012,** *13* (5), 632–650.

Phillipson, J. D. Medicinal Plants. *J. Biol. Educ.* (Soc. Biol.) **1999,** *31* (2), 109.

Pledgie-Tracy, A.; Sobolewski, M. D.; Davidson, N. E. Sulforaphane Induces Cell Type-Specific Apoptosis in Human Breast Cancer Cell Lines. *Mol. Cancer Ther.* **2007,** *6* (3), 1013–1021.

Pritzkuleit, R.; Beske, F.; Katalinic, A. Demographic Change and Cancer. *Onkologie* **2010,** *33* (Suppl. 7), 19–24.

Puchta, H.; Fauser, F. Synthetic Nucleases for Genome Engineering in Plants: Prospects for a Bright Future. *Plant J.* **2014,** *78* (5), 727–741.

Raees, M. A.; Hussain, H.; Al-Rawahi, A.; Csuk, R.; Muhammad, S. A.; Khan, H. Y.; Rehman, N. U.; Abbas, G.; Al-Broumi, M. A.; Green, I. R.; Elyassi, A.; Mahmood, T.; Al-Harrasi, A. Anti-Proliferative and Computational Studies of Two New Pregnane Glycosides From Desmidorchis Flava. *Bioorg. Chem.* **2016,** *67,* 95–104.

Research, B. Biologic Therapeutic Drugs: Technologies and Global Markets. BCC Research LLC: Wellesley, MA, 2013; pp 142.

Rischer, H.; Hakkinen, S. T.; Ritala, A.; Seppanen-Laakso, T.; Miralpeix, B.; Capell, T.; Christou, P.; Oksman-Caldentey, K. M. Plant Cells as Pharmaceutical Factories. *Curr. Pharm. Des.* **2013,** *19* (31), 5640–5660.

Rivera, A. L.; Gomez-Lim, M.; Fernandez, F.; Loske, A. M. Physical Methods for Genetic Plant Transformation. *Phys. Life Rev.* **2012,** *9* (3), 308–345.

Rosenberg, Y.; Sack, M.; Montefiori, D.; Forthal, D.; Mao, L. J.; Hernandez-Abanto, S.; Urban, L.; Landucci, G.; Fischer, R.; Jiang, X. M. Rapid High-Level Production of Functional HIV Broadly Neutralizing Monoclonal Antibodies in Transient Plant Expression Systems. *PloS One* **2013,** *8* (3), e58724.

Rottenberg, Y.; Barchana, M.; Liphshitz, I.; Peretz, T. The Changing Face of Cancer in the Elderly: Only a Demographic Change? *Arch. Gerontol. Geriatr.* **2010,** *50* (3), e59–62.

Sack, M.; Rademacher, T.; Spiegel, H.; Boes, A.; Hellwig, S.; Drossard, J.; Stoger, E.; Fischer, R. From Gene to Harvest: Insights Into Upstream Process Development for the GMP Production of a Monoclonal Antibody in Transgenic Tobacco Plants. *Plant Biotechnol. J.* **2015,** *13* (8), 1094–1105.

Schnekenburger, M.; Dicato, M.; Diederich, M. Plant-Derived Epigenetic Modulators for Cancer Treatment and Prevention. *Biotechnol. Adv.* **2014,** *32* (6), 1123–1132.

Schoffski, P.; Riggert, S.; Fumoleau, P.; Campone, M.; Bolte, O.; Marreaud, S.; Lacombe, D.; Baron, B.; Herold, M.; Zwierzina, H.; Wilhelm-Ogunbiyi, K.; Lentzen, H.; Twelves, C. European Organization for Treatment of Cancer New Drug Development, Phase I Trial of Intravenous Viscumin in Patients With Solid Tumors: A Study of the European Organization for Research and Treatment of Cancer New Drug Development Group. *Ann. Oncol.* **2004,** *15* (12), 1816–1824.

Schork, N. J. Personalized Medicine: Time for One-Person Trials. *Nature* **2015,** *520* (7549), 609–611.

Scott, A. M.; Wolchok, J. D.; Old, L. J. Antibody Therapy of Cancer. *Nat. Rev. Cancer* **2012,** *12* (4), 278–287.

Scotti, N.; Rybicki, E. P. Virus-Like Particles Produced in Plants as Potential Vaccines. *Expert Rev. Vaccines* **2013,** *12* (2), 211–224.

Selvi, B. R.; Pradhan, S. K.; Shandilya, J.; Das, C.; Sailaja, B. S.; Shankar, G. N.; Gadad, S. S.; Reddy, A.; Dasgupta, D.; Kundu, T. K. Sanguinarine Interacts With Chromatin, Modulates Epigenetic Modifications, and Transcription in the Context of Chromatin. *Chem. Biol.* **2009,** *16* (2), 203–216.

Shoji, Y.; Farrance, C. E.; Bautista, J.; Bi, H.; Musiychuk, K.; Horsey, A.; Park, H.; Jaje, J.; Green, B. J.; Shamloul, M.; Sharma, S.; Chichester, J. A.; Mett, V.; Yusibov, V. A Plant-Based System for Rapid Production of Influenza Vaccine Antigens. *Influenza Other Respir. Viruses* **2012,** *6* (3), 204–210.

Shukla, A. A.; Gottschalk, U. Single-Use Disposable Technologies for Biopharmaceutical Manufacturing. *Trends Biotechnol.* **2013,** *31* (3), 147–154.

Siddiqui, M.; Rajkumar, S. V. The High Cost of Cancer Drugs and What we can do About it. *Mayo Clin. Proc.* **2012,** *87* (10), 935–943.

Small, E.; Catling, P. M. Approaches Toward Production of Secondary Plant Metabolites. *J. Pharm. Bio. All. Sci.* **2018,** *4* (1), 10–20.

Solowey, E.; Lichtenstein, M., Sallo, S.; Paavilainen, H.; Solowet, E.; Lorberboum-Galski, H. Evaluating Medicinal Plants for Anticancer Activity. *Sci. World J.* **2014,** *2014,* 1–12.

Spiegel, H.; Boes, A.; Voepel, N.; Beiss, V.; Edgue, G.; Rademacher, T.; Sack, M.; Schillberg, S.; Reimann, A.; Fischer, R. Application of a Scalable Plant Transient Gene Expression Platform for Malaria Vaccine Development. *Front. Plant Sci.* **2015,** *6,* 1169.

Staniek, A.; Bouwmeester, H.; Fraser, P. D.; Kayser, O.; Martens, S.; Tissier, A.; Van der Krol, S.; Wessjohann, L.; Warzecha, H. Natural Products - Modifying Metabolite Pathways in Plants. *Biotechnol. J.* **2013,** *8* (10), 1159–1171.

Stoger, E.; Fischer, R.; Moloney, M.; Ma, J. K. C. Plant Molecular Pharming for the Treatment of Chronic and Infectious Diseases. *Annu. Rev. Plant Biol.* **2014,** *65* (1), 743–768.

Stoger, E.; Sack, M.; Perrin, Y.; Vaquero, C.; Torres, E.; Twyman, R. M.; Christou, P.; Fischer, R. Practical Considerations for Pharmaceutical Antibody Production in Different Crop Systems. *Mol. Breed.* **2002,** *9* (3), 149–158.

Strasser, R. Engineering of Human-Type O-glycosylation in Nicotiana Benthamiana Plants. *Bioengineered* **2013,** *4* (4), 191–196.

Strasser, R. Plant Protein Glycosylation. *Glycobiology* **2016,** *26* (9), 926–939.

Strasser, R.; Stadlmann, J.; Schahs, M.; Stiegler, G.; Quendler, H.; Mach, L.; Glossl, J.; Weterings, K.; Pabst, M.; Steinkellner, H. Generation of Glyco-engineered Nicotiana Benthamiana for the Production of Monoclonal Antibodies With a Homogeneous Human-Like N-glycan Structure. *Plant Biotechnol. J.* **2008,** *6* (4), 392–402.

Tabata, H. Paclitaxel Production by Plant-Cell-Culture Technology. *Adv. Biochem. Eng./ Biotechnol* **2004,** *87*, 1–23.

Takshak, S.; Agrawal, S. B. Defense Potential of Secondary Metabolites in Medicinal Plants Under UV-B Stress. *J. Photochem. Photobiol. B Biol* **2019,** *193,* 51–88.

The CMC, Biotech Working Group. A-Mab: a Case Study in Bioprocess Development, A-Mab: A Case Study in Bioprocess Development, 2.1 ed. CASSS – An International Separation Science Society: Emeryville, CA, USA, 2009; pp 1–278.

Twyman, R. M.; Stoger, E.; Schillberg, S.; Christou, P.; Fischer, R. Molecular Farming in Plants: Host Systems and Expression Technology. *Trends Biotechnol.* **2003,** *21* (12), 570–578.

Unnati, S.; Ripal, S.; Sanjeev, A.; Niyati A. Novel Anticancer Agents From Plant Sources. *Chinese J. Natl. Med.* **2013,** *11* (1), 0016–0023.

Valentine, L. *Agrobacterium Tumefaciens* and the Plant: The David and Goliath of Modern Genetics. *Plant Physiol.* **2003,** *133* (3), 948–955.

Vamvaka, E.; Arcalis, E.; Ramessar, K.; Evans, A.; O'Keefe, B. R.; Shattock, R. J.; Medina, V.; Stöger, E.; Christou, P.; Capell, T. Rice Endosperm is Cost-Effective for the Production of Recombinant Griffithsin With Potent Activity Against HIV. *Plant Biotechnol. J.* **2016,** *14* (6), 1427–1437.

Van Oppen, M. J.; Gates, R. D.; Blackall, L. L.; Cantin, N.; Chakravarti, L. J.; Chan, W. Y.; Cormick, C.; Crean, A.; Damjanovic, K.; Epstein, H.; Harrison, P. L.; Jones, T. A.; Miller, M.; Pears, R. J.; Peplow, L. M.; Raftos, D. A.; Schaffelke, B.; Stewart, K.; Torda, G.; Wachenfeld, D.; Weeks, A. R.; Putnam, H. M. Shifting Paradigms in Restoration of the World's Coral Reefs. *Global Change Biol* **2017,** *23* (9), 3437–3448.

Venuti, A.; Massa, S.; Mett, V.; Vedova, L. D.; Paolini, F.; Franconi, R.; Yusibov, V. An E7-Based Therapeutic Vaccine Protects Mice Against HPV16 Associated Cancer. Vaccine **2009,** *27* (25–26), 3395–3397.

Verpoorte, R.; Contin, A.; Memelink, J. Biotechnology for the Production of Plant Secondary Metabolites. *J. Phytochem. Rev.* **2002,** *1* (1), 13–25.

Von Hoff, D. D.; Ervin, T.; Arena, F. P.; Chiorean, E. G.; Infante, J.; Moore, M.; Seay, T.; Tjulandin, S. A.; Ma, W. W.; Saleh, M. N.; Harris, M.; Reni, M.; Dowden, S.; Laheru, D.; Bahary, N.; Ramanathan, R. K.; Tabernero, J.; Hidalgo, M.; Goldstein, D.; Van Cutsem, E.; Wei, X.; Iglesias, J.; Renschler, M. F. Increased Survival in Pancreatic Cancer With Nab-Paclitaxel Plus Gemcitabine. *N. Engl. J. Med.* **2013,** *369* (18), 1691–1703.

Wahl, O.; Oswald, M.; Tretzel, L.; Herres, E.; Arend, J.; Efferth, T. Inhibition of Tumor Angiogenesis by Antibodies, Synthetic Small Molecules and Natural Products. *Curr. Med. Chem.* **2011,** *18* (21), 3136–3155.

Wang, J. W.; Roden, R. B. S. Virus-Like Particles for the Prevention of Human Papillomavirus- Associated Malignancies. *Expert Rev. Vaccines* **2013,** *12* (2), 129–141.

Wani, M. C.; Horwitz, S. B. Nature as a Remarkable Chemist: A Personal Story of the Discovery and Development of Taxol. *Anticancer Drugs* **2014,** *25* (5), 482–487.

Wilson, S. A.; Roberts, S. C. Recent Advances Towards Development and Commercialization of Plant Cell Culture Processes for the Synthesis of Biomolecules. *Plant Biotechnol. J.* **2012,** *10* (3), 249–268.

Wirz, H.; Sauer-Budge, A. F.; Briggs, J.; Sharpe, A.; Shu, S. D.; Sharon, A. Automated Production of Plant-Based Vaccines and Pharmaceuticals. *J. Lab. Autom.* **2012,** *17* (6), 449–457.

Wurm, F. M. Production of Recombinant Protein Therapeutics in Cultivated Mammalian Cells. *Nat. Biotechnol.* **2004,** *22* (11), 1393–1398.

Yang, L.; Wen, K. S.; Ruan, X.; Zhao Y. X.; Wei F.; Wang Q. Response of Plant Secondary Metabolites to Environmental Factors. *Molecules* **2018,** *23* (4), E762. https://doi.org/10.3390/molecules23040762.

Yue, W.; Ming, Q. L.; Lin, B.; Rahman, K.; Zheng, C. J.; Han, T.; Qin, L. P. Medicinal Plant Cell Suspension Cultures: Pharmaceutical Applications and High-Yielding Strategies for the Desired Secondary Metabolites. *Crit. Rev. Biotechnol.* **2016,** *36* (2), 215–232.

Zarkovic, N.; Kalisnik, T.; Loncaric, I.; Borovic, S.; Mang, S.; Kissel, D.; Konitzer, M.; Jurin, M.; Grainza, S. Comparison of the Effects of Viscum Album Lectin ML-1 and Fresh Plant Extract (Isorel) on the Cell Growth in Vitro and Tumorigenicity of Melanoma B16F10. *Cancer Biother. Radiopharm.* **1998,** *13* (2), 121–131.

Zaynab, M.; Fatima, M.; Abbas, S.; Sharif, Y.; Umair, M.; Zafar, M. H.; Bahadar, K. Role of Secondary Metabolites in Plant Defense Against Pathogens. *Microb. Pathog.* **2018,** *124,* 198–202.

Zhong, J. J. Plant Cell Culture for Production of Paclitaxel and Other Taxanes. *J. Biosci. Bioeng.* **2002,** *94* (6), 591–599.

Zischewski, J.; Sack, M.; Fischer, R. Overcoming Low Yields of Plant-Made Antibodies by a Protein Engineering Approach. *Biotechnol. J.* **2015,** *11* (1), 107–116.

Zlotogorski, A.; Dayan, A.; Dayan, D.; Chaushu, G.; Salo, T.; Vered, M. Nutraceuticals as New Treatment Approaches for Oral Cancer: II. Green Tea Extracts and Resveratrol. *Oral Oncol.* **2013,** *49* (6), 502–506.

Zwierzina, H.; Bergmann, L.; Fiebig, H.; Aamdal, S.; Schoffski, P.; Witthohn, K.; Lentzen, H. The Preclinical and Clinical Activity of Aviscumine: A Potential Anticancer Drug. *Eur. J. Cancer* **2011,** *47* (10), 1450–1457.

CHAPTER 6

Genetic Engineering of Plants for Enhancing Secondary Metabolites with Anticancerous Properties

NILANJANA DAS[1] and ARYADEEP ROYCHOUDHURY[2]

[1]*Department of Biotechnology, St. Xavier's College (Autonomous), Kolkata, West Bengal, India*

[2]*Discipline of Life Sciences, School of Sciences, Indira Gandhi National Open University, New Delhi, India*

ABSTRACT

Cancer refers to a group of diseases where cells proliferate uncontrollably and abruptly followed by their migration into different parts of the body. It is considered as one of the leading causes of death in the world. Wide variety of medicines is coming up over the years for the treatment of different types of cancers. Metabolites derived from plants are being used by humans as medicines for the past 60,000 years. Secondary metabolites produced by plants modulate several molecules and pathways involved in the development of cancer. The advancement of genetic engineering technologies like CRISPR/Cas9 has enabled the route for the development of genetically modified plants, with enhanced secondary metabolites having anticancerous properties. In this chapter, we discuss about the different anticancerous secondary metabolites produced by plants and how plants are being genetically modified for the enhancement of these metabolites.

Plant-Derived Anticancer Drugs in the OMICS Era: Biosynthesis, Functions, and Applications.
Deepu Pandita, Anu Pandita (Eds.)

6.1 INTRODUCTION

Cancer refers to a group of diseases where cells in the body divide uncontrollably and can migrate to different parts of the body. It is one of the leading causes of death, thus decreasing the life expectancy all over the world. Mortality rate due to cancer is increasing rapidly, and in 112 countries, cancer is considered as the second leading cause of death before the age of 70 years (Bray et al., 2021). In 2020, there were approximately 19.3 million cases and 10 million deaths due to cancer. Breast cancer followed by lung, colorectal, prostate, and stomach cancers are the commonly diagnosed cancers. Lung cancer, followed by colorectal, liver, stomach, and breast cancers are the leading causes of death (Sung et al., 2021). Due to the heterogeneous nature of cancer, no unique treatment is available. Treatment of cancer includes surgery, chemotherapy, radiotherapy, and immunotherapy which are either used alone or are combined together. However, both diagnosis and prognosis of cancer are difficult and the quest to find biomarkers for early detection and potent drugs against cancer is going on. Thus, the fight against cancer requires more investment in finding out safe and effective anticancerous drugs.

Traditional medicines from indigenous plant cultivars are being used worldwide to treat different types of diseases. Secondary metabolites are a group of organic compounds which are not essential for growth, development, and reproduction, but mainly act for the survival purposes of the organism producing it. They play an important role in interaction of the plants with their environment and are mainly produced during stress responses. In plants, the secondary metabolites are named according to their chemical classification and the pathway via which they are synthesized. They are broadly classified into four groups: (1) phenolics containing aromatic rings with one or more hydroxyl groups are biosynthesized via the shikimic acid pathway; (2) terpenoids containing C5 isoprene units are biosynthesized via the mevalonic acid or methylerythritol phosphate pathway; (3) alkaloids are nitrogen-containing basic compounds mainly biosynthesized from L-amino acids like lysine, tyrosine, and phenylalanine (Delgoda and Murray, 2017; Kabera et al., 2014); and (4) glycosides containing a carbohydrate group attached to a noncarbohydrate group.

Secondary metabolites, produced by some fungi and bacteria like monensin produced by *Streptomyces cinnamonensis*, act as antibiotics. Secondary metabolites like auvericin produced by a fungus, *Beauveria bassiana*, exhibit insecticidal activity (Hamill et al., 1969). Toxic secondary metabolites produced by plants confer protection against animals. Secondary metabolites like forphenicine are found to have some immunological activity (Okura et al., 1986). Secondary metabolites from some organisms like a fungal phytotoxin, Aspergillomarasmine can act as inhibitor of certain metabolically important enzymes (Mikami and Suzuki, 1983). Secondary metabolites like pseudobactins produced by some *Pseudomonas* species act as mineral scavengers by scavenging iron (Schroth and Hancock, 1982). Pigmented secondary metabolites produced by some organisms can absorb light and protect the organisms against harmful radiations and radicals (Greenberg and Canale-Parola, 1975; Vining, 1990). Secondary metabolites obtained from plants are not enough to suffice the need of the pharmaceutical industries and require high cost as well as time. Nowadays, modern biotechnological methods like genetic engineering are alternative and preferable approaches for the production of biologically relevant molecules. Plants are now genetically engineered and used as an alternative system to microbial or cell culture methods for the production of products like vaccines, antibiotics, antibodies, oils, and bioplastics (Bauer, 2014). The advantages of using plants for the production of therapeutic proteins include high yield, less health risk, less contamination, low cost, and easy storage in organs like seeds (Ganz et al., 1996; Joshi and Sodhi, 2014). Plants can produce a wide variety of well-known anticancer drugs like taxol, camptothecin (CPT), and curcumin which are already in phase I/II clinical trials. In this chapter, we discuss about some of these anticancerous secondary metabolites and the genetic engineering approaches for enhancing their production.

6.2 SECONDARY METABOLITES FROM PLANTS WITH ANTICANCEROUS PROPERTIES

Secondary metabolites obtained from plants are known to exhibit a broad range of activities. Natural products obtained from plants are considered as more biological friendly and less toxic to cells (Mishra and Tiwari, 2011). Though many of these products are believed to have anticancer properties, using them directly is doubtful because of their low bioavailability and safety issues. Chemical modification of these natural products can increase their bioavailability, absorption, distribution, excretion, and can decrease the toxic and side effects, if any (Guo, 2017; Yao et al., 2017). Between 1940 and 2014, about 49% of small molecules approved for chemotherapy were natural products (Newman and Cragg, 2016). Secondary metabolites like alkaloids, polyphenols, terpenoids, and flavonoids from plants are reported to have anticancerous properties by targeting different metabolic pathways. A wide range of these metabolites have been tested for their anticancerous properties, but only a few have managed to reach the clinical trials because of certain limitations.

6.2.1 CURCUMIN

Curcumin is a hydrophobic polyphenolic compound synthesized via the phenylpropanoid pathway in the rhizome of turmeric (*Curcuma longa*). Curcumin exhibits antioxidant, anti-inflammatory, antimicrobial, chemotherapeutic, and wound-healing properties. It is known to target or modulate different cancer-related signaling pathways. Curcumin inhibits phosphorylation of NF-κB, impeding its translocation to the nucleus, thus preventing the transcription of oncogenes. Curcumin promotes apoptosis by downregulating AP-1, an anti-apoptotic protein (Shanmugam et al., 2015). Curcumin can also cause cell cycle arrest by regulation of the cell cycle inhibitors (Dasiram et al., 2017). It is known to inhibit JAK2/STAT3, PI3K, AKT, and MAPK signaling pathways preventing uncontrollable division of cells in several tumors (Mouhid et al., 2017; Wu et al., 2015; Schwertheim et al., 2017). Curcumin, either alone or with some other drugs is already under clinical trials for breast, prostate, cervical, and uterine cancers (Giordano and Tommonaro, 2019).

6.2.2 VINCRISTINE AND VINBLASTINE

Vincristine is an alkaloid derived from the leaves of the flowering plant, Madagascar periwinkle (*Catharanthus roseus*). Vinblastine is the reduced form of vincristine. Vincristine is used in the treatment of glioma, lymphoma, sarcoma, and neuroblastoma, whereas vinblastine is used in the treatment of breast and lung cancers, lymphosarcoma, neuroblastoma, choriocarcinoma, lymphocytic leukemia, and Hodgkin's lymphoma (Rai et al., 2014). Both of these *Catharanthus* alkaloids act as mitotic blockers, arresting the cells at metaphase. They bind to the β subunit of tubulin dimers, aggregating them and leading to the depolymerization of microtubules. This results in the destruction of the spindle fibers, arresting mitosis and preventing the cancer cells from actively dividing (Avendano and Menéndez, 2015; Wang et al., 2016). Food and Drug Administration (FDA) approved the use of vincristine (Marqibo) as a drug against acute lymphoblastic leukemia in 2012 (New Drug Application: 202497). Two semisynthetic derivatives of vinblastine, vindesine, and vinorelbine are known to be effective against different types of cancers. Vinorelbine is already approved by FDA for treating patients with lung cancer in the United States (Gregory and Smith, 2000).

6.2.3 RESVERATROL

Resveratrol (3,5,4′-trihydroxy-trans-stilbene), a nonflavonoid polyphenol, is a phytoalexin obtained from the roots of white hellebore (*Veratrum grandiflorum*). It is found in almost 70 species including grapes, peanuts, pines, and berries and is mainly produced in response to infection, radiation, or mechanical injury (Cucciolla et al., 2007). It is known to inhibit all the stages of cancer (initiation, promotion, and progression) (Varoni et al., 2016; Pezzuto, 2008). Resveratrol targets the components of several signaling pathways like EGFR, mTOR/AKT, JAK/STAT, PI3-kinase, p53, and Nrf2 signaling pathways. It upregulates the expression of pro-apoptotic proteins, induces the formation of ROS, and induces apoptosis and autophagy in cancer cells (Li et al., 2018). Resveratrol is known to inactivate NF-κB induced in the cancer cells which become chemotherapy-resistant in its presence, thus allowing chemotherapeutic agents to work properly at the target sites (Brisdelli et al., 2009; Shukla and Singh, 2011). It is known to have potential antitumor role against human cervical carcinoma, pancreatic cancer, breast cancer, skin cancer, prostate cancer, colorectal cancer, and lung cancer (Ko et al., 2017).

6.2.4 CYCLOPAMINE

Cyclopamine, a steroidal alkaloid obtained from corn lilies (*Veratrum californicum*), was first identified during the 1960s after an outbreak of cyclopia in lambs (Golden, 2009). Cyclopamine has been found to be the first inhibitor of Hedgehog signaling, dysregulation of which is responsible for different types of cancers like lung cancer, prostate cancer, pancreatic cancer, ovarian cancer, gastrointestinal cancer, and basal cell carcinoma (Karhadkar et al., 2004; Berman et al., 2003; Watkins et al., 2003; Jones et al., 2008; Bhattacharya et al., 2008; Stecca et al., 2007). Cyclopamine binds and targets smoothened, a G-protein-coupled receptor, the positive regulator of the Hedgehog-signaling pathway (Chen et al., 2002).

6.2.5 GLUCORAPHANIN

Glucoraphanin is a methionine-derived glucosinolate found in various *Brassica* species like *Brassica juncea*, *Brassica rapa*, and *Brassica oleracea*. The hydrolytic product of glucoraphanin, sulforaphane (SFN), is known to be a potent anticancerous metabolite and is known to modulate the development of several types of human cancers like gastric cancer, breast cancer, prostate cancer, colon cancer, and cervical cancer (Fahey et al., 2012; Clarke et al., 2011; Yanaka et al., 2009; Shapiro et al., 2001). SFN targets molecules involved in different cellular processes like differentiation, proliferation, cell cycle, and apoptosis. Treatment of prostate and colon cancer cells with SFN reduced the viability and induced G2/M cell cycle arrest (Cho et al., 2005; Jakubíková et al., 2005). SFN treatment of prostate and colon cancer cells also showed a decrease in the activity of NF-κB (Choi et al., 2007). SFN also inhibits angiogenesis by inhibiting the transcription factors, HIF-1α, and c-Myc which inhibits VEGF and MMP-9, reducing the metastatic potential (Bertl et al., 2006).

6.2.6 PACLITAXEL

Paclitaxel, sold under the brand name Taxol®, is a diterpenoid isolated from the bark of Pacific Yew trees (*Taxus brevifolia*) (Weaver, 2014). It is effective against a variety of cancers like ovarian cancer, breast cancer, neck cancer, bladder cancer, gastric cancer, and lung cancer (Bernabeu et al., 2017). It prevents the dynamic disassembly of microtubules by targeting β-tubulin, thereby preventing mitosis. It mainly kills the cancer cells by inducing mitotic arrest via activating the spindle assembly checkpoint (Weaver, 2014). It is also known to kill cancer cells at clinically relevant concentrations by inducing multipolar divisions which result due to the formation of abnormal spindle fibers segregating the chromosomes in different directions (Zasadil et al., 2014). It has been approved as a first-line drug against cancer by FDA (Fauzee, 2011).

6.2.7 INGENOL MEBUTATE

Ingenol mebutate is a biologically active macrocyclic diterpenoid compound, obtained from the milky latex of milkweed plant (*Euphorbia peplus*) (Rizk et al., 1985). It can also be isolated from other *Euphorbia* species like *Euphorbia helioscopia, Euphorbia myrsinites, Euphorbia paralias, Euphorbia palustris*, and *Euphorbia millii* (Butler et al., 2014; Béres et al., 2018). It is effective against skin cancers and is known to promote melanoma cell death by robust release of calcium from endoplasmic reticulum and mitochondria. It also exhibits its antitumor activity by increasing cytotoxic CD8+ cells and TNF-α related TRAIL ligand, thus inducing apoptosis (Le et al., 2009; Gillespie et al., 2004). It is known to have dual mode of actions where it causes necrosis as well as antibody-dependent cytotoxicity via neutrophils (Rosen et al., 2012). Ingenol mebutate participates in the signaling process via the PKC/MEK/ERK pathway in keratinocytes and induces interleukin decoy receptors, IL1R2 and IL13RA2 (Freiberger et al., 2015). In 2012, both EMA and FDA approved a gel formulation of ingenol mebutate for the treatment of actinic keratosis which if untreated can lead to squamous cell carcinoma (Doan et al., 2012; Tzogani et al., 2014).

6.2.8 BETULINIC ACID

Betulinic acid is a triterpenoid compound, obtained principally from the bark of white-barked birch trees (*Betula pubescens*) (Alakurtti et al., 2006). Betulinic acid is known to induce its anticancer effect by triggering the intrinsic pathway of apoptosis in cancer cells. It induces the generation of ROS, leading to the permeabilization of the outer mitochondrial membrane (Wick et al., 1999). Betulinic acid is also reported to modulate the activity of NF-κB in different cancer cell lines (Kasperczyk et al., 2005). Its anticancer activity has been reported against head and neck, neuroblastoma, breast, colon, lung, prostate, stomach, ovarian, pancreatic, bladder, hepatocellular, leukemia, and melanoma cancer cells (Thurnher et al., 2003; Schmidt et al., 1997; Ali et al., 2017; Fulda, 2008). Between 2006 and 2013, betulinic acid was in phase I/II clinical trial for the treatment of dysplastic melanocytic nevus, but due to lack of funds, such research was suspended (clinical trials database).

6.2.9 *CAMPTOTHECIN*

Camptothecin (CPT) is a monoterpenoid alkaloid obtained principally from the bark and stems of Chinese happy tree (*Camptotheca acuminata*). CPT binds to the topoisomerase I–DNA complex, preventing DNA from religating and creating a double-stranded break which causes apoptosis in the cancer cells (Hsiang et al., 1985). FDA approved two derivatives of CPT, topothecan, and irinothecan for the treatment of ovarian, cervical, small lung, and colorectal cancers in 1994 (Venditto and Simanek, 2010).

6.3 GENETIC ENGINEERING OF PLANTS WITH ENHANCED SECONDARY METABOLITES HAVING ANTICANCEROUS PROPERTIES

Secondary metabolites produced by plants are not enough to meet the needs of the pharmaceutical industries. Extraction of small amounts of metabolites from the plants is an expensive process. Researchers are trying to find out different strategies to increase the expression of these metabolites in order to overcome the needs. Due to the advancement of genetic engineering technologies, it is possible to produce them in higher amounts by regulation of their synthesis pathways. Overexpression of genes encoding enzymes and transcription factors can lead to the increased production of these secondary metabolites. The advantages of producing transgenic plants over using microorganisms are proper post-translational modifications, increase in disease and insect resistance, increase in yield and quality, easiness in growing, and reduced costs.

A current strategy to increase the production of secondary metabolites is genetic engineering to produce transgenic plants expressing the desired metabolite in higher amounts. This is done either by cloning the key genes of interest from a particular metabolic pathway or by knockdown of genes to redirect the pathway to desired metabolites. Stable plant lines are created mostly through *Agrobacterium*-mediated gene transformation. *Agrobacterium* is a microbe naturally occurring in soil and causes crown gall disease in plants. The disease-causing gene is replaced by the gene of interest and the desired plant species is infected by *Agrobacterium*. It stably delivers the gene of interest which gets integrated into the genetic material of the plant, thus creating a new transgenic line. DNA is also

TABLE 6.1 Sources and Functions of Some Anticancerous Drugs.

Compound	Source	Mechanism of action	Effective against
Curcumin	Rhizome of *Curcuma longa*	Induces apoptosis, inhibits activation of NF-κB, arrests cell cycle	Breast, prostate, cervical, and uterine cancers
Vincristine	Leaves of *Catharanthus roseus*	Interacts with tubulin, inhibits mitosis	Glioma, lymphoma, sarcoma, neuroblastoma, and nephroblastoma
Vinblastine	Leaves of *Catharanthus roseus*	Inhibits mitosis	Breast, lung cancer, lymphosarcoma, neuroblastoma, choriocarcinoma, lymphocytic leukemia, and Hodgkin's lymphoma
Resveratrol	Roots of *Veratrum grandiflorum*	Induces apoptosis, inhibits NF-κB	Cervical carcinoma, pancreatic, breast, skin, prostate, colorectal, and lung cancers
Cyclopamine	*Veratrum californicum*	Inhibits Hedgehog signaling	Lung, prostate, pancreatic, ovarian, gastrointestinal, and basal cell carcinoma
Glucoraphanin	*Brassica* sp.	Induces apoptosis, arrest cell cycle, inhibits angiogenesis	Gastric, breast, prostate, colon, and cervical cancers
Paclitaxel	Bark of *Taxus brevifolia*	Inhibits mitosis	Ovarian, breast, neck, bladder, gastric, and lung cancers
Ingenol mebutate	Latex of *Euphorbia peplus*	Induces apoptosis, necrosis, and antibody-dependent cellular cytotoxic (ADCC)	Squamous cell carcinoma
Betulinic acid	Bark of *Betula pubescens*	Induces apoptosis, modulate activity of NF-κB	Head and neck, neuroblastoma, breast, colon, lung, prostate, stomach, ovarian, pancreatic, bladder, hepatocellular, leukemia, and melanoma cancer
Camptothecin	Bark and stems of *Camptotheca acuminata*	Binds to topoisomerase I–DNA complex, induces apoptosis	Ovarian, cervical, small lung, and colorectal cancers

delivered physically by microprojectile bombardment method where the plant cells are shot with DNA adhered to gold particles (Klein et al., 1987). Electroporation is another method by which protoplasts are transformed with DNA of interest followed by generation of an electrical impulse which allows the DNA to enter into the cells by destabilizing the cell membrane. DNA can also be directly injected into the nucleus of the cells by the microinjection technique. However, there are certain limitations for each of these techniques and needs to be assessed properly before creating a transgenic plant (Masters, 2004).

6.3.1 PRODUCTION OF CURCUMIN

Low abundance of curcumin in plants makes it quite challenging for using it as a therapeutic agent. To increase the bioavailability of curcumin, a lot of strategies are being applied. Curcumin synthases are a group of enzymes which convert L-phenylalanine to curcuminoids. The content of curcumin depends on the expression of four enzymes: diketide-CoA synthase (DCS) and three curcumin synthases (CURS1, CURS2, and CURS3) (Li et al., 2015). Curcumin biosynthesis genes, *DCS* and *CURS2*, were introduced in *Arabidopsis thaliana* for enhancing the lignocellulosic biomass processing. The genes were placed under the control of promoter pCesA4 which restricts the expression of the genes to the lignifying walls (Oyarce et al., 2019). Three genes, *DCS* and *CURS3* from *C. amada* and glucosyl-transferase gene (CaUGT2) from *C. roseus* under the CaMV 35S promoter, were introduced through *Agrobacterium*-mediated transformation which resulted in the production of curcumin and its glucosides in hairy root cultures of *Atropa belladonna.* The clone expressing *DCS/CURS3* genes yielded about 180.62 ± 4.7 µg/g dry weight (DW) of curcumin, while the clones coexpressing *DCS* and *CURS3*, and that expressing *CaUGT2* genes yielded 67.89 ± 2.56 µg/g DW of curcumin and 32.63 ± 2.27 µg/g DW of curcumin, respectively (Singh et al., 2021).

6.3.2 PRODUCTION OF VINBLASTINE AND VINCRISTINE

Vinblastine is produced in low amounts by *C. roseus* plants. Vinblastine is produced via the MEP and shikimate pathway and is mainly stored in the vacuoles (Roytrakul and Verpoorte, 2007). Vinblastine is produced by the decarboxylation of tryptophan to tryptamine via tryptophan decarboxylase (Hashimoto and Yamada, 1994). ORCA3, a key transcription factor in the jasmonic acid-induced alkaloid pathway, is responsible for regulating few genes like *D4H*, *DXS*, *TDC*, *AS*, and *STR* in the alkaloid synthesis pathway (van der Fits and Memelink, 2000). G10H, a cytochrome P450 monooxygenase enzyme, is involved in conversion of geraniol to 10-hydroxygeraniol which is an initial step in the monoterpenoid synthesis pathway (Collu et al., 2001). Overexpression of ORCA3 and G10H in *C. roseus* increased the expression of vinblastine by 10.2-fold (Pan et al., 2012). Overexpression of two genes from *C. roseus tryptophan decarboxylase* (*CrTDC*), and *strictosidine synthase* (*CrSTR*) of alkaloid biosynthetic pathway was done in shoot and callus cultures of *C. roseus*. The genes were driven by CaMV35S promoter and were transformed using *Agrobacterium tumefaciens* which resulted in the increase of vinblastine in the transformed leaves, but not in callus cultures (Sharma et al., 2018).

Deacetylvindoline 4-*O*-acetyltransferase (*Cr*DAT) catalyzes the conversion of deacetylvindoline to vindoline, an important precursor of both vinblastine and vincristine. *Agrobacterium*-mediated transformation of *C. roseus* with *Cr*DAT increased the vincristine concentration by 1.63–2.48 fold (Pham et al., 2019).

6.3.3 PRODUCTION OF RESVERATROL

Genetic engineering of plants with stilbene synthase (STS), a polyketide synthase enzyme involved in the synthesis of phytoalexins via the phenylalanine or polymalonate pathway, is one of the current strategies used for the production of resveratrol. In 1990, *Nicotiana tabacum* was transformed with *STS* gene from *Arachis hypogea* for the production of *trans*-resveratrol (Hain et al., 1990). In 1993, transformation of *N. tabacum* with two grapevine *STS* genes (*Vst1 and Vst2*) yielded up to 400 μg/g fresh weight of *trans*-resveratrol (Hain et al., 1993). Following this, various crops including *Triticum aestivum, Vitis vinifera, Malus domestica, Lycopersicon esculentum, Rehmannia glutinosa, Lactuca sativa, Carica papaya, Brassica napus*, and *Humulus lupulus* were transformed using the *STS* gene under the control of different promoters (constitutive CaMV35S promoter, maize ubiquitin promoter, stress-responsive promoter Vst1, fungus inducible promoter *ms*PR10.1, seed-specific promoter p-nap) for the production of resveratrol (Fettig and Hess, 1999; Coutos-Thévenot et al., 2001; Szankowski et al., 2003; Giovinazzo et al., 2005; Lim et al., 2005; Liu et al., 2006; Zhu et al., 2004; Hüsken et al., 2005; Schwekendiek et al., 2007). For the improved expression of resveratrol, the use of enhancer elements like 35S enhancer element along with pVst1 promoter or the use of fused promoters like pPR10.1 promoter and the pVst1 promoter leads to an increased level of resveratrol (Serazetdinova et al., 2005; Leckband and Lörz, 1998). Transformation of *Vitis amurensis* callus culture with *rolB* oncogene of *Agrobacterium rhizogenes*, encoding a tyrosine phosphatase enzyme, increased the production of resveratrol by 100 times (Kiselev et al., 2007). Transformation of callus cultures of *V. amurensis* with *rolC* oncogene of *A. rhizogenes* increased the expression of phenylalanine ammonia-lyase and STS enzymes which increased resveratrol content by 3.7 and 11.9 times, respectively (Dubrovina et al., 2010).

6.3.4 PRODUCTION OF CYCLOPAMINE

V. californicum, the plant producing cyclopamine, is a slow-growing plant and is not suitable for cultivation. *Camelina sativa*, an oilseed crop, was used for the production of verazine, the precursor of cyclopamine. Four enzymes, namely, CYP90B27, CYP94N1, CYP90G1, and GABAT1 along with GAD2 enzyme from *Arabidopsis thaliana,* were cloned and transformed into *C. sativa* (Augustin et al., 2015; Turano and Fang, 1998). GAD2 enzyme was included to increase the concentration of GABA which is a cosubstrate used by GABAT1 enzyme. Three vectors were constructed: (1) first vector contained genes encoding CYP90B27 and CYP94N1 enzymes; (2) second vector contained genes encoding CYP90G1, GABAT1, and GAD2 enzymes; and (3) third vector contained genes encoding all the five enzymes. Cloning and transforming these four genes from *V. californicum* and GAD2 into *C. sativa* followed by analysis showed production of 41 ± 7 pg verazine/mg seed, 67 ± 13 pg verazine/mg seed, and 54 ± 6 pg verazine/mg in seeds in the first, second, and third transgenic lines, respectively (Augustin et al., 2017).

6.3.5 PRODUCTION OF GLUCORAPHANIN

Yield of glucoraphanin is low in most of the cultivable *Brassica* species due to the conversion of glucoraphanin to gluconapin by AOP2

(2-oxoglutarate-dependent dioxygenases) enzyme which is again converted to progoitrin by GSL–OH enzymes. These two metabolites are produced in high amounts in the *Brassica* species and are highly antinutritional in nature (Augustine et al., 2013). Thus, to reduce the accumulation of gluconapin and progoitrin, RNAi method was used to knock down *GSL-ALK* gene in *B. juncea*. They used *Agrobacterium*-mediated gene transformation method producing 29 T0 transgenic lines. After analysis, they found a reduction in the antinutritional glucosinolates and increased glucoraphanin content (43.11 μmol/seed) (Augustine and Bisht, 2015). RNAi method was also used to downregulate the expression of *GSK-ALK* genes in *B. napus* which reduced the progoitrin content by 65% and increased the glucoraphanin content (42.6 μmol/g seed) (Liu et al., 2012). In another study, the functional *AOP2* alleles (AOP2.2 and AOP2.3) were converted to their nonfunctional alleles through marker-assisted backcrossing in *B. rapa* which increased glucoraphanin content by 18 times, compared to the parent plant (Liu et al., 2017).

6.3.6 *PRODUCTION OF TAXOL*

Production of taxol is a challenging process due to the low content, high cost, and scarcity of *Taxus* trees (Tabata, 2004). In 1994, *T. brevifolia* and *T. baccata* were transformed using *Agrobacterium tumefaciens* (Han et al., 1994). Hairy root cultures of *Taxus* × *media* var. Hicksii, fed with precursors L-phenylalanine and *p*-amino benzoic acid in combination with methyl jasmonate, produced 221.8 μg/L of taxol (Syklowska-Baranek et al., 2009). In 2005, transgenic *T. mairei* plants were generated overexpressing genes encoding 10-deacetylbaccatin III-10-*O*-acetyltransferase (DBAT) and taxadiene synthase (TXS), the two most important enzymes in taxol biosynthesis pathway (Ho et al., 2005). Due to inefficient transformation of *Taxus* species, heterologous species were used for the production of taxol. Constitutive overexpression of *TXS* was performed in *A. thaliana* plants for the production of taxadiene, the first precursor of taxol. Using an inducible system like two-component glucocorticoid system, increased production of taxadiene by 30-fold was observed, as compared to the constitutively expressing transgenic lines (Besumbes et al., 2004). In another study, the redirection of geranyl geranyl diphosphate (GGDP) pool toward taxadiene production also resulted in the production of taxadiene in high amounts (160 mg/kg dried fruit) in transgenic tomato lines (Kovacs et al., 2007). Genetic transformation of cultured ginseng roots, *Nicotiana benthamiana* and *Artemisia annua* L. plant with *TXS* gene, also resulted in the production of high amounts of taxadiene (Cha et al., 2012; Hasan et al., 2014; Li et al., 2015). Another strategy of producing taxol was by overexpressing a gene in the ABA biosynthesis pathway in transgenic *T. chinensis* cells. Constitutive overexpression of 9-cis-epoxycarotenoid dioxygenase-1 (NCED1), the rate-limiting enzyme in ABA biosynthetic pathway, was performed in *T. chinensis* cell lines. Overexpression of *TcNCED1* increased the expression of the enzymes, TXS, DBAT, and 3-amino-3-phenylpropanoyltransferase, which increased the expression of taxol by 2.7-fold (Li et al., 2012).

6.3.7 PRODUCTION OF INGENOL MEBUTATE

Direct extraction from the *E. peplus* plants yielded only about 1.1 mg/kg of ingenol mebutate (Hohmann et al., 2000). To increase the production of an intermediate, jolkinolC, of ingenol mebutate, stable transformation of *N. benthamiana* was performed through *Agrobacterium*-mediated gene transfer where upregulation of the key genes of MEP pathway from *A. thaliana* plants led to increase in the production of diterpenoid precursor, geranylgeranyl pyrophosphate (GGPP). Coexpression of casbene synthase and two cytochrome P450 enzymes JcCYP726A20 and JcCYP71D495 from *Jatropha curcas* increased the production of casbene from GGPP, which was then converted to jolkinolC. From stable homozygous transformants, the function of alkenal reductase 3 enzyme was revealed which reduced the double bond at C12–C13 position of jolkinolC that can play an important role in the synthesis of ingenol mebutate (Forestier et al., 2021).

6.3.8 PRODUCTION OF BETULINIC ACID

Overexpression of *squalene synthase 1* (*PgSS1*) gene, involved in terpenoid biosynthesis, from *Panax ginseng* was performed in the hairy roots of transgenic *Senna obtusifolia*. Another line was constructed without the gene construct containing the *PgSS1* gene. Betulinic acid was found in a higher amount in the former (38.125 mg/g DW) compared to the latter (4.213 mg/g DW) (Kowalczyk et al., 2021).

6.3.9 PRODUCTION OF CAMPTOTHECIN

Due to high market value, a number of attempts have been made for the extensive production of CPT. The hairy roots of *C. acuminata* were transformed with *ORCA3* gene, a jasmonate-responsive transcription factor containing APETALA-2 domain isolated from *C. roseus.* In several other studies, ORCA3 overexpression enhanced the expression of the terpene biosynthetic genes. Constitutive expression of *ORCA3* gene using CaMV35S promoter increased the CPT content by 1.5-fold compared to the control (1.12 mg/g DW) (Ni et al., 2011). Strictosidine, the precursor of CPT, derived from the condensation of indoletryptamine and secologanin, is produced by the enzyme, strictosidine synthase (STR) (Lu et al., 2009). Geraniol 10-hydroxylase (G10H), a cytochrome P450 enzyme, catalyzes the committed step involved in the biosynthesis of secologanin (Collu et al., 2002). Introduction of both of these genes was done separately as well as together into the hairy roots of *Ophiorrhiza pumila.* The CPT content in two STR transgenic lines (S lines) was increased (average 1.04 mg/g DW) but decreased in two other S lines, compared to the wild type. The CPT content in all five G10H transgenic lines (G lines) were increased (average 1.27 mg/g) compared to the wild type. The CPT content in the transgenic lines (SG) overexpressing both the enzymes showed higher average CPT content (1.64 mg/g DW) than the S and G lines (Cui et al., 2015). Cell culture methods like hairy roots culture of *O. pumila* transformed with *A. rhizogenes* strain 15,834 which yielded CPT by 16-fold, are also a feasible method for the production of CPT (Saito et al., 2001).

6.4 CONCLUSION

Treatment of a complex disease like cancer is becoming one of the major concerns throughout the world. The drugs available for cancer therapy have several limitations and are often toxic to human health. Naturally derived drugs act as an alternative treatment for cancer. Secondary metabolites from plants act as a suitable choice due to their low toxicity and cost, many of which are already in clinical trials. However, the amounts of metabolites produced by plants are not enough to meet the needs of the industries. Nowadays, metabolic engineering of plants as well as microbes to enhance the production of the metabolites is a method of choice. It is now possible to engineer the whole pathway into plants to enhance the production of a particular metabolite. Optimization of pathways needs to be done to maximize the output of the desired product by overexpression of the key genes or by increasing the metabolic flux. Increased production of these metabolites results in their increased exploitation which ultimately causes risk to the biodiversity. However, there are certain limitations of creating transgenic plants and finding of new sustainable methods for the production of anticancerous secondary metabolites is needed.

ACKNOWLEDGMENTS

Financial assistance from the Science and Engineering Research Board, Government of India through the grant [EMR/2016/004799] and the Department of Higher Education, Science and Technology and Biotechnology, Government of West Bengal, through the grant [264(Sanc.)/ST/P/S&T/1G-80/2017] to Prof. Aryadeep Roychoudhury is gratefully acknowledged.

KEYWORDS

- **cancer**
- **genetic engineering**
- **secondary metabolites**
- **terpenoids**

REFERENCES

Alakurtti, S.; Mäkelä, T.; Koskimies, S.; Yli-Kauhaluoma, J. Pharmacological Properties of the Ubiquitous Natural Product Betulin. *Eur. J. Pharm. Sci.* **2006,** *29* (1), 1–13.

Ali, M. T. M.; Zahari, H.; Aliasak, A.; Lim, S. M.; Ramasamy, K.; Macabeoacabeo, A. P. G. Synthesis, Characterization and Cytotoxic Activity of Betulinic Acid and Sec-betulinic Acid Derivatives Against Human Colorectal Carcinoma. *Orient. J. Chem.* **2017,** *33,* 242–248.

Augustin, M. M.; Ruzicka, D. R.; Shukla, A. K., Augustin, J. M.; Starks, C. M.; O'Neil-Johnson, M.; McKain, M. R.; Evans, B. S.; Barrett, M. D.; Smithson, A.; Wong, G.

K. S.; Deyholos, M. K.; Edger, P. P; Pires, J. C.; Leebens-Mack, J. H.; Mann, D. A.; Kutchan, T. M. Elucidating Steroid Alkaloid Biosynthesis in *Veratrum californicum*: Production of Verazine in Sf9 Cells. *Plant J.* **2015,** *82* (6), 991–1003.

Augustin, M. M.; Shukla, A. K.; Starks, C. M.; O'Neil-Johnson, M.; Han, L.; Holland, C. K.; Kutchan, T. M. Biosynthesis of Veratrum Californicum Specialty Chemicals in *Camelina sativa* Seed. *Plant Biotechnol. Rep.* **2017,** *11* (1), 29–41.

Augustine, R.; Bisht, N. C. Biofortification of Oilseed *Brassica juncea* With the Anti-Cancer Compound Glucoraphanin by Suppressing *GSL-ALK* Gene Family. *Sci. Rep.* **2015,** *5* (1), 1–12.

Augustine, R.; Mukhopadhyay, A.; Bisht, N. C. Targeted Silencing of BjMYB28 Transcription Factor Gene Directs Development of Low Glucosinolate Lines in Oilseed *Brassica juncea*. *Plant Biotechnol. J.* **2013,** *11* (7), 855–866.

Avendano, C.; Menéndez, J. C. Anticancer Drugs Targeting Tubulin and Microtubules. Medicinal Chemistry of Anticancer Drugs; Elsevier: Boulevard, 2015; 359–387.

Bauer, A. Pharma Crops, State of Field Trials Worldwide. (accessed Oct 20, 2014).

Béres, T.; Dragull, K.; Pospíšil, J.; Tarkowská, D.; Dančák, M.; Bíba, O.; Tarkowski, P.; Doležal, K.; Strnad, M. Quantitative Analysis of Ingenol in *Euphorbia* Species Via Validated Isotope Dilution Ultra-high Performance Liquid Chromatography Tandem Mass Spectrometry. Phytochem. Anal. **2018,** *29* (1), 23–29.

Berman, D. M.; Karhadkar, S. S.; Maitra, A.; De Oca, R. M.; Gerstenblith, M. R.; Briggs, K.; Parker, A. R.; Shimada, Y.; Eshleman, J. R.; Watkins, D. N.; Beachy, P. A. Widespread Requirement for Hedgehog Ligand Stimulation in Growth of Digestive Tract Tumours. *Nature* **2003,** *425* (6960), 846–851.

Bernabeu, E.; Cagel, M.; Lagomarsino, E.; Moretton, M.; Chiappetta, D. A. Paclitaxel: What has Been Done and the Challenges Remain Ahead. *Int. J. Pharm.* **2017,** *526* (1–2), 474–495.

Bertl, E.; Bartsch, H.; Gerhäuser, C. Inhibition of Angiogenesis and Endothelial Cell Functions are Novel Sulforaphane-Mediated Mechanisms in Chemoprevention. *Mol. Cancer Ther.* **2006,** *5* (3), 575–585.

Besumbes, Ó.; Sauret-Güeto, S.; Phillips, M. A.; Imperial, S.; Rodríguez-Concepción, M.; Boronat, A. Metabolic Engineering of Isoprenoid Biosynthesis in *Arabidopsis* for the Production of Taxadiene, the First Committed Precursor of Taxol. *Biotechnol. Bioeng.* **2004,** *88* (2), 168–175.

Bhattacharya, R.; Kwon, J.; Ali, B.; Wang, E.; Patra, S.; Shridhar, V.; Mukherjee, P. Role of Hedgehog Signaling in Ovarian Cancer. *Clin. Cancer Res.* **2008,** *14* (23), 7659–7666.

Bray, F.; Laversanne, M.; Weiderpass, E.; Soerjomataram, I. The Ever-Increasing Importance of Cancer as a Leading Cause of Premature Death Worldwide. *Cancer* **2021.** 10.1002/cncr.33587.

Brisdelli, F.; D'Andrea, G.; Bozzi, A. Resveratrol: A Natural Polyphenol With Multiple Chemopreventive Properties. *Curr. Drug Metab.* **2009,** *10* (6), 530–546.

Butler, M. S.; Robertson, A. A.; Cooper, M. A. Natural Product and Natural Product Derived Drugs in Clinical Trials. *Nat. Prod. Rep.* **2014,** *31* (11), 1612–1661.

Cha, M.; Shim, S. H.; Kim, S. H.; Kim, O. T.; Lee, S. W.; Kwon, S. Y.; Baek, K. H. Production of Taxadiene From Cultured Ginseng Roots Transformed With Taxadiene Synthase Gene. *BMB Rep.* **2012,** *45* (10), 589–594.

Chen, J. K.; Taipale, J.; Cooper, M. K.; Beachy, P. A. Inhibition of Hedgehog Signaling by Direct Binding of Cyclopamine to Smoothened. *Genes Dev,* **2002,** *16* (21), 2743–2748.

Cho, S. D.; Li, G.; Hu, H.; Jiang, C.; Kang, K. S.; Lee, Y. S.; Kim, S. H.; Lu, J. Involvement of c-Jun N-Terminal Kinase in G2/M Arrest and Caspase-Mediated Apoptosis Induced by Sulforaphane in DU145 Prostate Cancer Cells. *Nutr. Cancer* 2005, *52* (2), 213–224.

Choi, S.; Lew, K. L.; Xiao, H.; Herman-Antosiewicz, A.; Xiao, D.; Brown, C. K.; Singh, S. V. D, L-Sulforaphane-Induced Cell Death in Human Prostate Cancer Cells is Regulated by Inhibitor of Apoptosis Family Proteins and Apaf-1. *Carcinogenesis* **2007,** *28* (1), 151–162.

Clarke, J. D.; Hsu, A.; Yu, Z.; Dashwood, R. H.; Ho, E. Differential Effects of Sulforaphane on Histone Deacetylases, Cell Cycle Arrest and Apoptosis in Normal Prostate Cells Versus Hyperplastic and Cancerous Prostate Cells. *Mol. Nutr. Food Res.* **2011,** *55* (7), 999–1009.

Collu, G.; Garcia, A. A.; van der Heijden, R.; Verpoorte, R. Activity of the Cytochrome P450 Enzyme Geraniol 10-Hydroxylase and Alkaloid Production in Plant Cell Cultures. *Plant Sci.* **2002,** *162* (1), 165–172.

Collu, G.; Unver, N.; Peltenburg-Looman, A. M.; van der Heijden, R.; Verpoorte, R.; Memelink, J. Geraniol 10-Hydroxylase1, a Cytochrome P450 Enzyme Involved in Terpenoid Indole Alkaloid Biosynthesis. *FEBS Lett.* **2001,** *508* (2), 215–220.

Coutos-Thévenot, P.; Poinssot, B.; Bonomelli, A.; Yean, H.; Breda, C.; Buffard, D.; Esnault, R.; Hain, R.; Boulay, M. In Vitro Tolerance to *Botrytis cinerea* of Grapevine 41B Rootstock in Transgenic Plants Expressing the Stilbene Synthase *Vst 1* Gene Under the Control of a Pathogen-Inducible PR 10 Promoter. *J. Exp. Bot.* **2001,** *52* (358), 901–910.

Cucciolla, V.; Borriello, A.; Oliva, A.; Galletti, P.; Zappia, V.; Ragione, F. D. Resveratrol: From Basic Science to the Clinic. *Cell Cycle* **2007,** *6* (20), 2495–2510.

Cui, L.; Ni, X.; Ji, Q.; Teng, X.; Yang, Y.; Wu, C.; Zekria, D.; Zhang, D.; Kai, G. Co-Overexpression of Geraniol-10-Hydroxylase and Strictosidine Synthase Improves Anti-Cancer Drug Camptothecin Accumulation in *Ophiorrhiza pumila. Sci. Rep.* **2015,** *5* (1), 1–9.

Dasiram, J. D.; Ganesan, R.; Kannan, J.; Kotteeswaran, V.; Sivalingam, N. Curcumin Inhibits Growth Potential by G1 Cell Cycle Arrest and Induces Apoptosis in p53-Mutated COLO 320DM Human Colon Adenocarcinoma Cells. *Biomed. Pharmacother.* **2017,** *86,* 373–380.

Delgoda, R.; Murray, J. E. Evolutionary Perspectives on the Role of Plant Secondary Metabolites. *Pharmacognosy* **2017,** 93–100.

Doan, H. Q.; Gulati, N.; Levis, W. R. Ingenol Mebutate: Potential for Further Development of Cancer Immunotherapy. *J. Drugs Dermatol.* **2012,** *11* (10), 1156.

Dubrovina, A. S.; Manyakhin, A. Y.; Zhuravlev, Y. N.; Kiselev, K. V. Resveratrol Content and Expression of Phenylalanine Ammonia-Lyase and Silbene Synthase Genes in rolC Transgenic Cell Cultures of *Vitis amurensis*. *Appl. Microbiol. Biotechnol.* **2010,** *88* (3), 727–736.

Fahey, J. W.; Wehage, S. L.; Holtzclaw, W. D.; Kensler, T. W.; Egner, P. A.; Shapiro, T. A.; Talalay, P. Protection of Humans by Plant Glucosinolates: Efficiency of Conversion of Glucosinolates to Isothiocyanates by the Gastrointestinal Microflora. *Cancer Prev. Res.* **2012,** *5* (4), 603–611.

Fauzee, N. J. S. Taxanes: Promising Anti-Cancer Drugs. *Asian Pac. J. Cancer Prev.* **2011,** *12,* 837–851.

Fettig, S.; Hess, D. Expression of a Chimeric Stilbene Synthase Gene in Transgenic Wheat Lines. *Transgenic Res.* **1999,** *8,* 179–189.

Forestier, E. C. F.; Czechowski, T.; Cording, A. C.; Gilday, A. D.; King, A. J.; Brown, G. D.; Graham, I. A. Developing a *Nicotiana benthamiana* Transgenic Platform for High-Value Diterpene Production and Candidate Gene Evaluation. *Plant Biotechnol. J.* **2021**.

Freiberger, S. N.; Cheng, P. F.; Iotzova-Weiss, G.; Neu, J.; Liu, Q.; Dziunycz, P.; Zibert, J. R.; Dummer, R.; Skak, K.; Levesque, M. P.; Hofbauer, G. F. Ingenol Mebutate Signals via PKC/MEK/ERK in Keratinocytes and Induces Interleukin Decoy Receptors IL1R2 and IL13RA2. *Mol. Cancer Ther.* **2015,** *14* (9), 2132–2142.

Fulda, S. Betulinic Acid for Cancer Treatment and Prevention. *Int. J. Mol. Sci.* **2008,** *9* (6), 1096–1107.

Ganz, P. R.; Dudani, A. K.; Tackaberry, E. S.; Sardana, R.; Sauder, C.; Cheng, X.; Altosaar, I. Expression of Human Blood Proteins in Transgenic Plants: The Cytokine GM-CSF as a Model Protein. In *Transgenic Plants: A Production System for Industrial and Pharmaceutical Proteins,* 1996; pp 281–297.

Gillespie, S. K.; Zhang, X. D.; Hersey, P. Ingenol 3-Angelate Induces Dual Modes of Cell Death and Differentially Regulates Tumor Necrosis Factor–Related Apoptosis-Inducing Ligand–Induced Apoptosis in Melanoma Cells. *Mol. Cancer Ther.* **2004,** *3* (12), 1651–1658.

Giordano, A.; Tommonaro, G. Curcumin and Cancer. *Nutrients* **2019,** *11* (10), 2376.

Giovinazzo, G.; D'Amico, L.; Paradisio, A.; Bollini, R.; Sparvoli, F.; DeGara, L. Antioxidant Metabolite Profiles in Tomato Fruit Constitutively Expressing the Grapevine Stilbene Synthase Gene. *Plant Biotechnol. J.* **2005,** *3* (1), 57–69.

Golden, J. A. Holoprosencephaly. In *Encyclopedia of Neuroscience*; Academic Press, 2009; 1181–1187.

Greenberg, E. P.; Canale-Parola, E. Carotenoid Pigments of Facultatively Anaerobic Spirochetes. *J. Bacteriol.* **1975,** *123* (3), 1006–1012.

Gregory, R. K.; Smith, I. E. Vinorelbine–A Clinical Review. *Br. J. Cancer* **2000,** *82* (12), 1907–1913.

Guo, Z. The Modification of Natural Products for Medical Use. *Acta Pharm. Sin. B* **2017,** *7* (2), 119–136.

Hain, R.; Bieseler, B.; Kindl, H.; Schröder, G.; Stöcker, R. Expression of a Stilbene Synthase Gene in *Nicotiana tabacum* Results in Synthesis of the Phytoalexin Resveratrol. *Plant Mol. Biol.* **1990,** *15,* 325–335.

Hain, R.; Reif, H. J.; Krause, E.; Langebartels, R.; Kindl, H.; Vornam, B.; Wiese, W.; Schmelzer, E.; Schreier, P.; Stöcker, R.; Stenzel, K. Disease Resistance Results From Foreign Phytoalexin Expression in a Novel Plant. *Nature* **1993,** *361,* 153–156.

Hamill, R. L.; Higgens, C. E.; Boaz, H. E.; Gonnan, M. The Structure of Beauvericin, A New Depsipeptide Antibiotic Toxic to *Artemia salina. Tetrahedron Lett.* **1969,** 4255–4258.

Han, K. H.; Fleming, P.; Walker, K.; Loper, M.; Chilton, W. S.; Mocek, U.; Gordon, M. P.; Floss, H. G. Genetic Transformation of Mature Taxus: An Approach to Genetically Control the In Vitro Production of the Anticancer Drug, Taxol. *Plant Sci.* **1994,** *95* (2), 187–196.

Hasan, M. M.; Kim, H. S.; Jeon, J. H.; Kim, S. H.; Moon, B.; Song, J. Y.; Shim, S. H.; Baek, K. H. Metabolic Engineering of *Nicotiana benthamiana* for the Increased Production of Taxadiene. *Plant Cell Rep.* **2014,** *33* (6), 895–904.

Hashimoto, T.; Yamada, Y. Alkaloid Biogenesis: Molecular Aspects. *Ann. Rev. Plant Biol.* **1994,** *45* (1), 257–285.

Ho, C. K.; Chang, S. H.; Lung, J.; Tsai, C. J.; Chen, K. P. The Strategies to Increase Taxol Production by Using *Taxus mairei* Cells Transformed With TS and DBAT Genes. *Int. J. Appl. Sci. Eng.* **2005,** *3* (3), 179–185.

Hohmann, J.; Evanics, F.; Berta, L.; Bartók, T. Diterpenoids From *Euphorbia peplus*. *Planta Med.* **2000,** *66* (03), 291–294.

Hsiang, Y. H.; Hertzberg, R.; Hecht, S.; Liu, L. F. Camptothecin Induces Protein-Linked DNA Breaks Via Mammalian DNA Topoisomerase I. *J. Biol. Chem.* **1985,** *260* (27), 14873–14878.

Hüsken, A.; Baumert, A.; Milkowski, C.; Becker, H. C.; Strack, D.; Möllers, C. Resveratrol Glucoside (Piceid) Synthesis in Seeds of Transgenic Oilseed Rape (*Brassica napus* L.). *Theor. Appl. Genet.* **2005,** *111* (8), 1553–1562.

Jakubíková, J.; Sedlák, J.; Mithen, R.; Bao, Y. Role of PI3K/Akt and MEK/ERK Signaling Pathways in Sulforaphane-and Erucin-Induced Phase II Enzymes and MRP2 Transcription, G2/M Arrest and Cell Death in Caco-2 Cells. *Biochem. Pharmacol.* **2005,** *69* (11), 1543–1552.

Jones, S.; Zhang, X.; Parsons, D. W.; Lin, J. C. H.; Leary, R. J.; Angenendt P, Mankoo, P.; Carter, H.; Kamiyama, H.; Jimeno, A.; Hong, S. M.; Fu, B.; Lin, M. T.; Calhoun, E. S.; Kamiyama, M.; Walter, K.; Nikolskaya, T.; Nikolsky, Y.; Hartigan, J.; Smith, D. R.; Hidalgo, M.; Leach, S. D.; Klein, A. P.; Jaffee, E. M.; Goggins, M.; Maitra, A.; Iacobuzio-Donahue, C.; Eshleman, J. R.; Kern, S. E.; Hruban, R. H.; Karchin, R.; Papadopoulos, N.; Parmigiani, G.; Vogelstein, B.; Velculescu, V. E.; Kinzler, K. W. Core Signaling Pathways in Human Pancreatic Cancers Revealed by Global Genomic Analyses. *Science* **2008,** *321* (5897), 1801–1806.

Joshi, M.; Sodhi, K. S. Transgenic Plants as Sole Source Biopharmaceuticals. *Int. J. Recent Trends Sci. Technol.* **2014,** *13* (1), 97–106.

Kabera, J. N.; Semana, E.; Mussa, A. R.; He, X. Plant Secondary Metabolites: Biosynthesis, Classification, Function and Pharmacological Properties. *J. Pharm. Pharmacol.* **2014,** *2*, 377–392.

Karhadkar, S. S.; Bova, G. S.; Abdallah, N.; Dhara, S.; Gardner, D.; Maitra, A.; Isaacs, J. T.; Berman, D. M.; Beachy, P. A. Hedgehog Signalling in Prostate Regeneration, Neoplasia and Metastasis. *Nature* **2004,** *431* (7009), 707–712.

Kasperczyk, H.; La Ferla-Brühl, K.; Westhoff., M. A.; Behrend, L.; Zwacka, R. M.; Debatin, K. M.; Fulda, S. Betulinic Acid as New Activator of NF-κ B: Molecular Mechanisms and Implications for Cancer Therapy. *Oncogene* **2005,** *24* (46), 6945–6956.

Kiselev, K. V.; Dubrovina, A. S.; Veselova, M. V.; Bulgakov, V. P.; Fedoreyev, S. A.; Zhuravlev, Y. N. The rolB Gene-Induced Overproduction of Resveratrol in *Vitis amurensis* Transformed Cells. *J. Biotechnol.* **2007,** *128* (3), 681–692.

Klein, T. M.; Wolf, E. D.; Wu, R.; Sanford, J. C. High Velocity Microprojectiles for Delivering Nucleic Acids Into Living Cells. *Nature* **1987,** *327*, 70–73.

Ko, J. H.; Sethi, G.; Um, J. Y.; Shanmugam, M. K.; Arfuso, F.; Kumar, A. P.; Bishayee, A.; Ahn, K. S. The Role of Resveratrol in Cancer Therapy. *Int. J. Mol. Sci.* **2017,** *18* (12), 2589.

Kovacs, K.; Zhang, L.; Linforth, R. S.; Whittaker, B.; Hayes, C. J.; Fray, R. G. Redirection of Carotenoid Metabolism for the Efficient Production of Taxadiene [taxa-4 (5), 11 (12)-diene] in Transgenic Tomato Fruit. *Transgenic Res.* **2007,** *16* (1), 121–126.

Kowalczy, K. T.; Sitare, K. P.; Toma, M.; Rijo P, Domínguez-Martíne, E.; Falcó, .; Sánchez, G.; Śliwiński, T. Enhanced Accumulation of Betulinic Acid in Transgenic Hairy Roots of *Senna obtusifolia* Growing in the Sprinkle Bioreactor and Evaluation of Their Biological Properties in Various Biological Models. In *Chemistry & Biodiversity,* 2021.

Le, T. T.; Gardner, J.; Hoang-Le, D.; Schmidt, C. W.; MacDonald, K. P.; Lambley, E.; Schroder, W. A.; Ogbourne, S. M.; Suhrbier, A. Immunostimulatory Cancer Chemotherapy Using Local Ingenol-3-Angelate and Synergy With Immunotherapies. *Vaccine* **2009,** *27* (23), 3053–3062.

Leckband, G.; Lörz, H. Transformation and Expression of a Stilbene Synthase Gene of *Vitis Vinifera* L. in Barley and Wheat for Increased Fungal Resistance. *Theor. Appl. Genet.* **1998,** *96* (8), 1004–1012.

Li, S. T.; Fu, C. H.; Zhang, M.; Zhang, Y.; Xie, S.; Yul, J. Enhancing Taxol Biosynthesis by Overexpressing a 9-cis-epoxycarotenoid Dioxygenase Gene in Transgenic Cell Lines of *Taxus chinensis*. *Plant Mol. Biol. Repr.* **2012,** *30* (5), 1125–1130.

Li, M.; Jiang, F.; Yu, X.; Miao, Z. Engineering Isoprenoid Biosynthesis in *Artemisia Annua* L. for the Production of Taxadiene: A Key Intermediate of Taxol. *Biomed. Res. Int.* **2015,** *2015*, 504932.

Li, D.; Ono, N.; Sato, T.; Sugiura, T.; Altaf-Ul-Amin, M.; Ohta, D.; Suzuki, H.; Arita, M.; Tanaka, K.; Ma, Z.; Kanaya, S. Targeted Integration of RNA-Seq and Metabolite Data to Elucidate Curcuminoid Biosynthesis in Four *Curcuma* Species. *Plant Cell Physiol.* **2015,** *56* (5), 843–851.

Li, L.; Qiu, R. L.; Lin, Y.; Cai, Y.; Bian, Y.; Fan, Y.; Gao, X. J. Resveratrol Suppresses Human Cervical Carcinoma Cell Proliferation and Elevates Apoptosis Via the Mitochondrial and p53 Signaling Pathways. *Oncol. Lett.* **2018,** *15* (6), 9845–9851.

Lim, J. D.; Yun, S. J.; Chung, I. M.; Yu, C. Y. Resveratrol Synthase Transgene Expression and Accumulation of Resveratrol Glycoside in *Rehmannia glutinosa*. *Mol. Breed.* **2005,** *16* (3), 219–233.

Liu, Z.; Hirani, A. H.; McVetty, P. B.; Daayf, F.; Quiros, C. F.; Li, G. Reducing Progoitrin and Enriching Glucoraphanin in *Braasica Napus* Seeds Through Silencing of the *GSL-ALK* Gene Family. *Plant Mol. Biol.* **2012,** *79* (1), 179–189.

Liu, S.; Hu, Y.; Wang, X.; Zhong, J.; Lin, Z. High Content of Resveratrol in Lettuce Transformed With a Stilbene Synthase Gene of *Parthenocissus Henryana*. *J. Agric. Food Chem.* **2006,** *54* (21), 8082–8085.

Liu, Z.; Liang, J.; Zheng, S.; Zhang, J.; Wu, J.; Cheng, F.; Yang, W.; Wang, X. Enriching Glucoraphanin in *Brassica Rapa* Through Replacement of BrAOP2.2/BrAOP2.3 With Non-functional Genes. *Front. Plant Sci.* **2017,** *8*, 1329.

Lu, Y.; Wang, H.; Wang, W.; Qian, Z.; Li, L.; Wang, J.; Zhou, G.; Kai, G. Molecular Characterization and Expression Analysis of a New cDNA Encoding Strictosidine Synthase From *Ophiorrhiza japonica*. *Mol. Biol. Rep.* **2009,** *36* (7), 1845–1852.

Masters, B. S. Safety of Genetically Engineered Foods: Approaches to Assessing Unintended Health Effects; The National Academies of Sciences: Washington, DC, 2004.

Mikami, Y.; Suzuki, T. Novel Microbial Inhibitors of Angiotensin Converting Enzyme, Aspergillomarasmines A and B. *Agric. Bioi. Chem.* **1983,** *47,* 2693–2695.

Mishra, B. B.; Tiwari, V. K. Natural Products: An Evolving Role in Future Drug Discovery. *Eur. J. Med. Chem.* **2011,** *46* (10), 4769–4807.

Mouhid, L.; Corzo-Martínez, M.; Torres, C.; Vázquez, L.; Reglero, G.; Fornari, T.; Ramírez de Molina, A. Improving in Vivo Efficacy of Bioactive Molecules: An Overview of Potentially Antitumor Phytochemicals and Currently Available Lipid-Based Delivery Systems. *J. Oncol.* **2017,** *2017,* 7351976.

Newman, D. J.; Cragg, G. M. Natural Products as Sources of New Drugs From 1981 to 2014. *J. Nat. Prod.* **2016,** *79* (3), 629–661.

Ni, X.; Wen, S.; Wang, W.; Wang, X.; Xu, H.; Kai, G. Enhancement of Camptothecin Production in *Camptotheca acuminata* Hairy Roots by Overexpressing *ORCA3* Gene. *J. Appl. Pharm. Sci.* **2011,** *1* (8), 85.

Okura, A.; Arakawa, H.; Yoshinari, T.; Naito, K.; Ishizuka, M.; Takeuchi, T.; Umezawa, H. Effect of Forphenicinol on the Production of Ia-Positive Macrophages in Mice With or Without L1210 Leukemia and on the Growth of L1210 in Immunized Mice. *J. Antibiot.* **1986,** *39* (4), 575–580.

Oyarce P, De Meester B, Fonseca F, de Vries L, Goeminne G, Pallidis A, Rycke, R. D.; Tsuji, Y.; Li, Y.; Van den Bosch, S.; Sels, B.; Ralph, J.; Vanholme, R.; Boerjan, S. W. Introducing Curcumin Biosynthesis in Arabidopsis Enhances Lignocellulosic Biomass Processing. *Nature Plants* **2019,** *5* (2), 225–237.

Pan, Q.; Wang, Q.; Yuan, F.; Xing, S.; Zhao, J.; Choi YH, Verpoorte, R.; Tian, Y.; Wang, G.; Tang, K. Overexpression of *ORCA3* and *G10H* in *Catharanthus roseus* Plants Regulated Alkaloid Biosynthesis and Metabolism Revealed by NMR-Metabolomics. *PLoS One* **2012,** *7* (8), e43038.

Pezzuto, J. M. Resveratrol as an Inhibitor of Carcinogenesis. *Pharm. Biol.* **2008,** *46* (7–8), 443–573.

Pham, T. T. N.; Nguyen, T. N. L.; Bui, T. H.; Nguyen, H. Q.; Nguyen, T. T.; Le, V.S.; Chu, H. M. *Agrobacterium*-Mediated Transformation of the *CrDAT* Gene and Selection of Transgenic Periwinkle Lines With a High Vincristine Accumulation. *J. Hortic. Sci. Biotechnol.* **2019,** *94* (5), 591–598.

Rai, V.; Tandon, P. K.; Khatoon, S. Effect of Chromium on Antioxidant Potential of *Catharanthus roseus* Varieties and Production of Their Anticancer Alkaloids: Vincristine and Vinblastine. *Biomed. Res. Int.* **2014,** *2014,* 934182.

Rizk, A. M.; Hammouda, F. M.; El-Missiry, M. M.; Radwan, H. M.; Evans, F. J. Biologically Active Diterpene Esters From *Euphorbia peplus. Phytochemistry* **1985,** *24* (7), 1605–1606.

Rosen, R. H.; Gupta, A. K.; Tyring, S. K. Dual Mechanism of Action of Ingenol Mebutate Gel for Topical Treatment of Actinic Keratoses: Rapid Lesion Necrosis Followed by Lesion-Specific Immune Response. *J. Am. Acad. Dermatol.* **2012,** *66* (3), 486–493.

Roytrakul, S.; Verpoorte, R. Role of Vacuolar Transporter Proteins in Plant Secondary Metabolism: *Catharanthus roseus* Cell Culture. *Phytochem. Rev.* **2007,** *6* (2), 383–396.

Saito, K.; Sudo, H.; Yamazaki, M.; Koseki-Nakamura, M.; Kitajima, M.; Takayama, H.; Aimi, N. Feasible Production of Camptothecin by Hairy Root Culture of *Ophiorrhiza pumila. Plant Cell Rep.* **2001,** *20* (3), 267–271.

Schmidt, M. L.; Kuzmanoff, K. L.; Ling-Indeck, L.; Pezzuto, J. M. Betulinic Acid Induces Apoptosis in Human Neuroblastoma Cell Lines. *Eur. J. Cancer* **1997,** *33* (12), 2007–2010.

Schroth, M. N.; Hancock, J. G. Disease Suppressive Soil and Root-Colonizing Bacteria. *Science* **1982,** *216* (4553), 1376–1381.

Schwekendiek, A.; Spring, O.; Heyerick, A.; Pickel, B.; Pitsch, N. T.; Peschke, F.; De Keukeleire, D.; Weber, G. Constitutive Expression of a Grapevine Stilbene Synthase Gene in Transgenic Hop (*Humulus lupulus* L.) Yields Resveratrol and its Derivatives in Substantial Quantities. *J. Agric. Food Chem.* **2007,** *55* (17), 7002–7009.

Schwertheim, S.; Wein, F.; Lennartz, K.; Worm, K.; Schmid, K. W.; Sheu-Grabellus, S. Y. Curcumin Induces G2/M Arrest, Apoptosis, NF-κB Inhibition, and Expression of Differentiation Genes in Thyroid Carcinoma Cells. *J. Cancer Res. Clin. Oncol.* **2017,** *143* (7), 1143–1154.

Serazetdinova, L.; Oldach, K. H.; Lörz, H. Expression of Transgenic Stilbene Synthases in Wheat Causes the Accumulation of Unknown Stilbene Derivatives With Antifungal Activity. *J. Plant Physiol.* **2005,** *162* (9), 985–1002.

Shanmugam, M. K.; Rane, G.; Kanchi, M. M.; Arfuso, F.; Chinnathambi, A.; Zayed, M. E.; Alharbi, S. A.; Tan, B. K.; Kumar, A. P.; Sethi, G. The Multifaceted Role of Curcumin in Cancer Prevention and Treatment. *Molecules* **2015,** *20* (2), 2728–2769.

Shapiro, T. A.; Fahey, J. W.; Wade, K. L.; Stephenson, K. K.; Talalay, P. Chemoprotective Glucosinolates and Isothiocyanates of Broccoli Sprouts: Metabolism and Excretion in Humans. *Cancer Epidemiol. Prev. Biomarkers* **2001,** *10* (5), 501–508.

Sharma, A.; Verma, P.; Mathur, A.; Mathur, A. K. Genetic Engineering Approach Using Early Vinca Alkaloid Biosynthesis Genes Led to Increased Tryptamine and Terpenoid Indole Alkaloids Biosynthesis in Differentiating Cultures of *Catharanthus roseus*. *Protoplasma* **2018,** *255* (1), 425–435.

Shukla, Y.; Singh, R. Resveratrol and Cellular Mechanisms of Cancer Prevention. *Ann. N Y Acad. Sci.* **2011,** *1215* (1), 1–8.

Singh, S.; Pandey, P.; Akhtar, M. Q.; Negi, A. S.; Banerjee, S. A New Synthetic Biology Approach for the Production of Curcumin and its Glucoside in *Atropa belladonna* Hairy Roots. *J. Biotechnol.* **2021,** 328, 23–33.

Stecca, B.; Mas, C.; Clement, V.; Zbinden, M.; Correa, R.; Piguet, V.; et al. Melanomas Require HEDGEHOG-GLI Signaling Regulated by Interactions Between GLI1 and the RAS-MEK/AKT Pathways. *Proc. Natl. Acad. Sci. U. S. A.* **2007,** *104* (14), 5895–900.

Sung, H.; Ferlay, J.; Siegel, R. L.; Laversanne, M.; Soerjomataram, I.; Jemal, A.; Bray, F. Global Cancer Statistics 2020: GLOBOCAN Estimates of Incidence and Mortality Worldwide for 36 Cancers in 185 Countries. *CA Cancer J. Clin.* **2021,** *71* (3), 209–249.

Syklowska-Baranek, K.; Pietrosiuk, A.; Kokoszka, A.; Furmanowa, M. Enhancement of Taxane Production in Hairy Root Culture of *Taxus* × *media* var. Hicksii. *J. Plant Physiol.* **2009,** *166* (17), 1950–1954.

Szankowski, I.; Briviba, K.; Fleschhut, J.; Schönherr, J.; Jacobsen, H. J.; Kiesecker, H. Transformation of Apple (*Malus domestica* Borkh.) With the Stilbene Synthase Gene From Grapevine (*Vitis vinifera* L.) and a PGIP Gene From Kiwi (*Actinidia deliciosa*). *Plant Cell Rep.* **2003,** *22* (2), 141–149.

Tabata, H. Paclitaxel Production by Plant-Cell-Culture Technology. *Biomanufacturing* **2004,** 1–23.

Thurnher, D.; Turhani, D.; Pelzmann, M.; Wannemacher, B.; Knerer, B.; Formanek, M.; Wacheck, V.; Selzer, E. Betulinic Acid: A New Cytotoxic Compound Against Malignant Head and Neck Cancer Cells. *Head Neck J. Sci. Spec. Head Neck* **2003,** *25* (9), 732–740.

Turano, F. J.; Fang, T. K. Characterization of Two Glutamate Decarboxylase cDNA Clones From Arabidopsis. *Plant Physiol.* **1998,** *117,* 1411–1421.

Tzogani, K.; Nagercoil, N.; Hemmings, R. J.; Samir, B.; Gardette, J.; Demolis, P.; Salmonson, T.; Pignatti, F. The European Medicines Agency Approval of Ingenol Mebutate (Picato) for the Cutaneous Treatment of Non-hyperkeratotic, Non-hypertrophic Actinic Keratosis in Adults: Summary of the Scientific Assessment of the Committee for Medicinal Products for Human Use (CHMP). *Eur. J. Dermatol.* **2014,** *24* (4), 457–463.

Van der Fits, L.; Memelink, J. ORCA3, A Jasmonate-Responsive Transcriptional Regulator of Plant Primary and Secondary Metabolism. *Science* **2000,** *289,* 295–297.

Varoni, E. M.; Lo Faro, A. F.; Sharifi-Rad, J.; Iriti, M. Anticancer Molecular Mechanisms of Resveratrol. *Front. Nutr.* **2016,** *3,* 8.

Venditto, V. J.; Simanek, E. E. Cancer Therapies Utilizing the Camptothecins: A Review of the in Vivo Literature. *Mol. Pharm.* **2010,** *7* (2), 307–349.

Vining, L. C. Functions of Secondary Metabolites. *Ann. Rev. Microbiol.* **1990,** *44* (1), 395–427.

Wang, X.; Song, Y.; Su, Y.; Tian, Q.; Li, B.; Quan, J.; Deng, Y. Are PEGylated Liposomes Better Than Conventional Liposomes? A Special Case for Vincristine. *Drug Delivery* **2016,** *23* (4), 1092–1100.

Watkins, D. N.; Berman, D. M.; Burkholder, S. G.; Wang, B.; Beachy, P. A.; Baylin, S. B. Hedgehog Signalling Within Airway Epithelial Progenitors and in Small-Cell Lung Cancer. *Nature* **2003,** *422* (6929), 313–317.

Weaver, B. A. How Taxol/Paclitaxel Kills Cancer Cells. *Mol. Biol. Cell* **2014,** *25* (18), 2677–2681.

Wick, W.; Grimmel, C.; Wagenknecht, B.; Dichgans, J.; Weller, M. Betulinic Acid-Induced Apoptosis in Glioma Cells: A Sequential Requirement for New Protein Synthesis, Formation of Reactive Oxygen Species, and Caspase Processing. *J. Pharmacol. Exp. Ther.* **1999,** *289* (3), 1306–1312.

Wu, L.; Guo, L.; Liang, Y.; Liu, X.; Jiang, L.; Wang, L. Curcumin Suppresses Stem-Like Traits of Lung Cancer Cells Via Inhibiting the JAK2/STAT3 Signaling Pathway. *Oncol. Rep.* **2015,** *34* (6), 3311–3317.

Yanaka, A.; Fahey, J. W.; Fukumoto, A.; Nakayama, M.; Inoue, S.; Zhang S, Tauchi, M.; Suzuki, H.; Hyodo, I.; Yamamoto, M. Dietary Sulforaphane-Rich Broccoli Sprouts Reduce Colonization and Attenuate Gastritis in *Helicobacter pylori*-Infected Mice and Humans. *Cancer Prev. Res.* **2009,** *2* (4), 353–360.

Yao, H.; Liu, J.; Xu, S.; Zhu, Z.; Xu, J. The Structural Modification of Natural Products for Novel Drug Discovery. *Expert Opin. Drug Discov.* **2017,** *12* (2), 121–140.

Zasadil, L. M.; Andersen, K. A.; Yeum, D.; Rocque, G. B.; Wilke, L. G.; Tevaarwerk, A. J.; Raines, R. T.; Mark E Burkard, M. E.; Weaver, B. A. Cytotoxicity of Paclitaxel in Breast Cancer is Due to Chromosome Missegregation on Multipolar Spindles. *Sci. Transl. Med.* **2014,** *6* (229), 229ra43–229ra43.

Zhu, Y. J.; Agbayani, R.; Jackson, M. C.; Tang, C. S.; Moore, P. H. Expression of the Grapevine *Stilbene Synthase* Gene VST 1 in Papaya Provides Increased Resistance Against Diseases Caused by *Phytophthora palmivora. Planta* **2004,** *220* (2), 241–250.

CHAPTER 7

Genomics of Plants with Anticancer Properties: Breaking New Ground in Cancer Therapy

MUBASSHIRA MOHAMMED MAZHAR-UL-HAQUE[1], LEKHA BHAGTANEY[1], and PRIYA SUNDARRAJAN[2]

[1]*Caius Research Laboratory, St. Xavier's College (Autonomous), Mumbai, India*

[2]*Department of Life Science and Biochemistry and Director, Caius Research Laboratory, St. Xavier's College (Autonomous), Mumbai, India*

ABSTRACT

A comprehensive study of biomolecules can be achieved with the employment of omics technologies. Integration of such a multidimensional technology with bioinformatics can focus on high-throughput sequencing and identification of phytochemicals, metabolites, proteins, RNA, and genes which can further be coupled with pharmacology for therapeutic purposes. The study of the whole genome of an organism is known as genomics. Genomics allows us to examine and comprehend genomes so as to lessen the existing gap between genotypes and phenotypes. Currently, one of the major contributors to mortality worldwide is cancer. Clinical therapies for cancer involve chemotherapy, radiotherapy, surgery, and targeted therapy. Every day there are new advancements in these therapies however, the complete cure for this disease remains a challenge. Most of these therapies have presented many side effects along with the impairment of normal

Plant-Derived Anticancer Drugs in the OMICS Era: Biosynthesis, Functions, and Applications.
Deepu Pandita, Anu Pandita (Eds.)

cells. Due to this, novel compounds derived from plants have been gaining interest for their effective activity against cancerous cells with minimal side effects. Natural products derived from plants sources such as taxol, etoposide, irinotecan, topotecan, withaferin A, with anolides, vincristine, vinblastine, and camptothecin are being utilized as a part of cancer therapy. With whole genome analysis of a particular plant, we can identify the genes and metabolic pathways associated with secondary metabolites that are ultimately utilized as anticancer agents. The production of important secondary metabolites with anticancer properties can be significantly improved with the latest tools of genomics. In addition to this, methods of combinatorial biochemistry assisted by genomics can synthesize novel compounds. Drug discovery and development originating from anticancer plants can be strengthened with the use of phylogenomics and molecular phylogeny by estimating chemo diversity and bioprospecting. Advancements in the field of genomic technology can aid in medicinal plant breeding thereby allowing for the efficient production of medicinal compounds which have anticancer properties. Metabolic engineering or molecular breeding of medicinal plants can reduce the excessive utilization of plants for pharmaceutical compounds. Such methodologies support sustainable use of medicinal plants.

7.1 INTRODUCTION

Cancer is a disease characterized by unregulated cell proliferation. Some cancers also have the property of "metastasis" where they can spread to other parts of the body. Environmental factors or hereditary/somatic mutations are usually the cause of this multifarious disease. The difficulty in prescribing a single treatment for cancer stems is because of the fact that various factors are involved in the modification of normal cell growth. The key concern in cancer therapy is the resistance of tumors to current treatment alternatives. As a result, research is now focused on the discovery of novel compounds in cancer treatment that tumors are highly sensitive to (Akhtar and Swami, 2018).

Cancer treatment employs a wide range of techniques, from traditional to modern. The techniques utilized include surgery, radiation therapy, chemotherapy, or targeted therapy, however, each of them has some drawbacks. The use of traditional chemicals has negative and harmful effects. As a result, new and enhanced cancer treatments are required. Anticancer compounds derived from plants are being explored as they are easily accessible, non-toxic, and harmless. Moreover, it is believed that the impact on the body due to a disease is neutralized by the use of medicinal plant compounds. The secondary metabolites derived from the plants having anticancer properties can trigger apoptosis in cancer cells. These metabolites are also crucial in the development of cancer as they can prevent the transformation to a malignant state. Compounds derived from plants such as camptothecin, podophyllotoxin, and vinca alkaloids are utilized in the treatment of cancer (Khan et al., 2019). Additionally, compounds such as topotecan, vinblastine, taxol among many others have been successfully studied as anticancer drugs in clinical trials (Ashraf, 2020).

7.2 OVERVIEW OF MEDICINAL PLANTS HAVING ANTICANCER PROPERTIES

Several plants with anticancer properties and their phytochemicals have been shown to curb the development of cancer. Bark, leaf, stem, embryo, rhizomes, roots, seeds, fruits, sprouts, and flowers are the various parts of plants that have presence of different phytochemicals which are known for their biological activity. The secondary metabolites, biomolecules, and other plant compounds show anticancer properties by induction of antioxidant activity, promotion of the synthesis of protective enzymes, activation of DNA repair pathways, or inhibition of activator proteins/signaling pathways/enzymes in cancer cells (Iqbal et al., 2017).

Several phytochemicals have been extracted from plants and have been shown to be effective in the treatment of cancer (Table 7.1). Vinblastine and vincristine are drugs originating from a class of phytochemicals known as vinca alkaloids extracted from *Catharanthus roseus*. These drugs have been used as an anticancer treatment in cancers like Kaposi's sarcoma, breast cancer, lung cancer, testicular cancer, lymphoma, and leukemia. Phytochemicals extracted from *Taxus brevifolia* Nutt. led to the discovery of paclitaxel. This drug is also an example of a significant discovery made from traditional medicinal plant knowledge of the Native American Tribes. Another drug efficient in the treatment of acute myelogenous leukemia is homoharringtonine which was extracted from a tree found in China called *Cephalotaxus harringtonia* var. drupacea. A homoharringtonine and harringtonine racemate are given as treatment for cancer in China. A medicinal plant, *Bleekeria vitensis* A. C. Sm., which is native to Fiji was used to extract elliptinium. It is used for the treatment of breast cancer (Ashraf, 2020).

TABLE 7.1 List of Phytochemicals obtained from Plants That Are Used to Cure Cancer.

Medicinal plant	Phytochemical	Treatment of cancer	Reference
C. roseus	Vinca alkaloids (vincristine, vinblastine)	Kaposi's sarcoma, breast cancer, lung cancer, testicular cancer, lymphoma, and leukemia	Ashraf, 2020
T. brevifolia Nutt.	Taxol (paclitaxel)	Kaposi's sarcoma, lung cancer, breast cancer, ovarian cancer	Weaver, 2014; Ashraf, 2020
C. harringtonia var. drupacea	Homoharringtonine	Acute myelogenous leukemia	Ashraf, 2020
B. vitensis A. C. Sm.	Elliptinium	Breast cancer	Ashraf, 2020
Curcuma longa	Curcumin	Prostate cancer, oral cancer, colon cancer, breast cancer	Akhtar and Swami, 2018
Polygonum cuspidatum	Resveratrol	Liver cancer, skin cancer, colorectal cancer	Iqbal et al., 2017
Artemisia annua	Artemisinin	Liver cancer, breast cancer, pancreatic cancer	Khan et al., 2019; Iqbal et al., 2017
Camelia sinesis	Epigallocatechin gallate	Breast cancer, prostate cancer, skin cancer, bladder cancer, lung cancer	Akhtar and Swami, 2018; Iqbal et al., 2017

The following sections will highlight some of the most well-known plants with anticancer characteristics and phytochemicals that have the potential to be employed as cancer treatments (Table 7.1).

C. longa belongs to the Zingiberaceae (ginger) family and is a perennial herbaceous plant. Pharmacological activities like anti-bacterial, nematocidal, anti-oxidant, and anti-inflammatory have been exhibited by *C. longa*. The therapeutic action of *C. longa* is attributed to the phytochemical curcumin. Several studies have noted the anticancer and anti-inflammatory properties of curcumin (Khan et al., 2019). The use of curcumin in studies involving animal models have demonstrated its ability to retard tumor growth and in cancer cell lines it has demonstrated the ability to cause cell death. Several cancers like prostate, oral, colon, and breast have been suppressed by curcumin. The chemical nature of curcumin which shows a *β*-diketone component in the center and methoxy group containing unsaturated side chain attached to a benzene ring is mainly responsible for the anticancer activities. This chemical nature of curcumin intervenes with the cell division signaling pathways of the cells by engaging directly or regulating the gene expression cascades (Akhtar and Swami, 2018).

The roots of *P. cuspidatum* contain the phytochemical resveratrol, a polyphenolic phytoalexine compound that is naturally occurring. Resveratrol has successfully been tested on various cancer cell lines for its anticancer properties and has shown its potential by regulating various molecular targets. It has wide-ranging anticancer effects such as on intestinal flora, metabolism, immunity, apoptosis, metastasis, invasion, and cancer cell proliferation (Wu et al., 2018). Resveratrol originating from *P. cuspidatum* has shown suppression of liver, skin, and colorectal cancer (Iqbal et al., 2017).

A. annua derived artemisinin is a 1, 2-trioxane compound. Many studies, both in vitro and in vivo, have ascertained that artemisinin is a promising anticancer compound. Arteether, artemether, and artesunate are artemisinin derived semi-synthetic compounds. On further research, it was found that artesunate is highly effective against cancer of colon and leukemia. Another observation was that artesunate is more effective against these cancers as compared to other drugs commonly used. 1, 8-cineole, and scopoletin are two other compounds extracted from *A. annua* (Khan et al., 2019).

C. sinesis has high amounts of catechins out of which epigallocatechin gallate is in the highest concentration. When epigallocatechin gallate and other catechins found in *C. sinesis* were analyzed, cancer development was considerably inhibited, and treated cells released TNF-alpha. This may be attributed to its property of scavenging for free radicals. A synergistic effect is observed when epigallocatechin gallate and ginseng were given together in case of colon cancer cells where the anticancer property was enhanced. Theobromine is another compound derived from

C. sinesis that induces apoptosis and inhibits cancer cell proliferation. Epigallocatechin gallate and other tea polyphenols have shown significant anticancer activity against nasopharyngeal carcinoma, laryngeal squamous carcinoma, epidermoid carcinoma, osteogenic sarcoma, prostate cancer, breast cancer, and ovarian cancer (Akhtar and Swami, 2018).

Plant genome sequencing has proven to be a solid method for delving into a wide range of concepts with clinical relevance. Medicinal plant genomic research lags behind that of model plants and significant crop varieties. The genomic studies unveil important data about heredity, physiology, evolution, and origin of the plant. This information aids in understanding a plant's chemodiversity, which includes identifying the valuable secondary metabolites. The sequencing of medicinal plants' genomes facilitates the elucidation of secondary metabolite biosynthesis pathways and regulatory factors. It also promotes the molecular breeding of high-yielding medicinal plants and the cultivation of transgenic medicinal plants (Hao and Xiao, 2015).

7.3 GENOMICS OF PLANTS HAVING COMPOUNDS WITH ANTICANCER PROPERTIES

Sequencing and assembling a complete plant genome is a very tremendous task. Whole-genome sequencing can aid in genome-wide investigations into fundamental evolutionary questions, as well as give hundreds of nuclear markers for population-level and phylogenetic research (Li and Harkness, 2018). Genome sequencing provides critical information at the microscopic level regarding the plant origin, development as well as epigenomic regulation. Anticancer drugs' biosynthesis processes and secondary metabolites can be identified using high throughput sequencing technology in medicine. (Mehta and Hasija, 2018). It is of great help to explore the genetic variability among or within any kind of species. In cancer research, these technologies have made significant discoveries (Duitama et al., 2014).

Some criteria that need to be considered while selecting a particular medicinal plant for the whole genome sequencing are as follows:

1. Source of plants (including key chemical drugs that are in heavy demand)

2. Characteristics of plants from the huge medicinal genus/family [e.g. *Glycyrrhiza uralensis* (Chinese liquorice; Fabaceae) and *Lycium chinense* (Chinese boxthorn; Solanaceae)] should be known
3. Medicinal plants whose genetic makeup is already known, etc. (Hao and Xiao, 2015)

The "Herb Genome Program" was started with the goal of sequencing the genomes of numerous medicinal plants and performing post-genomic functional analyzes of secondary metabolite biosynthesis pathways. However, only a few plant genomes have been assembled till today probably because of their complexity (Chakraborty, 2018). *Ganoderma lucidum*, *Salvia miltiorrihiza*, and *C. roseus* are three plants whose genomes have been sequenced and have emerged as excellent models for studying genetics and metabolic activities of herbs. For example, in one of the studies, the whole-genome shotgun sequencing strategy of haploid G. lucidum 260125 was performed. *G. lucidum* contains a 43.3 Mb genome and 16,113 predicted genes, according to next-generation sequencing and optical mapping techniques. Secondary metabolism is aided by sequence analysis of genes encoding cytochrome P450s (CYP), transporters, and regulatory proteins. *G. lucidum* often known as "mushroom of immortality" and "the symbol of traditional Chinese medicine" is one of the well-known medicinal macro-fungi in the world (Chen et al., 2012).

The approach that can be used to determine the heterozygosity of the genome is RAD Seq (restriction-site associated DNA sequencing). It is an effective tool for constructing the RAD library. Genetic and physical maps are essential tools for assembling complex plant genomes and conducting functional genomic research. The outcome is suitable for map-based cloning. The information gained from the RAD-Seq and genotyping by sequencing can be utilized to figure out where anticancer plants came from and where they are now. (Hao and Xiao, 2015).

Some other medicinal plants in which genome sequencing has also been determined are *Mitragyna speciosa (Kratom), Gelsemium sempervirens, Calotropis gigantean, Camptotheca acuminate, C. roseus.* The genome sequencing of the above-mentioned medicinal plants can be downloaded from (Medicinal Plant Genomics resource, n.d.). Example: Whole-genome shotgun sequencing of *M. speciosa (Kratom)* was undertaken, resulting in a 523 Mb assembly with an N50 scaffold size of 26.2 Kbp. The genome of

M. speciose can be downloaded from Dryad Digital Repository. Similarly, for other plants, genome sequences can be downloaded like this too.

In another study, *Ocimum tenuiflorum* (Tulsi) was subjected to whole-genome sequencing, which revealed amino acid alterations present at the loci of genes involved in biosynthesis. It confers some pharmaceutical properties to the loci. Ursolic acid, luteolin, apigenin, taxol, oleanolic acid, sitosterol, and eugenol are secondary metabolites generated by this plant that have anticancer properties. Specific genes that aid in the treatment of cancer can be identified through whole-genome sequencing, which can aid in the development of targeted drugs. (Mehta and Hasija, 2018).

Molecular tools (e.g. microsatellite markers or Simple Sequence Repeats) are significantly effective because of their good genome coverage, co-dominant inheritance, relative abundance as well as high reproducibility. In comparison to the original lineages, DNA sequence analysis employing microsatellite markers can identify changes in repetitive motifs (Valdiani et al., 2013). The semiparasitic medicinal herb *Viscum coloratum* (Santalaceae) is well-known for its anticancer effects. In addition, 19 new polymorphic microsatellites markers were created to enhance population genetic studies and ecological conservation of the plant. (Kim et al., 2017). The examples of genomic techniques used for genomic analysis of plants with anticancer properties are given in Table 7.2.

TABLE 7.2 Examples of Genomic Techniques That Are Used for Genomic Analysis of Anticancer Plants.

Genomic techniques	Plants
Whole genome sequencing	*M. speciosa (Kratom), G. sempervirens, C. gigantean, C. acuminate, C. roseus, O. tenuiflorum, G. uralensis*
Simple Sequence Repeats	*V. coloratum* (Santalaceae)
Genome Assembly	*C. gigantea*
Illumina sequencing technology	*P. cuspidatum*

Medicinal plants and herbal remedies provide a lot of information to modern medicine and could also provide a great deal to sound as well as science-based solutions of the future. Unfortunately, due to their complexity, only a few well-assembled herbal genomes have been revealed till date. The genomes of certain common herbs, such as *G. lucidum*, *S. miltiorrihiza*, and *C. roseus*, have already been sequenced, and they have shown to be useful models for researching herb genetics and metabolism.

7.4 ANALYSIS OF GENOMES OF ANTICANCER PLANTS USING BIOINFORMATICS APPROACHES

The different biotechnological approaches used for genomic applications of plants with anticancer properties have been summarized in Table 7.3.

TABLE 7.3 Genomic Analysis of Anticancer Plants Using Biotechnological Approach.

Genomic application	Biotechnological methods
Whole-Genome Sequence Analysis	Rmap, Seqmap, Zoom, Maq, Ngsep, Sam Tools
Genome Assembly	Phrap, Cap, Cap3, Bac Card I, Soap Denovo, Velvet
Search for homology in nucleotide sequences	Blastn, Blastp, Tblastx
Nucleotide	
Comparative Genome Visualization	Syn Browse, Cmap, and Cmap3d Cmap
(Rad-Seq) Pyrad	STACKS, RADIS
Protein-Coding Gene Prediction	Exonerate, AUGUSTUS

7.5 USE OF BIOINFORMATICS APPROACHES FOR WHOLE-GENOME SEQUENCE ANALYSIS

The whole-genome sequencing platform is selected based on financial constraints and a preliminary assessment of candidate genomes.

7.5.1 RMAP

It reads mapping paired-end from next-generation sequencing technologies effectively. It employs more advanced quality scores for probability indicators. It can scan base pairs with a length of 20–64 bits per second. The user can fit as many mismatches as possible between a read and the location it is mapping to. (Mehta and Hasija, 2018).

7.5.2 SEQMAP

It uses an index filtering algorithm. It is used to map millions of small sequences to billions of nucleotides in a genome. It detects the positions of sequences in the reference genome, as well as various nucleotide base changes, insertions, and deletions. For high-throughput sequencing analysis, this is crucial. (Mehta and Hasija, 2018).

7.5.3 ZILLIONS OF OLIGOS MAPPED (ZOOM)

It is a next-generation technology and it produces billions of short reads. Faster software is required to map resequencing and personalized medicine sequencing to a reference genome in order to find SNPs or uncommon transcripts. In one CPU, it can map illumine/Solexa reads of around 15X coverage of the human genome against the reference human genome, even with two mismatches at full sensitivity (Lin et al., 2008).

7.5.4 MAQ (MAPPING AND ASSEMBLY WITH QUALITY)

It is an alignment software and is quite different from the existing software because: (1) it measures the probability of the alignment being wrong as well as mapping quality for each alignment. This helps in accurate variant calling. (2) It has a low mapping score however, it maps every read that has a match and replaces the repetitive reads among the equally good alternatives instead of discarding them. This helps to avoid any ambiguity in defining the "unique", and thus provides more data for further analysis. (3) In a sliding window, MAQ aligns mate-pair can be read, examine the proper paired positions and if their mates have unique regions then it allows read in repeats that can be aligned with high confidence. Also, a Phred-like quality, allows the user to control the sensitivity/specificity trade-off and thus facilitates the use of MAQ calls in downstream analysis (Li et al., 2008)

7.5.5 NGSEP (NEXT GENERATION SEQUENCING ECLIPSE PROGRAM)

It is a bioinformatics tool that is used to carry out the accurate analysis of high throughput sequencing reads with different deployment alternatives to the end-users. The functions of NGSEP involve the genetic mapping of complex traits, alignment sorting, functional annotation, format conversation, a variant detector which helps us to make the simultaneous discovery of SNVs (Single nucleotide Variants), indels and CNV(Copy number Variation), and several other features. It has the potential to play a significant role in anticancer plant genetic improvement and genomic selection (Tello et al., 2019; Mehta and Hasija, 2018).

7.5.6 SAM TOOLS

It is an important program that interacts with high-throughput data. BAM, CRAM, and SAM can be used to read DNA sequence alignments. It is a format that stores large nucleotide sequence alignments in the generic format. The DNA sequence is one of their key goals. With the help of the given tools, read alignments may be inspected, stored, and indexed; they're also interconvertible and small in size, allowing most of the alignment's actions to be performed on a stream. It is extremely versatile; it can hold all of the alignment data produced by other alignment programs. It enables files that need to be indexed by genomic position to obtain all reads aligning to a locus efficiently (Mehta and Hasija, 2018; SAM tools, n.d.).

7.6 GENOME ASSEMBLY

7.6.1 PHRAP

It is a shotgun sequencing strategy program that handles large datasets. It allows massive sets of DNA sequences to be compared, aligned, and assembled quickly. It employs a pairwise comparison of the input sequences. It permits the entire read to be used rather than just the high-quality bits that have been cut. When the repeats are available, it improves the assembly process by simply combining the user-supplied and then internally computed high-quality data. It also provides information regarding trouble-shooting programs successfully (De la Bastide and McCombie, 2017).

7.6.2 CONTIG ASSEMBLY PROGRAM (CAP) AND CAP3

The Contig Assembly Program identifies a set of fragments' shortest common superstring. With the use of a filter, it helps DNA shotgun sequencing by removing DNA fragment pairings that cannot overlap. The maximal-scoring overlapping alignment is computed for the remaining fragments. The pieces are then put together in order of alignment scores. The CAP3 program is an upgraded version of CAP sequence assembly program. It employs forward-reverse constraints to correct assembly errors and connect contigs, as well as base quality values to compute overlaps between sequence reads, produce multiple read alignments, and generate consensus sequences. CAP3 can also automatically trim readings with poor 5' and 3' regions. It performs better than Phrap with forward-reverse constraints for generating scaffolds on low-pass data (CAP3-Contig Assembly Program, n.d.).

7.6.3 BAC CARD I

This program can be used to validate whole-genome shotgun assemblies and integrate various forms of genomic data. It looks for misassembles, calculates contig scaffolding, and performs an intergenomic comparison of related strains (Mehta and Hasija, 2018).

7.6.4 SOAP DENOVO AND SOAP DENOVO 2

It is a unique short read assembly method that can generate a de novo draft assembly for genomes, particularly using illumina GA short reads. It is utilized to conduct precise assessments of yet-to-be-explored plant genomes. For the approach to be more efficient, some adjustments are required. SOAP 2 Denovo benefits from a new algorithm design that minimizes memory usage in graph construction. It solves the problem of more repetition areas in contig assembly, enhances gap closing, and optimizes for big genomes by increasing the length and coverage of scaffolds (Luo et al., 2012).

7.6.5 VELVET

It is a unique de novo assembly process. It may be used to swiftly construct lengthy continuous sequences or contigs, as well as gapped scaffold assemblies, using short-read datasets generated by next-generation sequencing technologies. This plays an important role in studying the data from the new organism for which reference genomes have not been assembled yet, or during the determination of the origin of unmapped reads (Zerbino, 2010).

7.7 NUCLEOTIDE SEQUENCE HOMOLOGY SEARCH NUCLEOTIDE

7.7.1 *NUCLEOTIDE BASIC LOCAL ALIGNMENT SEARCH TOOL (BLASTN)*

The nucleotide sequence is specified. It searches for comparable regions in biological sequences. This program searches sequence databases for nucleotide or protein sequences and determines statistical significance (Basic Local Alignment Search Tools, n.d.).

7.7.2 *NUCLEOTIDE 6-FRAME TRANSLATION-NUCLEOTIDE 6-FRAME TRANSLATION (TBLASTX)*

It involves a complex algorithm, that is why it is one of the slowest programs in the BLAST family. It is a nucleotide sequence that is specified. It compares a six-frame translation of the nucleotide sequence database with all of the queries translated in all six available frames. For each comparison between the query and target sequences in the database, this program performs 36 comparisons. This is the reason why it takes longer to complete the analysis. This helps to detect the distant relationships between nucleotide sequences (Genomics and comparative genomics, n.d.).

7.7.3 *PROTEIN-PROTEIN BASIC LOCAL ALIGNMENT SEARCH TOOL (BLASTP)*

It specifies the sequence of the protein. It compares the protein query to the protein sequence database. (Mehta and Hasija, 2018).

7.7.4 *PROTEIN-NUCLEOTIDE 6-FRAME TRANSLATION (TBLASTN)*

It specifies the sequence of the protein. This program compares the query sequence to the nucleotide sequence database's six reading frames. It is used when direct comparisons need to be done, and does not involve translations. It identifies proteins in uncharacterized genomes (Mehta and Hasija, 2018).

7.8 COMPARATIVE GENOME VISUALIZATION

7.8.1 SYN BROWSE

It is a program for analyzing and visualizing genomic alignments within and between species. It is primarily used to compare genetic sequences. It can be used to investigate microsynteny, macrosynteny, and homologous genes in different sequences. It helps to identify unspecified genes and putative regulatory elements in comparison with the reference genome (Pan et al., 2005).

7.8.2 CONNECTIVITY MAP (CMAP) AND CMAP3D

It is an extremely effective tool for comparing genetic maps and sequenced genomes. It is made up of three primary parts: The cMapDB database, which may be used for a variety of mapping applications, the user interface, and a data retriever. The locations, placements, and linkage groups are all specified. It has a limitation in terms of comparing nearby aligned maps. Also, if there is any modification in the view, a reload and redraw of maps are required. CMap3D has been developed to overcome these limitations. It allows the comparison of many genetic maps or data in three-dimensional space (Duran et al., 2010).

7.9 RESTRICTION SITE-ASSOCIATED DNA SEQUENCING ANALYSIS (RAD-SEQ) PYRAD

It is used to put together de novo RAD seq loci. Its goal is to maximize coverage across phylogenetic datasets. It's a pipeline that wraps an alignment-clustering technique in a wrapper. PyRAD has an advantage over STACKS since indels do not break homologous locus clusters. (Eaton, 2014).

7.9.1 RADIS

For phylogenetic inference, RADIS can be used to handle huge volumes of data obtained through illumine sequencing. Users specify various parameter values that need to be checked as well as routes to other applications in this software (configuration: RADIS.cfg). The user-specified directory in which the output files and required subdirectories are produced automatically. The exploration of RAD-seq data becomes more straightforward and efficient. STACKS, on the other hand, are necessary to remove PCR duplicates, establish loci, and separate data from multiple systems (Cruaud, 2016).

7.9.2 STACKS

It is used to convert short-read sequences to specific loci that are produced by the illumine platform. The aim of developing the stack was to build the genetic maps from the RAD-tag Illumina sequence data but can also apply to population studies and phylogeography. It is a flexible program that can be used to look at anticancer plants with or without reference genomes. A web-based user interface and a relational database are used. This interface aids data display, user-directed alterations, and genetic hypothesis corrections. It can also be used to study wild plankton adaption through population genetics (Catchen et al., 2011; Catchen et al., 2013).

7.10 PROTEIN-CODING GENE PREDICTION

7.10.1 AUGUSTUS

It's a generalized Hidden Markov Model-based eukaryotic gene prediction tool. It integrates the evidence from EST's, proteomics, RNA-Seq, etc., as well as predicts the genes ab initio. The extension to AUGUSTUS (PPX) helps to find out the new member of the family in a genome when protein sequence multiple sequence alignment as an input is provided. In one of the studies, for the de novo prediction of the gene in P. cuspidatum, the transposable element (TE)-masked genome was used in conjunction with the AUGUSTUS software (AUGUSTUS, n.d.; Zhang et al., 2019).

7.10.2 EXONERATE

It's a tool for comparing pairwise sequences in general. It's a tool for predicting protein-coding genes. It aligns sequences using several alignment models, including dynamic programming and heuristics. It utilizes the C4 dynamic programming library. It is general and fast. It produces either gapped or ungapped alignments depending upon the variety of different alignment models. It enables the user to align sequences using a variety of alignment models, including dynamic programming and other heuristics (Vertebrate genomic team, n.d.) Many alternative techniques, including PolySSR, SA-SSR, poly, SyMAP, SynChro, and others, can be used to find anticancer genes in plants.

A summary of the various genome analysis techniques used for plants with anticancer properties is provided in Figure 7.1.

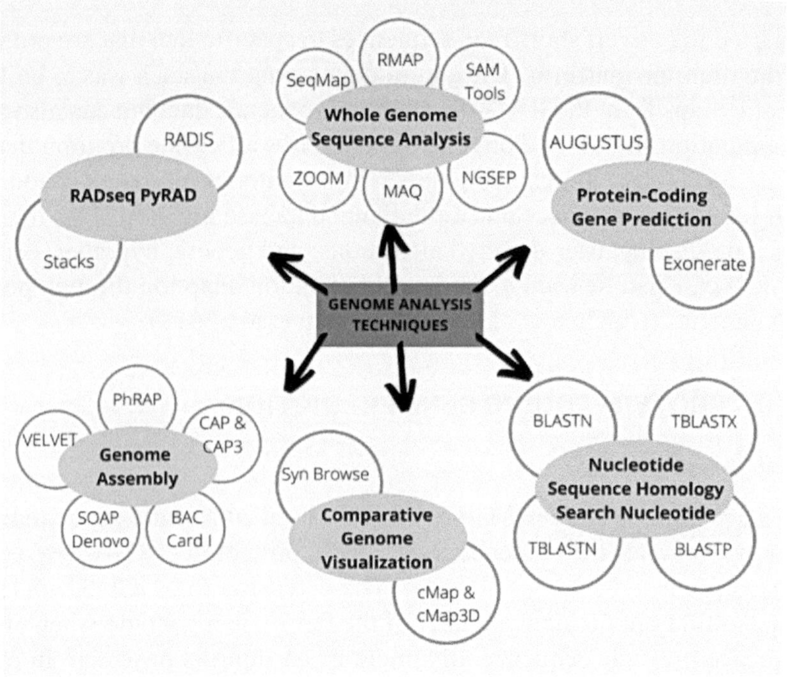

FIGURE 7.1 Genome analysis techniques.

7.11 CONCLUSION

Cancer is a big problem across the world. Synthetic drugs are mostly being used to treat cancer however their usage is limited because of the toxic effects associated with them. Hence, there is a need for an alternative to synthetic drugs for the treatment of cancer. Plant-based natural products are a valuable resource for many drug development methods. Plant-derived chemicals have a complicated structure and biological activity, implying that there is still more to learn. Secondary metabolites present in the plant are responsible for anticancer activity and have contributed to the development of new drugs. There is so much more to learn about the genetic and epigenetic mechanisms of medicinal plants. Modern sequencing platforms help to understand the unique structural organization of genes and the regulatory mechanisms that have expression patterns thus allowing the generation of catalogs of specialized metabolism in a way that is immeasurable to the herbalists who first identified their healing properties long back.

KEYWORDS

- **genomics**
- **anticancer properties**
- **medicinal plants**
- **secondary metabolite**

REFERENCES

Akhtar, M. S.; Swamy, M. K. Eds. *Anticancer Plants: Mechanisms and Molecular Interactions*; Springer: Singapore, 2018.

Ashraf, M. A. Phytochemicals as Potential Anticancer Drugs: Time to Ponder Nature's Bounty. *Biomed Res. Int.* **2020,** *2020*, 8602879.

AUGUSTUS. https://bio.tools/AUGUSTUS (accessed June 4, 2021)

Basic Local Alignment Search Tools. https://blast.ncbi.nlm.nih.gov/Blast.cgi (accessed June 2, 2021)

CAP3-Contig Assembly Program. https://www.msi.umn.edu/sw/cap3-contig-assembly-program (accessed June 2, 2021)

Catchen, J.; Amores, A.; Hohenlohe, P.; Cresko, W.; Postlethwait, J. *Stacks: Building and Genotyping Loci de novo from Short-read Sequences. G3: Genes, Genomes. Genetics.* **2011,** *1*, 171–182.

Catchen, J.; Hohenlohe, P. A.; Bassham, S.; Amores, A.; Cresko, W. A. Stacks: An Analysis Tool Set for Population Genomics. *Mol. Ecol.* **2013,** *22* (11), 3124–3140.

Chakraborty, P. Herbal Genomics as Tools for Dissecting New Metabolic Pathways of Unexplored Medicinal Plants and Drug Discovery. *Biochim. Open.* **2018,** *6*, 9–16.

Chen, S.; Xu, J.; Liu, C.; Zhu, Y.; Nelson, D. R.; Zhou, S.; Sun, C. Genome Sequence of the Model Medicinal Mushroom Ganoderma lucidum. *Nat. Commun.* **2012,** *3* (1), 1–9.

Cruaud, A.; Gautier, M.; Rossi, J. P.; Rasplus, J. Y.; Gouzy, J. RADIS: Analysis of RAD-seq Data for Interspecific Phylogeny. *Bioinform.* **2016,** *32* (19), 3027–3028.

De la Bastide, M.; McCombie, W. R. Assembling Genomic DNA Sequences with PHRAP. *Curr. Protoc. Bioinform.* **2007,** *17* (1), 11–4.

Duitama, J.; Quintero, J. C.; Cruz, D. F.; Quintero, C.; Hubmann, G.; Foulquie-Moreno, M. R.; Tohme, J. An Integrated Framework for Discovery and Genotyping of Genomic Variants from High-throughput Sequencing Experiments. *Nucleic Acids Res.* **2014,** *42* (6), e44–e44.

Duran, C.; Boskovic, Z.; Imelfort, M.; Batley, J.; Hamilton, N. A.; Edwards, D. CMap3D: A 3D Visualization Tool for Comparative Genetic Maps. *Bioinform.* **2010,** *26* (2), 273–274.

Eaton, D. A. PyRAD: Assembly of De Novo RADseq Loci for Phylogenetic Analyses. *Bioinform.* **2014,** *30* (13), 1844–1849.

Genomics and Comparative Genomics. https://www.integratedbreeding.net/courses/genomics-and-comparative-genomics/www.generationcp.org/genomics/indexba4f.html?page=1177 (accessed June 2, 2021)

Hao, D. C.; Xiao, P. G. Genomics and Evolution in Traditional Medicinal Plants: Road to a Healthier life. *Evol. Bioinform.* **2015,** *11*, EBO–S31326.

Iqbal, J.; Abbasi, B. A.; Mahmood, T.; Kanwal, S.; Ali, B.; Shah, S. A.; Khalil, A. T. Plant-derived Anticancer Agents: A Green Anticancer Approach. *Asian Pac. J. Trop. Biomed.* **2017,** *7* (12), 1129–1150.

Khan, T.; Ali, M.; Khan, A.; Nisar, P.; Jan, S. A.; Afridi, S.; Shinwari, Z. K. Anticancer Plants: A Review of the Active Phytochemicals, Applications in Animal Models, and Regulatory Aspects. *Biomolecules.* **2019,** *10* (1), 47.

Kim, B. Y.; Park, H. S.; Kim, S.; Kim, Y. D. Development of microsatellite markers for Viscum coloratum (Santalaceae) and their Application to Wild Populations. *Appl. Plant Sci.* **2017,** *5* (1), 1600102.

Li, F.W.; Harkess, A. A Guide to Sequence your Favorite Plant Genomes. *Appl. Plant Sci.* **2018,** *6* (3), 1030. DOI: 10.1002/aps3.1030.

Li, H.; Ruan, J.; Durbin, R. *Maq: Mapping and Assembly with Qualities*; 2008, Version 0.6,3, 508.

Lin, H.; Zhang, Z.; Zhang, M. Q.; Ma, B.; Li, M. ZOOM! Zillions of Oligos Mapped. *Bioinform.* **2008,** *24* (21), 2431–2437.

Luo, R.; Liu, B.; Xie, Y.; Li, Z.; Huang, W.; Yuan, J.; Wang, J. SOAPdenovo2: An Empirically Improved Memory-efficient Short-read De Novo Assembler. *Gigascience.* **2012,** *1* (1), 2047–217X.

Medicinal Plant Genomics resource. http://medicinalplantgenomics.msu.edu/ (accessed June 2, 2021)

Mehta, A.; Hasija, Y. Bioinformatics Approaches for Genomics and Post Genomics Applications of Anticancer Plants. In *Anticancer Plants: Mechanisms and Molecular Interactions*. Springer: 2018; 238–317.

Mining Plant Genomes. A Modern Approach to Herbal Healing. https://www.ddw-online.com/mining-plant-genomes-a-modern-approach-to-herbal-healing-1018-201904/ (accessed May 29, 2021)

Moumbock, A. F.; Simoben, C. V.; Wessjohann, L.; Sippl, W.; Günther, S.; Ntie-Kang, F.; Badria, F. A. Computational Studies and Biosynthesis of Natural Products with Promising Anticancer Properties. *Natural Products and Cancer Drug Discovery. Intech Open, Rijeka.* **2017,** 257–285.

Pan, X.; Stein, L.; Brendel, V. SynBrowse: A Synteny Browser for Comparative Sequence Analysis. *Bioinform.* **2005,** *21* (17), 3461–3468.

SAM tools. http://samtools.sourceforge.net/ (accessed June 2, 2021)

Tello, D.; Gil, J.; Loaiza, C. D.; Riascos, J. J.; Cardozo, N.; Duitama, J. NGSEP3: Accurate Variant Calling across Species and Sequencing Protocols. *Bioinform.* **2019,** *35* (22), 4716–4723.

Valdiani, A.; Javanmard, A.; Talei, D.; Tan, S. G.; Nikzad, S.; Kadir, M. A.; Abdullah, S. N. A. Microsatellite-based Evidences of Genetic Bottlenecks in the Cryptic Species "Andrographis Paniculata Nees": A Potential Anticancer Agent. *Mol. Biol. Rep.* **2013,** *40* (2), 1775–1784.

Vertebrate Genomic Team. https://www.ebi.ac.uk/about/vertebrate-genomics/software/exonerate (accessed June 8, 2021)

Weaver, B. A. How Taxol/Paclitaxel Kills Cancer Cells. *Mol. Biol. Cell.* **2014,** *25* (18), 2677–2681.

Wu, X.; Li, Q.; Feng, Y.; Ji, Q. Antitumor Research of the Active Ingredients from Traditional Chinese Medical Plant Polygonum Cuspidatum. *Evid.-Based. Complement. Altern. Med.* **2018,** *2018*, 2313021.

Zerbino, D. R. Using the Velvet De Novo Assembler for Short-read Sequencing Technologies. *Curr. Protoc. Bioinform.* **2010,** *31* (1), 11–5.

Zhang, Y.; Zheng, L.; Zheng, Y.; Zhou, C.; Huang, P.; Xiao, X.; Li, C. Assembly and Annotation of a Draft Genome of the Medicinal Plant Polygonum Cuspidatum. *Front. Plant Sci.* **2019,** *10*, 1274.

[illegible] Plant Resources [illegible]
com [illegible] (accessed [illegible]).

[illegible] Natural Products with Anticancer Properties. *Natural Products and Cancer Drug Discovery* [illegible] 2017, 257–285.

Pan, X.; Stein, L.; Brendel, V. SynBrowse: A Synteny Browser for Comparative Sequence Analysis. *Bioinformatics* 2005, 21 (17), 3461–3468.

[illegible] (accessed June 2, 2021).

[illegible] Calling [illegible] and Sequencing Protocols. [illegible] 2019, 35 (22), [illegible]

[illegible] Based Evidence [illegible] 2017.

CHAPTER 8

Metabolomics of Anticancer Plants

S. RUTH ASSUMI[1], KHANMI KASOMVA[2], and POOJA BHADRECHA[3]

[1]*Division of System Research and Engineering, ICAR Research Complex for NEH Region, Meghalaya, India*

[2]*Functional Genomics Laboratory, School of Biotechnology, Jawaharlal Nehru University, New Delhi, India*

[3]*University Institute of Biotechnology, Chandigarh University, Chandigarh, Punjab, India*

ABSTRACT

Millions of people lose their lives to cancer per year. Various treatments have been invented and employed to cure cancer and give promising results, but they also lead to severe side-effects. Hence, researchers have been turning toward the utilization of natural sources, like herbal plant extracts, to cure this deadly disease. Implementation of some latest omics-techniques to grab the best potential from nature's treasuries have given outstanding results. In this chapter, we have discussed the bioactive compounds present in some herbal plant extracts and the applications of metabolomic tools. Anticancer properties of plants like *Artemisia annua*, *Tinospora cordifolia*, *Ziziphus nummularia*, *Phyllanthus emblica*, and *Centella asiatica* have been discussed in detail. The chapter also enlightens the utilization of metabolomic tools like mass spectrometry, nuclear magnetic resonance, gas chromatography-mass spectrometry, liquid chromatography-mass spectrometry, and METLIN for exploring metabolite profiles of these extracts.

Plant-Derived Anticancer Drugs in the OMICS Era: Biosynthesis, Functions, and Applications.
Deepu Pandita, Anu Pandita (Eds.)

8.1 INTRODUCTION

Unfortunately, in this digital era whether it is a developed or developing nation, we are still fighting with cancer epidemic as one of the public health and economic disasters. More than nineteen million new cases of cancer were recorded in the year 2020, with almost 10 million people losing their life. Such alarming statistics since last few decades have popularized research areas focussing on the detection and treatment of cancer. Exclusive technologies like gene therapy, chemotherapy, and radiation therapy are employed world-wide to treat cancer. Several conventional as well as advanced techniques developed against cancer cells. Though they stand promising as a treatment, many side-effects are associated with these therapies. Moreover, highly metastatic and aggressive cancer patients commonly develop chemotherapy and radiation therapy resistance (Sung et al., 2021; Khan et al., 2020). As this problem persists in the treatment, new approaches or therapeutic drugs are needed for the control of the disease.

The irrepressible and complicated disease "cancer" has been defined as an unbeatable proliferation of cells, which leads to the formation of tumor which eventually exaggerates to organs and/or lead to metastasis. Heredity, alterations at the level of oncogenes, regulatory systems for cell cycles, and cell death are considered the major possibilities for such uncontrolled cell divisions. Other factors like ionizing radiations, reactive oxidative species (ROS), somatic mutations, and various other chemical and biological agents have been identified and classified as major carcinogens by the WHO. Ionizing radiation alters the hydrogen double bonds present in nucleic acids, modifying their chemical structure, which affects genetic expression and regulation. Bacterial, fungal, and viral infections have been recorded to lead to cancer formation as the after-effects, for example, HPV (human papilloma virus) is known to be a reason behind cervical cancer, the hepatitis B and hepatitis C to liver cancer, *Salmonella* infections to colon or gallbladder cancer, etc. (Valent et al., 2012; Fernald and Kurokawa et al., 2013; Stewart and Wild, 2014; Narayanan and Saladi, 2010; Zhao et al., 2016; Martin and Gutkind, 2008). Figure 8.1 represents the general carcinogens, as per WHO (Garcia-Oliveira et al., 2021).

Though hydrogen peroxide and other hydroxyl radicals are the general metabolic products, they may arise as ROSs on contact with oxygen and may elicit membrane alterations and disruptions in nucleic acids and proteins, and hence ROSs result in proliferation of tumorous cells. Significant carcinogens of chemical origin, like hydrocarbons which are

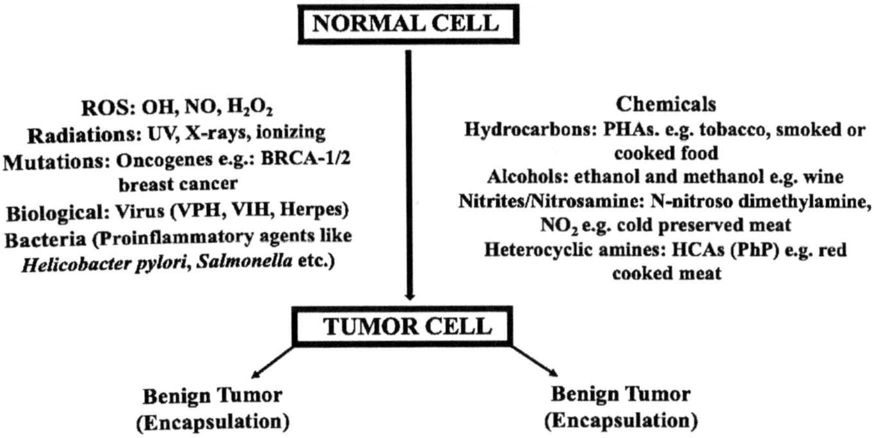

FIGURE 8.1 Cancer-causing agents.

polycyclic aromatic (PAHs), alcohol, compounds of N-nitroso, and amines which are heterocyclic in nature (HCAs) are present in the diet. Examples include anthracenes (PAHs), 2-amino-1-methyl-6-phenylimidazo-4,5-bi-pyridine (HCAs), N-nitrosedimethylamine, ethanol, and other alcohols present in beverages (Hansen et al., 2010; Reuter et al., 2010; Shen et al., 2014; Bansal and Kim, 2015; Song et al., 2015).

8.2 ANTICANCER PLANTS

Traditionally, herbs are utilized since hundreds of years because they possess the capability of neutralizing and diminishing diseases. Chemical compounds extracted from herbal medicines have proved efficient and harmless in treating cancer and are also easily accessible. Plant metabolites with anticancer properties cause apoptosis and hinder proliferation of cancerous cells, for example, anticancer medicinal plants such as *Phaleria macrocarpa*, *Fagonia indica* are well documented to contain active compounds with anticancer properties. The fruits of *P. macrocarpa* contain gallic acid which is well-studied for stimulation of programmed cell deaths in case of leukemia and adenocarcinoma cell lines. Several other compounds like vinca alkaloids, camptothecin, and podophyllotoxin extracted from plants have been documented for their potential as anticarcinogens (Khan et al., 2020). Major anticancer components of plant origin have been classified as the derivatives of camptothecin, epipodophyllotoxins, taxanes, and vinca alkalids. The exclusive examples of camptothecin derivatives include camptotecin and irinotecan; examples of epipodophyllotoxins are etoposide and teniposide; examples of taxanes are docetaxel as well as paclitaxel; whereas the examples of vinca alkaloids include vinblastine, vincristine, and vindesine, all of which are recorded with anticancerous properties (Desai et al., 2008).

Herbal plants have been well-known and studied from various decades for their outstanding medicinal values. Hence, they are actively under investigation for some promising anticancerous potentials. Several extracts from herbal plants have been documented to possess some splendid potentials for curing different types of cancer (Figure 8.2) (Khan et al., 2020). Examples of some herbal plants reported to be potential anticancer agents have been listed in Table 8.1. (Figure 8.3) presents a schematic illustration of plant extracts with the anticancer properties they possess (Khan et al., 2020).

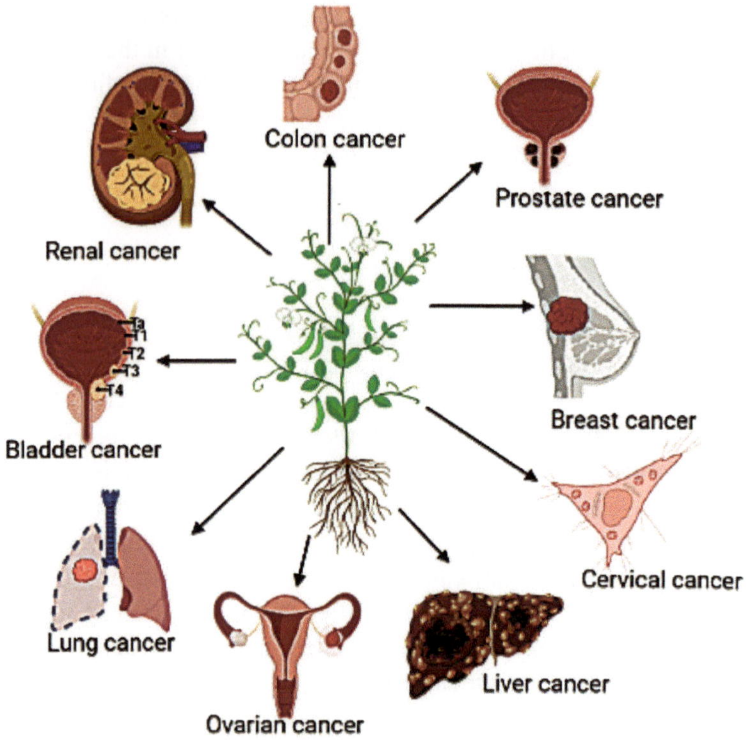

FIGURE 8.2 Anticancer properties of plant metabolites.

Source: Adapted from Khan et al., 2020.

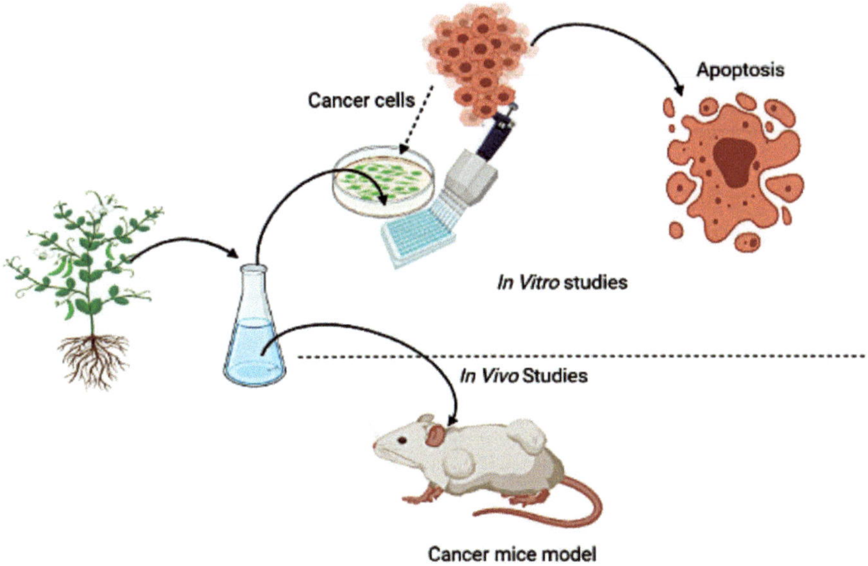

FIGURE 8.3 Illustration for plant extracts' anticancer activities.
Source: Adapted from Khan et al., 2020.

In the following section, we have discussed about different plants which have been exclusively explored for anticancerous potentials.

8.2.1 *ARTEMISIA ANNUA*

A. annua is an herbal plant from China that is popular as "sweet wormwood," has amazing medicinal values and hence has been used traditionally to treat malaria, jaundice, and hepatitis in Asian and African countries and has been reported to be very helpful in medical conditions like headache, nausea, excessive sweating, and infections. A compound termed as Artemisinin (ART) is present in extracts of *A. annua*, which has a sesquiterpene lactone structure with a bridge of peroxide in their (Cangcang et al., 2020; Lang et al., 2019; Slezakova et al., 2017; Khan et al., 2020). ART as well as its derivatives such as artemether, arteether, sodium artesunate, and sodium artelinate are enlisted as artemisinin compounds (Cangcang et al., 2020), which are generally hydrophobic and mainly act within the cell's membrane system and organelles like endoplasmic reticulum, vacuoles, mitochondrion, etc. ART's central mechanisms of action enlist

TABLE 8.1 List of Herbal Plants with Active Compounds They Possess as Anticancer Agents.

Sr. No.	Name of plant	Parts used	Solvent used	Active compounds	Cancer cell line used	Animal model used
1.	*A annua* (Rassias et al., 2019)	Leaves	Methylene chloride	Artemisinin, dried leaves of *A. annua*	NSCLC cell lines A549, H1299, and PC9	Xenograft murine
2.	*T. cordifolia* (Mishra et al., 2015)	Stem	aqueous ethanolic extract	Betulin, Betulinic acid	IMR-32 human neuroblastoma cell line	
3	*P. amarus Schum.* and *Thonn* (Mohamed et al., 2021)	Whole plant parts, leaves, roots, and shoots	80% ethanolic	Phyllanthin, hypophyllahtin, nirtetralin, phyltetralin	HCT116 Human Colon Cancer Cells	
4	*P. emblica* (Mahata et al., 2013)	Fruit	aqueous extract	Corilagin, chebulagic acid, diterpenes, ellagic acid, and gallic acid	SiHa cells and HeLa cells	
5	*C. asiatica* (Naidoo et al., 2017; Babykutty et al., 2008; Hussin et al., 2014)	Whole parts	ethanolic extract methanolic extract juice	Asiatic acid, madecassic acid, asiaticoside, madecassoside, and madecassic acid	MCF-7, PBMC, and THP-1 cells	
6	*F. schweinfurthii* (Pareek et al., 2013)	Whole plant	ethanolic extract	Carbon tetrachloride	HepG2 cell line	Rats
7	*Garcinia Preussii* (Biloa Messi B et al., 2014)	Plant's fruits and leaves	Meohextract	Benzophenones	Du145, hela, ht-29, and a431 cell lines	
8	*Morus nigra* (Turan et al., 2017)	Airy parts of the plant	Extract with dimethyl sulfoxide	Ascorbic acid, chlorogenic acid, and other phenolic compounds	Human prostate adenocarcinoma (PC-3)	
9	*Nitraria retusa* (Boubaker et al., 2018)	Leaves	Chloroform extract	B-sitosterol and palmitic acid	B16-f10 cells lines	Balb/c mice

TABLE 8.1 *(Continued)*

Sr. No.	Name of plant	Parts used	Solvent used	Active compounds	Cancer cell line used	Animal model used
10	*Paris polyphylla* (Li et al., 2013)	Rhizomes	Methanol extract	Steroidal saponins	A549 cell line	Tumor-bearing mice c57bl/6
11	*Perilla frutescens* (Wang et al., 2012)	Plant leaves	Methanol extract	Isoegomaketone	Huh-7 hepatoma cell carcinoma	Tumor-xenograft nude mice
12	*Scutellaria baicalensis* (Sato et al., 2013)	Root	Aqueous extract	Baicalin	Cell line of human oral squamous cell carcinoma (OSCC)	
13	*Tussilago farfara* (Jo et al., 2008)	Flowers' buds	Methanolic extract	Quercetin-glycosides	Human colon cancer cells (Ht-29)	
14	*Wedelia chinensis* (Manjamalai et al., 2012)	Plant's Leaves	Essential oils form the plant	Carvocrol and trans-caryophyllene	Melanoma metastatic cell line (B16f-10)	C57bl/6 mice
15	*Platycodon grandifloras* (Manjamalai et al., 2012)	Root	Platycodin d was dissolved In Phosphate-buffered saline	Platycodin D	Human breast cancer cell line, mcf-7	

the generation of ROS, arresting the cell cycles at G_0/G_1 phases, apoptosis, suppression of angiogenesis, and ferroptosis. The synthetic compounds such as scopoletin and 1,8-cineole are synthesized from *A. annua*. Several artemisinin derivatives are well-documented for anticancer potentials; examples include arteether, artemether, and artesunate. Amongst these compounds, the effect of artesunate has been evaluated in different tumor cells including leukemia, glioblastoma, T-cell lymphoma, neuroblastoma, melanoma, embryonal rhabdomyosarcoma cells, and other cancers like breast, ovary, colon, hepatocellular, and renal cancer (Cangcang et al., 2020; Crespo-Ortiz et al., 2012; Krishna et al., 2008; Efferth, 2008).

Oncosis-non-apoptotic mode of cell death is described as rapid swelling of cells, organelles, problems related to permeability of cell membranes and cell lysis. Moreover, oncosis results in heightened ROS generation, swelling of mitochondrion, depleted ATP content, failed Ca^{2+} homeostasis, stimulation of some harmful proteases like calpains and cathepsins, disrupted lysosomes, and eventual breaching of the plasma membrane. Studies have shown that artesunate and plasma membrane rupture brings about cell lysis (oncosis-like) in case of cancer associated with the pancreas and renal cancer. Further, artesunate promotes cell oncosis by suppressing the VEGF (i.e. vascular endothelial growth factor) and heightening calcium contents by activation of calpain-2 in gastric cancer (Cangcang et al., 2020; Du et al., 2010; Jeong et al., 2015; Zhou et al., 2013). Moreover, artesunate induces caspase-mediated cell death and arrest of the cell cycle, through the decrease of Bcl 2 protein, as well as, enhancing the expression of Bax protein. In case of lung cancer, cancer cells are supressed by artesunate via regulating the potential of mitochondrial membrane, as well as, inducing programmed cell death through this mechanism (Zhao et al., 2020). Acetonitrile maceration enhanced the activity of *A. annua* extract-derived compounds, by inhibiting the viability of cells by the action of MDA-MB-231 and MCF-7 in breast cancer, MIA PaCa-2 in cases of pancreatic cancer, PC-3 for prostate cancer, A459 for the non-small cell lung cancer cells, and normal mammary epithelial cells, lymphocytes. The extract treatment elevated cell number during S and G2/M phases of the cell cycle, resulting in cell proliferation which eventually leads to deprivation in the potential of mitochondrial membrane and also the regulation of caspase3 activation, both of which contribute to generating apoptotic hypodiploid cell population. Furthermore, treatment using the plant's extracts supressed cell proliferation, diminished development of tumor and stimulated cell death in case of TNBC (triple-negative breast cancer) by MDA-MB-231 xenografts cultivated at CAM (chick chorioallantoic membrane) and nude mice (Lang et al., 2019). The mentioned phenomenon indicated artemisinin and its derivatives are promising therapeutic potential in the treatment of cancers.

8.2.2 *TINOSPORA CORDIFOLIA*

T. cordifolia is a common shrub found in India, Myanmar, Shri Lanka, and China; are from the family *Menispermaceae* and is popular as "guduchi," "giloya," and "heartleaf moonseed" in Sanskrit, Hindi, and English, respectively. The plant's stems are enriched with essential alkaloids and are hence the most popularly employed plant part for medicinal uses. It's potential as an effective cure for diabetes, inflammations, arthritis, allergies, stress, leprosy, malaria, and as an immunomodulators have spotlighted it as a significant plant for pharmacological applications. Similarly, the extracts have shown antiproliferative and antimetastasis effects against various cancers like prostate, liver, cervical, and against glioblastoma and neuroblastoma. The extracts of *T. cordifolia* have radioprotective and chemopreventive properties and have been reported to stimulate radio sensitization, differentiation, senescence, damage of DNA, and suppression of cells that are cancer stem-like in nature. The extracts' chemopreventive characteristic induces the antioxidant system in the body, whereas the radioprotective characteristic is credited by free radical scavenging system (Mishra et al., 2013; Sharma et al., 2019; Ansari et al., 2017; Mishra et al., 2015).

T. cordifolia 50% of ethanol extract has significantly reduced cell multiplication and stimulated differentiation of the glioblastoma cells. Reductions in cell proliferation have been reported to enhance senescence marker and mortalin's expression, and regulate their transfer between perinuclear and pancytoplasmic regions. Its major potential lies in quelling the production and availability of cyclin D1 protein which is a G_1/S phase-specific protein and the Bcl-xL proteins which are antiapoptotic in nature, which results in halting the target cells in cell cycle phases G_0/G_1 and G_2/M. Further cell migration as well as invasion is hacked by reducing the NCAM (neural cell adhesion molecule) plasticity markers, PSA-NCAM (polysialic acid neural cell adhesion molecule) along with matrix metalloproteinases-2(MMP-2) and 9. Similarly, the *T. cordifolia* hexane extracts and chloroform extracts significantly reduced cell proliferation and induced differentiation, enhanced the regulation of stress markers HSP70 and Mortalin as well as stimulated senescence. Moreover, the chloroform and hexane extract diminished the expression of NCAM, hence suppressing the transfer of U87MG glioblastoma and IMR-32 neuroblastoma. The extracted contents are harmless to healthy cells, which is an add-on significance for liability (Mishra et al., 2013; Sharma et al., 2019).

8.2.3 *ZIZIPHUS NUMMULARIA*

Z. nummularia is a common shrub in India that is thorny and belongs to the family of *Rhamnaceae*. It is popularly employed for treating cutaneous disorders, cough cold, typhoid, and pain. *Z. nummularia* presents important phytochemical such as tannins, flavonoids, steroids, glycosides, and alkaloids. It is well-documented for medicinal potentials like antioxidant, antipyretic, antinociceptive, anti-inflammation, analgesic, and effective in case of inflammation (Fardoun et al., 2017; Padalia et al., 2017). Compounds betulin and betulinic acid present in the plant's bark and stem extracts have shown antitumor activities (Desai et al., 2008). Betulin derivatives are utilized in cancer therapy since they possess exclusive selection properties for cancerous cells. These compounds target the mitochondrion membranes and alter their permeability which affects their potential across the membranes and discharge the soluble apoptotic factors (e.g. cytochrome C and AIF-apoptosis inducing factor) in cytoplasm. These compounds have been reporter trigger caspases and lead to the generation of ROS, an important process for cell death. Biased participation of p38 signaling in apoptosis is also proposed due to the phosphorylated pro-apoptotic mitogen-activated protein kinases (MAPKs) (Csuk et al., 2010; Fulda et al., 2005). Betulinic acid is reported to induce apoptosis via production of ROS, devastation of topoisomerase I, stimulation of MAPK cascade, angiogenesis suppression, modulation of pro-growth activators (transcription) along with altering aminopeptidase-N's activity. Additionally, induction of cell death by betulinic acid is brought about via p53- and CD95-independent mechanism. Such processes grant chemotherapeutic properties to betulinic acid, enabling them to kill cancerous cells (Eiznhamer et al., 2004; Desai et al., 2008).

8.2.4 PHYLLANTHUS AMARUS SCHUM. AND THONN

The popular herb *P. amarus Schum.* and *Thonn* from the *Euphorbiaceae* family grow exclusively subtropical and tropical regions of Asia, Africa, South America, and West Indies. The entire plant, including the leaves, roots, and shoots, was discovered to have medicinal properties, imparted by magnificent compounds like alkaloid, flavonoid, lignan, polyphenol, sterol, tannin, triterpene, and several volatile oils. *P. amarus* extracts comprise of lignan compounds like corilagnin, ellagic acid, gallic acid, nirtetralin, phyllanthin, phyltetralin, and polyphenols. The plant is documented for its medical potentials like ethano-pharmacological activities, effectiveness against inflammation, liver problems, neural diseases, cancer, kidney problems; and for being a good antioxidant with effective activities against virus, bacteria, hyperglycemic, and hypercholesterolemia. This plant possesses chemoprotective characteristics since it inhibits carcinogen activation, induce the arrest of cell cycles and hinders DNA repair which is possible due to its potential against carcinogenic compounds, stimulation of metabolism, arrest of cell cycles and disturbance caused while DNA repair (Desai et al., 2008; Harikrishnan et al., 2018; Jantan et al., 2016).

Around 80% of ethanol extracts from this plant display strong actions against inflammation. Some major examples documented are as follow: This plant's extracts possess TNF and interleukin, which are well-known pro-inflammatory cytokines; the plant's extracts increase regulation of lipopolysaccharide (LPS)-induced U937 macrophages; whereas cells pre-treated in LPS-induced U937 macrophages showed significant down-regulated increase in TNF and interleukin transcription. This mechanism supressed nuclear factor-kappa B (NF-κB), IκBα and IKKα/β's phosphorylation, along with re-established IκBα degradation, the expression of Akt, JNK, ERK, as well as protein kinase (MAPKs) activation by p38 mitogen. The extracts were also recorder to supress upstream signaling molecule's expressions (such as TLR4 and MyD88), that have important functions for activating NF-κB, MAPK, and PI3K-Akt signaling pathways. Similarly, an 80% ethanolic extract from plant *P. amarus* diminished growth as well as expansion in HCT116 cancer cells from human colon, while having no toxicity effect on normal human fibroblast CCD-18Co. Its phyllanthin and gallic acid extracts stimulated phosphatidylserine induced cell death by Caspases 3/7, 8, and 9(Mohamed et al., 2021; Harikrishnan et al., 2018). Besides that, the hexane extracts from *P. amarus* are rich in lignin and have proved efficient to inhibit P-glycoprotein (P-gp) function in vitro (Leite et al., 2006).

Furthermore, the compounds ethyl-8-hydroxy-8-methyl-tridecanoate and 1,7,8-trihydroxy-2-naphtaldehyde present in *P. amarus* extracts inhibited nitric oxide production significantly. These extracts are procured through an extraction method which utilizes n-hexane, ethyl acetate, and methanol. In a similar manner of isolation, compounds such as corilagin and geranii demonstrated strong activity of inhibition on interleukin-1β and tumor necrosis factor-α, which regulates lymphocyte proliferation, as well as release of cytokine from phagocytes (Jantan et al., 2016).

8.2.5 *PHYLLANTHUS EMBLICA*

The plant *P. emblica*, which has also been popularly known as *Emblica officinalis*, is called as "Indian Gooseberry" or "Amla." It refers to a subtropical and tropical fruit tree indigenous to China, India, Indonesia, the Malay Peninsula, and other South-East Asian countries. Several traditional medical lineages, including Chinese herbal medicines, Egyptian medicines, Tibetan medicines, Ayurvedic medicines, and others, make extensive use of the fruits of *P. emblica.* It is well documented for its antioxidant, hypolipidemic, hypoglycemic, antimicrobial, antiseptic, anti-inflammatory and antitumor properties. The fruit has huge contents of vitamin C (ascorbic acid), it contains a chemical compound of diterpenes such as gibberellins, triterpene lupeol, flavonoids, and polyphenols which possess cancer-preventative as well as antitumor activities (Mahata et al., 2013; Zhao et al., 2015; Liu et al., 2012). Mahat et al. (2013) demonstrated action mechanism of *P. emblica* fruit extract (PE) on activator protein-1(AP-1) activity and HPV (human papillomavirus) transcription, necessary for the tumorigenicity of cervical cancer cells. Binding of DNA was affected by the PE in HPV16-positive (SiHa) as well as HPV18-positive (HeLa) cervical cancer cells. PE-induced suppression of AP-1 is regulated by down-regulation of AP-1 constituent proteins (c-Jun, JunB, JunD, and c-Fos). This mechanism to inhibit AP-1 by PE suppresses viral transcription, which affects the growth as well as cell death of the cervical cancer cells (Mahata et al., 2013). The ripened fruit from *P. emblica L*, known as "*Fructus phyllanthi*," is dried and possesses several significant characteristics like anti-inflammatory as well as antitumor properties. The *F. phyllanthi* tannin fraction (PTF) refers to an extract preparation of dry fruits *F. phyllanthi*, that consist of high fractions of tannins, composed of chebulagic acid, corilagin, ellagic acid, as well as gallic acid. PTF from

P. emblica stimulated apoptosis in human lung squamous carcinoma cells (NCI-H1703) by suppressing p-ERK1/2 and MMP-2/9's expression while increasing p-JNK expression. Furthermore, *P. emblica* PTF induced cell death via the MAPK/MMP pathways (Zhao et al., 2015; Tang et al., 2020).

8.2.6 *CENTELLA ASIATICA*

C. asiatica, also known as "Gotu kola," "Asiatic pennywort", and "tiger herb" is a creeper found primarily in wetlands in India, Australia, China, Madagascar, Sri Lanka, South Africa, the South United States, South East Asia and along continental tropical America. Because of its diverse chemical properties, the entire plant has traditionally been used for formulating Ayurvedic and Chinese traditional medicines. The plant's extracts have been widely utilized for wound healing, insanity, asthma, leprosy, ulcers, and eczema, and also possess antidiabetic, anti-inflammatory, antioxidant, antitumor, cardio-protective, and hepato-protective properties. Triterpene saponosides and triterpene glycosides found in *C. asiatica* include asiatic acid, madecassic acid, asiaticoside, centellasaponin, madecassoside, sceffoleoside, and madecassic acid. Several other essential compounds of great medicinal values, like flavonoid derivatives, minerals, phenolic acids, polysaccharides, sterols, and vitamins are also present. In many types of cancer, the *C. asiatica* extract demonstrated anti-inflammatory, antioxidant, chemopreventive, and antiproliferative activity. Asiaticoside, the most abundant Triterpen glycoside compound extracted from C. asiatica, can be converted into Asiatic acid. By inducing apoptosis in cancer cells, this compound implements cytotoxicity on fibroblast cells (Babykutty et al., 2008; Hussin et al., 2014; Naidoo et al., 2017). Similarly, asiatic acid compounds can stimulate lung cancer cells via interference of mitochondrial activities (Wu et al., 2017).

C. asiatica's ethanolic leaf extracts' consequences on leukemic THP-1 cells and PBMCs (i.e., normal peripheral blood mononuclear cells) revealed that the extract can significantly reduce PBMC as well as THP-1 cell viability while increasing oxidant scavenging activity. This demonstrates that cytokine downregulation, like interleukin 1, 6, 10 and TNF, modulates inflammation in PBMC and THP-1 cells. In addition, suppressed activity of caspase-9,-3/7 activated apoptotic cell death (Naidoo et al., 2017). Similarly, *C. asiatica* juice had the potential of cytotoxic effects on cancer cells from liver via programmed cell death and DNA alterations. In addition, it could reduce the expression of c-mcy gene while increasing the gene expression (c-fos and c-erbB2) in tumor cells (Hussin et al., 2014). *C. asiatica* methanolic extracts stimulated cell death of MCF-7 cells of breast cancer, leading to condensation of the nucleus, lost membrane potential of mitochondrial, and DNA damage (Babykutty et al., 2008).

8.3 METABOLOMICS

The comprehensive study of metabolites, encompassing their molecular, structural and functional diversity, is referred as "metabolomics." These tiny molecules are elusive to explore because there's a wide spectrum of physicochemical properties that need to be considered for analysis. There are three steps involved in metabolomics analysis: Collection of data, preprocessing of the collected data and recognition of possible patterns. A combination of updated and advanced analytical techniques along with pattern recognition, represents significant factors for research in metabolomics (Clayton et al., 2006). Table 8.2 enlists some metabolomics tools which are available free of cost (Piasecka et al., 2019).

TABLE 8.2 Free of Cost Metabolomics Tools.

Tool	Reference
XCMS online	https://xcmsonline.scripps.edu/
MeltDB	https://meltdb.cebitec.uni-bielefeld.de/
PRIMe	http://prime.psc.riken.jp/
Workflow4Metabolics (W4M)	http://workflow4metabolomics.org/
MetaboAnalyst	https://www.metaboanalyst.ca/
MetFrag	http://c-ruttkies.github.io/MetFrag

Separation technologies utilized for analysis of metabolites include liquid chromatography (LC), gas chromatography (GC), HPLC-mass spectroscopy (HPLC-MS), UHPLC-MS, GC-MS, microscale separation, SFC-MS, CE-MS and supercritical fluid chromatography. Analysis of metabolites employs several techniques like NMR, GC-MS and LC-MS. In case of NMR technique, either a hydrogen spectrum (1 H NMR), a carbon spectrum (13C NMR), or a phosphorus spectrum (31P NMR) are popularly utilized, and among these 1 H NMR is the most widely employed method (Segers et al., 2019, Zhang et al., 2019; Zhang et al., 2013; Dong et al., 2012; Larive et al., 2015). Sample quality to be analyzed, and its characteristics like the sample matrix, physicochemical properties and concentration are the major perspectives to choose analytical techniques for metabolite samples (Segers et al., 2019). Metabolites are identified and analyzed via several databases for metabolome analysis, including the METLIN and NIST (Guijas et al., 2018; Domingo-Almenara et al., 2019). Figure 8.4 represents scheme to procure data analysis in studies dedicated to explore the metabolome.

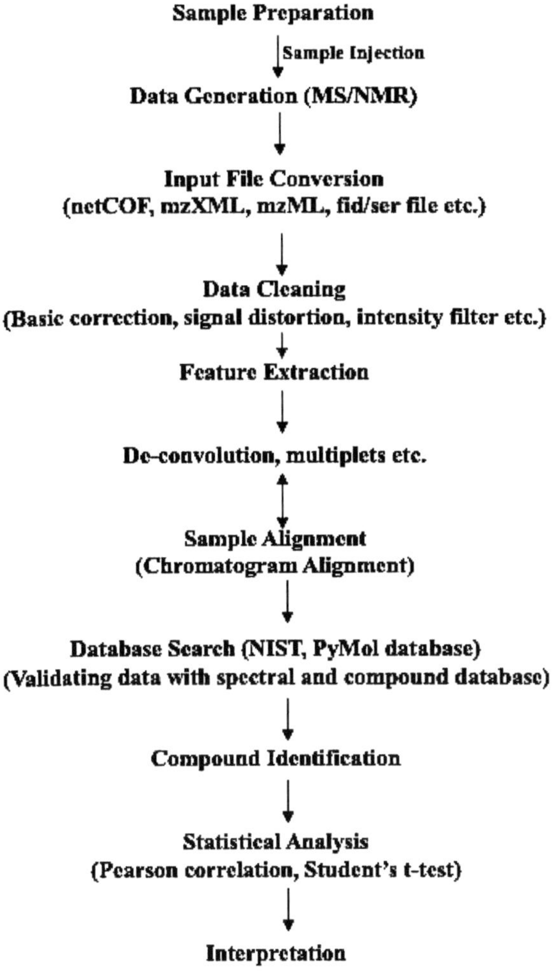

FIGURE 8.4 Scheme for data collection and analysis in metabolomics studies (Kumar et al., 2017).

Regular advancements in techniques available for the analysis of metabolites provide enable exclusive exploration of the biological processes at cellular and molecular levels, that too, at various growth stages, as a response to distinct stimuli and/or in case of several diseases/disorders and also acts as molecular signatures for identification of cell types. A mere exhibitor of phenotype which enables in-depth investigations of cellular metabolism of the normal as well as diseased tissues, discovery of biomarkers and formulation of personalized medicines, is referred as "metabolome". Still, extensive analysis and identification of metabolite pools, which are quite complex, remains disputed because the lendable methodologies demand a huge spectrum of parameters to be optimized (Scheubert et al., 2017). A comparative analysis of the most widely employed metabolomics tools is presented in Table 8.3 (Gomez-Casati et al., 2013).

TABLE 8.3 Distinct Feature of Some Commonly Used Techniques in Metabolomics.

Techniques	Uses	Characters
HPLC-MS	metabolite target analysis, metabolite profiling, metabolomics	Highly sensitive, it can detect and analyze the non-volatile metabolites, it is costly
GC-MS	metabolite target analysis, metabolomics	Highly sensitive, only the analysis of volatile metabolites is possible, non-expensive
NMR	metabolite profiling, metabolites flux analysis, metabolic fingerprinting	The method is safe and can be employed for metabolites which are abundant; method has lower sensitivity and is quite reproducible
MS	Analysis of targeted metabolites, generation of metabolite profiles, metabolomic studies, metabolites flux analysis, metabolic fingerprinting	Highly sensitive, mostly collaborated with other techniques
Raman spectroscopy	metabolic fingerprinting	Resolution and sensitivity are lower, the method is automated and high throughput

Few latest technological advances include integration of CSI:FingerID in SIRIUS4 to identify compounds; use of Chemoinformatic strategies for multi-level annotations to classify the sample compound and determine number of carbon (Duhrkop et al., 2019; Tsugawa et al., 2019). Platforms like MetaboAnalyst 4.0 are exploited for integrative metabolism, whereas annotations are based on the metabolic reaction's networks (Chong et al., 2018; Shen et al., 2019). Genome-scale metabolic standards aid the modeling of microbiome and hence use of different creative applications are utilized to analyze the metagenomic data and to detect the presence and identify the available metabolites which tend to modulate phenotypes (Garza et al., 2018; Guijas et al., 2018). As metabolomics is in a developing stage and expanding its horizons with all the excellence, a major credit relies on combinations of different -omics data which promises studies designed in upgraded sophisticated manners for general and specific analysis of data (Singh, 2020). Table 8.4 gives a glimpse of comparison of analytical techniques like NMR, with mass spectrometry techniques including HPLC-, SPC-, CE- and GC-mass spectrometry, and these all are popularly employed in metabolic profiling (Segers et al., 2019).

Table 8.5 represents a well-defined profile for the analysis of several metabolomics tools and techniques, highlighting their pros, cons, and areas of application (Panda et al., 2018). It is followed by the section where we discuss about few techniques like mass spectrometry, nuclear magnetic resonance, GC-MS, LC-MS and METLIN, which have been widely employed for metabolome analysis.

8.3.1 MASS SPECTROMETRY TECHNOLOGY

When it comes to metabolite profiling, the lead role is played by mass spectrometry and it is considered the most widely employed analytical tool because it offers profound specificity and high sensitivity, spotlighting it as one of the most reliable technique (Nakabayashi and Saito, 2013). The consistent upgradation of mass spectrometry techniques and its combinations with other -omics methodologies present it as one of the most trustworthy methodologies, utilized for a wide spectrum of analytical procedures (Sun et al., 2019; Sun et al., 2013). Consecutive advancements in analysis spectrum and applications of the technique permits better insights in understanding the pathogenesis of various infectious diseases and discovering various putative disease biomarkers. For applications in the field of plant science, various considerations involved are the ease for hyphenation of spectrometers with the desired separation methodologies (either gas chromatography or liquid chromatography, along

TABLE 8.4 Comparison of the Analytical Techniques for Metabolic Profiling

Property	Techniques					
	NMR	**HPLC-MS**	**UHPLC-MS**	**SFC-MS**	**CE-MS**	**GC-MS**
Sensitivity	-	++	+++	+++	+	+++
Reproducibility	High			Lower than NMR		
Resolution	Low			Higher than NMR		
Quantification	Yes			Yes; internal standard needed		
Amount of sample preparation	Low	Meduim	Medium	Medium	Medium	Extensive
Amount of sample requireed for injection	100-200 μl	± 10 μl	± 2-10 μl	± 1- 10 μl	1-20 nl	±1-2 μl
Range of metabolites	Polar and nonpolar	RPLC: Nonpolar HILIC: Polar		Polar and nonpolar	Polar	Volatile polar and nonpolar
Identification of metabolites	Easy		Difficult (database need to be improved)		Easy (spectral libraries)	

HILIC: Hydrophilic-interaction liquid chromatography; RPLC: Reversed-phase liquid chromatography; SFC-MS: Supercritical fluid chromatography mass spectrometry; UHPLC-MS: Ultrahigh-performance liquid chromatography mass spectometry

TABLE 8.5 Metabolomics Tools: Advantages, Disadvantages, and Applications.

Sr. No.	Analytical platform	Advantages	Disadvantages	Applications
1.	GC-MS (Hagel and Facchini, 2008; Ernst et al., 2014)	Volatile compounds are directly analyzed; databases are available; suitable for analysis of mixed samples	Recommended only for volatile and thermos-stable metabolites; demands derivatization depending on the sample; derivatization can interrupt the results	Low-molecular-weight hydrophobic compounds (essential oils, hydrocarbons, esters)
2.	LC-MS (Allwood and Goodacre, 2010; Ernst et al., 2014)	Demand for derivatization is surpassed; analysis of thermos-unstable metabolites	Technique is limited to targeted analysis only	Appropriate to analyze polar compounds
3.				
3.1	FT-ICR-MS (Ernst et al., 2014)	Trapping of ions by strong magnetic fields; stable calibration of instrument; detection is non-destructive; a complex mixture can be easily analyzed for thousands of components	Acquisition time is longer; not effective for isomers; not cost-effective; the dynamic range is short	Analysis of ions, high resolution MALDI, characterization of surfaces
3.2	TOF (Fuchs et al., 2009)	Highly sensitive; favorable for MALDI's pulsed ion generation	Dynamic range can be hindered using fast digitizer; restricted selectivity for the precursor ion	Applications in coordination with MALDI and GC-MS systems
4.	NMR (Kim et al., 2011)	Sample preparation is not complicated; fast analysis; quantification is easier; stereochemical data generates structural information	Inferior sensitivity; complex spectra for example in plant samples, result in overlapped signals	Analysis of various metabolites from fluid samples and microorganisms
4.1	1D NMR (Farag et al., 2012)	Less time for acquisition; prior separation not necessary	Signal overlap	Detection of metabolites, and distinction among two samples

TABLE 8.5 *(Continued)*

Sr. No.	Analytical platform	Advantages	Disadvantages	Applications
4.2	2D NMR (Forseth and Schroeder, 2011)	Resonance is spread in a different dimension and hence signal overlapping is suppressed	Longer acquisition time	Detection of metabolites, and distinction among two samples
4.3	Isotope- labeled NMR (Fan and Lane, 2011; Bothwell and Griffin, 2011)	Quantification of low concentration metabolites in biological samples; increase sensitivity and resolution of NMR	Isotope labels are too expensive; restricted potential for larger metabolites	Detection of metabolite pathway by tracing metabolites
4.4	Microcoil NMR (Cloarec et al., 2007; Gowda and Raftery, 2014)	Analysis of very small amounts of LC-MS samples possible; coinciding analysis of metabolites possible via NMR as well as MS from a single sample	Analysis gets interrupted by presence of high salt and protein content	Liquid-state NMR spectroscopy of tiny molecules; structural biology and genomics
4.5	HR-MASNMR (Bharti et al., 2011)	Information about the structure is procured in four-dimensional multitudes; minimal sample is required	Fruitful implementation, yet to be practiced	Detection and analysis of several classes of metabolites; chemotype variation study
4.6	NMRI (Borisjuk et al., 2013; As and Duynhoven, 2013; Sumner et al.,2015)	Paramagnetic nuclei's resonance intensity is employed to create images of metabolites present in the sample	Lower sensitivity, longer time duration for scanning, not cost-effective	Analysis of lipids inside seeds, study of C-allocation
5	HSQC (Ye et al., 2010; Tayyari et al., 2013)	Rapid detection of presence or absence of suspects in samples; less time requirements to analyze the data	Acquisition time spam may be longer and the spectrum recovered is in single dimension	Various types of samples can be detected and characterized

TABLE 8.5 *(Continued)*

Sr. No.	Analytical platform	Advantages	Disadvantages	Applications
6	J-resolved (Ludwig and Viant, 2010)	Distinct effects of chemical shift and J-coupling in two dimensions that are non-related, which reduces spectral crowding, as well as high resolution spectra on intact biological samples	Bigger size of file is produced, which has longer spectra acquisition time, and detection of metabolites is limited to systems that are homogenous	Detects metabolites that have a better resolution
7	SOFAST-^{1}H-^{15}N HMQ (Motta et al., 2010)	Monitoring metabolic pathway in real time	Single-dimension data acquisition	Pathway analysis

with capillary electrophoresis) and affirmable applications of various physical phenomena to ionize the molecules that are analyzed, and also, the separation of generated entities. These facts provide ample sensitivity, versatility, and reproducibility. The intense complexity in the case of sample mixtures of biological origin demands exclusive analysis which is successfully availed by MS analytical methodologies engaging LC, GC, and CE. These combinations yield exclusive separation and enhanced detection of metabolites, as depicted in Figure 8.5. Nevertheless, it's not just the advantages offered here. Their challenges and shortcomings are also bonded with these techniques. The major bottleneck in the evolution of this technology is the lack of comparative and correlative perspectives of data generated by the same samples by distinct research groups (Yang et al., 2019).

MS with its great sensitivity allow for attaining wide coverage of metabolome. This allows for the identification of biomarkers and molecules that can be used for construction of metabolic pathways (Kumar et al., 2017). As per the desired requirements, sample analysis may be organized in a targeted or untargeted manner. For targeted analysis, the test samples solid phase extraction methods are employed to improve samples quality in a distinct class of compounds, and this uses various solid phases in the employed cartridges with different solvents to elute the sample (Hou et al., 2008; Ma et al., 2008). Metabolite profiling for supervising quantitative and qualitative alterations in the composition of samples of biological origins is procured via untargeted approaches which allow analysis of samples that have undergone various environmental stress conditions. Sample preparation for this approach is quite elementary which requires extraction of biological entities utilizing water or other solvents that are organic. For analysis via mass spectrometry, the samples are either directly infused inside the chamber for ionization, or the separation is performed chromatographically before the mass spectrometry records, both of which promise high-resolution analysis (Piasecka et al., 2019; Prinsloo and Vervoort, 2018; Nakabayashi and Saito, 2013). For profiling the structural characteristics of natural products in the sample mixture, various MS techniques are applicable for analysis in a targeted manner. As the present compounds are analyzed, elucidation of structural data becomes possible in a single analysis (Kachlicki et al., 2016; Aliferis et al., 2014). Though mass spectrometry provides enough information regarding the identification and annotation of each compound, it doesn't promise elaborate structural

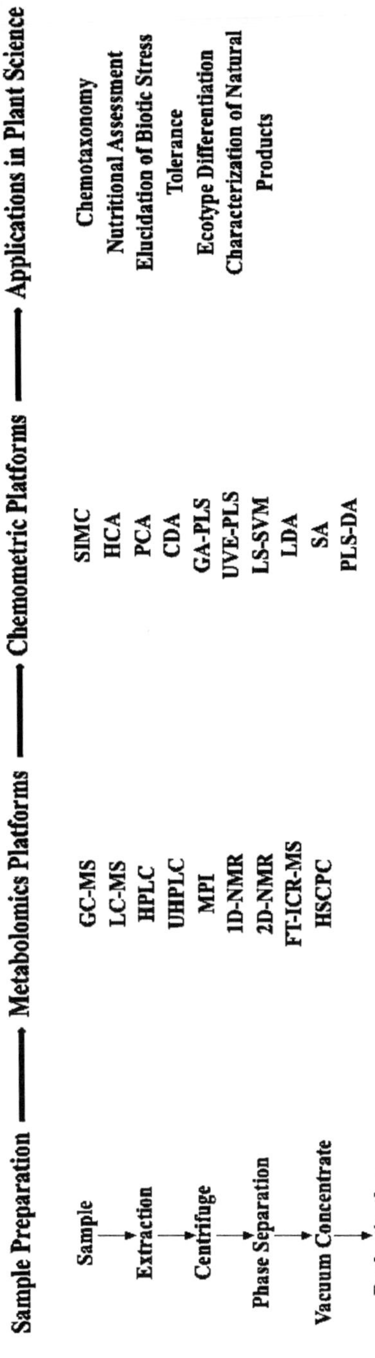

FIGURE 8.5 Standard pattern for metabolomics of plant samples

Source: Panda et al., 2018

analysis or excusive identification results of each natural product in the samples, which has been analyzed. Other methodologies offered by mass spectrometry include detailed profiling of a molecule's elementary composition which is extracted by ions' m/z measurements in high resolutions and accuracies (<5 ppm error-fourth decimal point accuracy), which must be aided via calculation of the isotopic patterns of protonated/deprotonated molecules. CID MS/MS (i.e., Collisional induced dissociation mass spectra) provides fragmentation patterns which permits the detection of several functional groups which might be present in the sample molecules. For the procedure of annotation, the chromatographic characters of the analyzed compounds must be considered. Few mass spectrometers rely on ion mobility spectroscopy (IMS) which allows separation of ions from compounds that co-elute during chromatography. In case of high molecular weight compounds which are widely distributed in the world of plants, the annotation of compounds doesn't just rely on the elemental composition of ions which though, have been recorded with high accuracy (error <1 ppm) (Kind and Fiehn, 2006). The additive data generated by targeted profiling of metabolites through CID MS/MS via mobility spectroscopy acquainted with mass analyzer, warranties better analyze selectivity (Gabelica and Matklund, 2018). As compounds vary in terms of their physicochemical characteristics, they have distinct ionization efficiency, which makes the interpretation of mass spectrometry data troublesome. In case of opting for ionization techniques like ESI (i.e., electrospray ionization) or APCI (i.e., atmospheric pressure chemical ionization), different proton affinities or deprotonation may occur. If the compound concentration exceeds five magnitude orders, additive issues occur in the dynamic range of mass analyzers, for example in case of hormones procured from plants, the samples fall in the spectrum of range lower than picomoles and millimoles. Such cases demand specialized strategies with optimized processing of metabolomic data (Kachlicki et al., 2016). Mass spectrometry technique is widely utilized for revealing the sample's metabolomics wherein the deciphering of metabolite patterns in plant tissues or cells becomes possible. The MALDI (i.e., matrix-assisted laser desorption ionization) and DESI (i.e., desorption electrospray ionization mass spectrometry) techniques are employed ionization of the metabolites (Wiseman et al., 2006; Boughton et al., 2016; Heyman and Dubery, 2016). Several techniques are implemented with mass spectrometry to study the metabolome. Table 8.6 presents several such techniques (Panda et al., 2018).

TABLE 8.6 Various Ionizing Techniques for Analysis of Metabolites.

Ionization technique	Mass	Advantages	Disadvantages	Applications
Electron Ionization/ Impact (Mirsaleh-Kohan et al. 2008; Castro et al., 2010; Abate et al., 2010)	<1000 Da	Used for volatile compounds, has duplicable mass spectra; and provides with the samples' structural information	Thermally volatile and stable samples can be analyzed	Elemental composition; quality assessment of natural products
Chemical Ionization (Munson, 2000)	<1000 Da	Detection of molecular weight is done using the ions; produces a simplified mass spectrum; as compared to EI, fragmentation is lesser	Volatile and stable metabolites can be detected; the fragment patterns are less informative	Commonly used for the analysis of cholesterol esters of fatty acid
Desorption Chemical Ionization (Vincenti, 2001)	<1500 Da	Reduced thermal decomposition; faster analysis; simpler instrumentation	Not particularly reproducible; fast heating is necessary for fast scanning; not suitable for large and heat-labile compounds	Characterization of large volatile molecules and nonpolar polymers
Negative Chemical Ionization (Raina and Hall, 2008)	<1000 Da	High sensitivity; efficient ionization; lesser fragmentation as compared to electron and chemical ionization	Poor duplicability	Very popular and efficient for analysis of environmental samples
Electrospray Ionization (Banerjee and Mazumdar, 2012)	<200,000 Da	Method efficient for detection of high molecular mass compounds; quadrupole mass analyzers allow accurate mass detection of samples	Cannot analyze the mixture very well, multiple charges that are attached to the molecular ions can interfere with spectral data	Extensively used to produce gas phase with fragmentation for heat-labile large supra-molecules
Desorption Electrospray Ionization (Dill et al., 2009; Harris et al., 2011)	<1000 Da	Collaborated analysis via electrospray and desorption ionization	Ionization is limited by the compound that is ionized by ESI	Chemical composition of atmospheric aerosols; identification of secondary metabolites

TABLE 8.6 *(Continued)*

Ionization technique	Mass	Advantages	Disadvantages	Applications
Desorption Corona Beam Ionization (Wang et al., 2010)	<600 Da	Pre-treatment of metabolites is not necessary; better localization of sampling area is received; congestion in mass spectra is lowered	Higher molecular weight compounds can't be analyzed; analysis is dependent on the sample's volatility	Mass spectra for pesticides, veterinary drugs, and natural drugs
Desorption Electrospray/ Metastable-Induced Ionization (Nyadong et al., 2009; Galhena, 2010)	<1000 Da	Wide polarity range; DART; multiple operational mode	Limited use in direct MSI due to the production of reactive stream	Multi-mode detection of intact drug
Easy Ambient Sonic-Spray Ionization (Haddad et al., 2006; Lalli et al., 2010; Porcari et al., 2016)	<1000 Da	A simple ion source is required; low charge density of the droplets decreases solvent chemical noise	Spatial resolution of analytes gets altered	Identification and inks; analysis of surface-modification brought about by polymers; complex matrix can be analyzed in a targeted manner; vegetable oils and drugs can be precisely analyzed
Probe Electrospray Ionization (Mandal et al., 2010; Harris et al., 2011)	<1000 Da	This technique employs a solid needle which solves the issue of clogging. High salt and urea contents are also tolerated, and it has higher ionization efficiency		Metabolites present as content of a high salt concentration solution can be detected
Fast Atom Bombardment (Ljung et al., 2010)	300-6000 Da	This fast and simplified technique is favorable for stable compounds which have higher mass and are stable in terms of thermodynamics. It is even suitable for nanomolar samples	This method is not advisable for compounds with multiple charges; Method offers low sensitivity	Plant hormone analysis

TABLE 8.6 *(Continued)*

Ionization technique	Mass	Advantages	Disadvantages	Applications
Secondary Ion Mass Spectrometry (Passarelli and Winograd, 2011)	300-13,000 Da	Similar to fast atom bombardment except for improved sensitivity	Target can get more heated due to more energetic primary beams; ion source requires more maintenance	Lipid imaging, polymer analysis, application in plants yet to be functionally elucidated
Atmospheric Pressure Chemical Ionization (Portoles et al., 2010)	<2000 Da	An appropriate method for compounds with lesser polarity; the LC/MS interface collaborates perfectly	Specific instruments are required and hence it becomes costly	Metabolite profiling, pesticide residue analysis
Matrix-Assisted Laser Disruption/Ionization (Harada et al., 2009; Miura et al., 2012)	<500,000 Da	The method is very fast and exclusive to detect mass	Availability of mass analyzers which have compatibility with pulsed ionization technique is essential	Analysis of small molecules; plant metabolomics study in response, natural drug discovery; protein analysis

8.3.2 NUCLEAR MAGNETIC RESONANCE

Nuclear magnetic resonance, commonly referred to as NMR, is another reliable technique for metabolomic analysis (Bayer et al., 1982; Jaroszewski, 2005a; Jaroszewski, 2005b). NMR results are reproducible and provide an unbiased metabolite profile. Moreover, NMR offers the opportunity to deliver additional structural information, in other words, about the presence of chemical functional groups and spatial decomposition of the chemical groups and to elucidate biochemical pathways (Lane and Fan, 2017; Agin et al., 2016). The detection sensitivity in NMR does not depend on acid-base properties nor on hydrophobicity of the metabolite, allowing a broader metabolome coverage in a single run than MS coupled to chromatographic techniques (Agin et al., 2016). Because of the simple sample preparation and short analysis times, NMR is suitable for high-throughput untargeted metabolomics but is nevertheless less applied than MS (Marx et al., 2018). Though quantitative comparability of the compounds analyzed is possible with NMR, it has lower sensitivity. And hence, for enriched results, NMR, and MS methods can be utilized in a collaborative manner (Prinsloo and Vervoort, 2018). NMR relies on employing the magnetic potential in the atoms' nuclei present at the magnetic field and refers to a non-destructive method followed to detect smaller metabolites (<50kD). It is use for profiling, finger printing, etc. but has low sensitivity. Commonly utilized spectrums for NMR analysis are 1H NMR (hydrogen spectrum), 13C NMR (carbon spectrum) and 31P NMR (phosphorus spectrum), but the most widely employed spectrum is the 1H NMR (Segers et al., 2019; Larive et al., 2015). NMR is a spectroscopic technique that is rapid as well as duplicable, which is dependent on the absorption of energy and re-emission from the atom's nuclei caused by alterations in magnetic field (Bothwell and Griffin, 2011) and distinct metabolomic records are generated which rely upon the nuclei targeted by the magnetic fields. Since it is omnipresent in biological samples, hydrogen has been a widely targeted nucleus (as in 1H-NMR) for analysis of samples of biological origin. Although less frequent, other atoms are also looked for NMR, including carbon (13C-NMR), and phosphorus (31P NMR), which offer additive information regarding specific metabolites (Reo, 2002). Sample analysis by NMR demands information regarding pH and ionic strength, distinct from that required for mass spectrometry. The spectral data generated via NMR allows for quantification of concentration of metabolites, along with presenting the records of sample's chemical structure (Alonso et al., 2015).

The main application of NMR in vivo is procuring detailed anatomical images from the human body by MRI, which is also referred as MRS (magnetic resonance spectroscopy), a technique that is non-invasive as well as, it can be applied in living organisms (van der Graaf, 2010). Another non-destructive and real-time NMR technique, like MRS, is HR-MAS (high-resolution magic angle spinning). This method represents the advantage of NMR, in solid-phase as well as liquid-phase (Gogiashvili, 2019). Higher resolution is obtained with both in liquid NMR and HR-MAS compared with MRS. HR-MAS was introduced in 1996 for the analysis of intact tissue specimens for cancer research. In that study, the gel-like nature of the tissue samples resulted in many variations in liquid NMR, due to the matrix. Therefore, it was necessary to work with 2D NMR, but still, the acquisition time was excessive, resulting in sample degradation. HR-MAS, on the other hand, allows analyzing the intact tissue samples with a high spectral resolution (Gogiashvili, 2019; Dinges et al., 2019). The method was applied for different research purposes, such as for database development of biopsy specimens (Ruhland et al., 2019), cancer research (Gogiashvili, 2019; Dinges et al., 2019; Cheng et al., 2019) and biomarker discovery for drug-resistant epilepsy (Detour et al., 2018). Verhoeven et al. (2017, 2018) developed a model that can directly quantify metabolites in 1D NMR spectra without deconvolution. This method was used for biofluids such as serum and plasma, but it will also be feasible for several biofluids which possess stable constitution and pH, for example, cerebrospinal fluid and cell extracts.

8.3.3 GC-MS, LC-MS

Gas chromatography-mass spectrometry is widely utilized for analysis to be done in an untargeted manner (Dutta et al., 2012) and it requires derivatization of test samples which results in generation of volatile compounds; however, it results in unnoticed underivatized compounds (except hydrocarbon). Use of GC X GC-TOF-mass spectrometry (Gas chromatography and time-of-flight) has effectively enhanced the distinction of co-eluting peaks as well as, it has allowed better sample analysis (Ralston-Hooper et al., 2008). LC-mass spectrometry generally employs

Electrospray ionization (ESI) along with atmospheric pressure chemical ionization (APCI) for targeted as well as non-targeted approaches in identifying both primary and secondary metabolites of a higher mass (Turner et al., 2016). Also, combining UPLC with Quadrupole time-of-flight mass spectrometry (QTOF-MS) enhances the resolution of peaks, accuracy in terms of mass and faster detection of several metabolites in a smaller time duration (Chawla and Ranjan, 2016). CE- mass spectrometry separates distinct classes of analyzes at a very précised scale, as per their charges, whether the analysis is targeted or untargeted (Ramautar and de Jong, 2014). Fourier transform ion cyclotron resonance mass spectrometry (FT-ICR-MS) mass analysis is a high-resolution technique that offers high accuracy determination to detect metabolites at large-scale (Brown et al., 2005), which may be collaborated with techniques specific for separation, for resolving "very complex matrices" (Schrader and Klein, 2004) as well as attaining other perspectives like ion separation (Lopes et al., 2017). Additionally, high-field asymmetric waveform ion mobility spectrometry (known as FAIMS) and differential mobility spectrometry (DMS) refer to the electrophoretic technique coupled with MS, which is based on ion mobility. FAIMS technology has also been employed to detect the production of any volatile compounds during the growth phase of bacterial population (Zrodnikov and Davis, 2012). GC/MS and LC/MS, effectively provide a scientific basis of resolving any problem related to metabolite research and elucidating metabolic pathways. Figure 8.6 represents the standard pathway followed for analysis of untargeted metabolites in biological samples.

8.3.4 METLIN

The identification and characterization of known, as well as unknown molecules present in sample mixtures has become possible by combination of MS/MS generated data with METLIN. METLIN aims at overcoming the issues generated while sample analysis for metagenomics, activity screening, experimentations to trace isotopes, and facilitating use of metabolomic procedures in guiding data interpretation for system biology. The most popular feature of Fragment Similarity Search is to characterize the unknowns, which id developed by increasing the concentration of recently incorporated, known compounds, with the mass spectrometry/

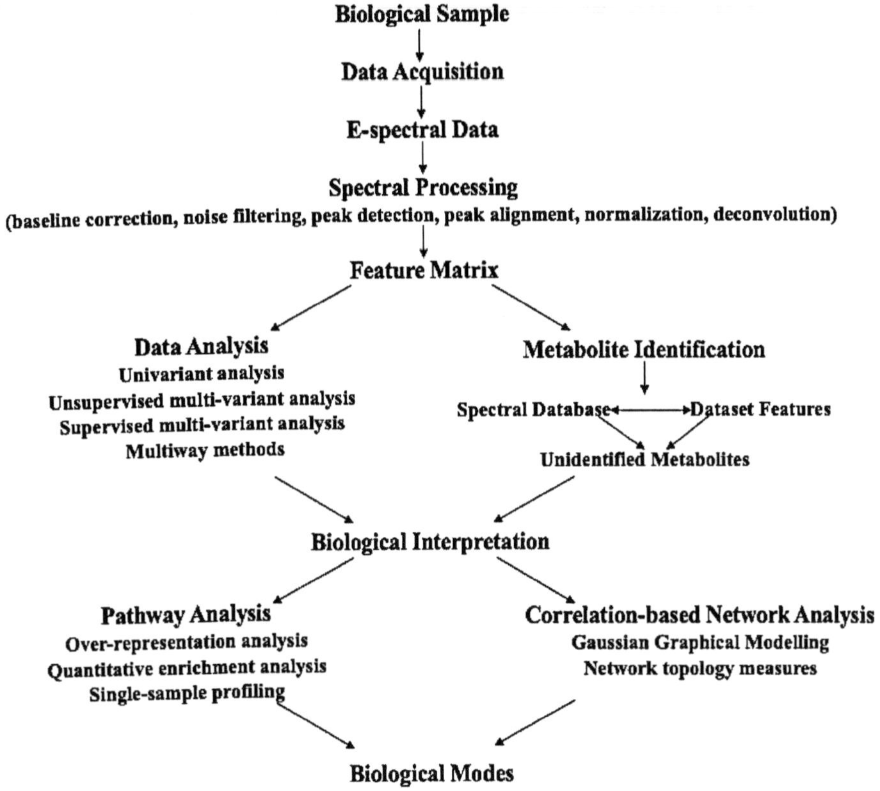

FIGURE 8.6 Metabolic analysis of untargeted metabolomic studies (Alonso et al., 2015).

mass spectrometry records. METLIN keeps integrating within cloud-based XCMS bioinformatic platform, which permits detection of documented molecules, as well as identification of the unknown molecules, and since there are such provisions offered by this technique, it has been exclusively utilized worldwide and has been consistently upgraded and expanding. While the sample is undergoing analysis, the METLIN data is collected in negative and positive ionization modes, that too at multiple collision energies. It has been successfully implemented among multiple tandem MS instruments, by providing a high-resolution spectrum, which has been developed and is curated from the standard values and their respective stable isotope analogs, manually. Several databases that secure data procured from electron impact (EI) or nuclear MR (NMR) studies are complementary to METLIN data records (Kind et al., 2017;

Vinaixa et al., 2016; Wishart et al., 2007). Fagged records collected via tools with outstanding performances, further refined on data processing platforms, tools, and resources like Allocator, ChromaTOF, MET-Align, MET-COFEA, MET-XAlign, MS-Assisted Resolution of Signals (MARS) (Zhang et al., 2014, 2015; Pegasus, 2003; Misra and van der Hooft, 2016; Ma et al., 2016; Kessler et al., 2014; Lommen et al., 2012). The identified metabolites get further subjected to statistical analysis for correlation mapping, analysis of boxplot, heatmap, K-means clustering, partial least squares, principal component as well as reconstruction of the metabolic pathways, using online tools like MetaboAnalyst, Cytoscape, Statistical analysis tool and so on (Tsugawa et al., 2015; Xie et al., 2015).

KEYWORDS

- **metabolomics**
- **mass spectrometry (MS)**
- **nuclear magnetic resonance (NMR)**
- **gc-ms, lc-ms**
- **metlin**
- **anticancer plants**
- ***Artemisia annua***
- ***Tinospora cordifolia***
- ***Ziziphus nummularia***

REFERENCES

Abate, S.; Ahn, Y. G.; Kind, T.; Cataldi, T. R. I.; Fiehn, O. Determination of Elemental Compositions by Gas Chromatography/time-of-flight Mass Spectrometry using Chemical and Electron Ionization. *Rapid Commun. Mass Spectrom.* **2010,** *24,* 1172–1180.

Agin, A.; Heintz, D.; Ruhland, E.; Chao de la Barca, J. M.; Zumsteg, J.; Moal, V.; Gauchez, A. S.; Namer, I. J. Metabolomics–An Overview. From Basic Principles to Potential Biomarkers (Part 1). *Med. Nucleaire.* **2016,** *40* (1), 4–10.

Aliferis, K. A.; Faubert, D.; Jabaji, S. A. Metabolic Profiling Strategy for the Dissection of Plant Defence against Fungal Pathogens. *PLoS One.* **2014,** *9,* e111930.

Allwood, J. W.; Goodacre, R. An Introduction to Liquid Chromatography-mass Spectrometry Instrumentation Applied in Plant Metabolomic Analyses. *Phytochem. Anal.* **2010,** *21*, 33–47.

Alonso, A.; Marsal, S.; Julia, A. Analytical Methods in Untargeted Metabolomics: State of the Art in 2015. *Front. Bioeng. Biotechnol.* **2015,** *3*, 23.

Ansari, J. A.; Rastogi, N.; Ahmad, M. K.; Mahdi, A. A.; Khan, A. R.; Thakur, R.; Srivastava, V. K.; Mishra, D. P.; Fatima, N.; Khan, H. J.; Waseem, M. ROS Mediated Pro-apoptotic Effects of *Tinospora cordifolia* on Breast Cancer Cells. *Front. Biosci.* (Elite Ed). **2017,** *9*, 89–100.

As, H. V.; and Duynhoven, J. V. MRI of Plants and Foods. *J. Magn. Reson.* **2013,** *229*, 25–34.

Babykutty, S.; Padikkala, J.; Sathiadevan, P. P.; Vijayakurup, V.; Azis, T. K.; Srinivas, P.; Gopala, S. Apoptosis Induction of *Centella asiatica* on Human Breast Cancer Cells. *Afr. J. Tradit. Complement Altern. Med.* **2008,** *6* (1), 9–16.

Banerjee, S.; Mazumdar, S. Electrospray Ionizationmass Spectrometry: a Technique to Access the Information beyond the Molecular Weight of the Analyte. *Int. J. Anal. Chem.* **2012,** 1–40.

Bansal, V.; Kim, K. H. Review of PAH Contamination in Food Products and their Health Hazards. *Environ. Int.* **2015,** *84*, 26–38.

Bayer, E.; Albert, K.; Nieder, M.; Grome, E.; Wolff, G.; Rindlisbacher, M. Online Coupling of Liquid Chromatography and High Field Nuclear Magnetic Resonance Spectrometry. *Anal. Chem.* **1982,** *54*, 1747–1750.

Bharti, S. K.; Bhatia, A.; Tewari, S. K.; Sidhu, O. P.; Roy, R. Application of HR-MAS NMR Spectroscopy for Studying Chemotype Variations of *Withania somenifera (L.) Dunal. Magn. Reson. Chem.* **2011,** *49*, 659–667.

Biloa Messi, B.; Ho, R.; Meli Lannang, A.; Cressend, D.; Perron, K.; Nkengfack, A. E.; Carrupt, P. A.; Hostettmann, K.; Cuendet, M. Isolation and Biological Activity of Compounds from *Garcinia preussii. Pharm. Biol.* **2014,** *52* (6), 706–11.

Borisjuk, L.; Rolletschek, H.; Neuberger, T. Nuclear Magnetic Resonance Imaging of Lipid in Living Plants. *Prog. Lipid. Res.* **2013,** *52*, 465–487.

Bothwell, J. H. F.; Griffin, J. L. An Introduction to Biological Nuclear Magnetic Resonance Spectroscopy. *Biol. Rev. Camb. Philos. Soc.* **2011,** *86*, 493–510.

Boubaker, J.; Ben Toumia I.; Sassi, A.; Bzouich-Mokded, I.; Ghoul Mazgar, S.; Sioud, F.; Bedoui, A.; Safta Skhiri, S.; Ghedira, K.; Chekir-Ghedira, L. Antitumoral Potency by Immunomodulation of Chloroform Extract from Leaves of *Nitraria retusa*, Tunisian Medicinal Plant, Via its Major Compounds β-sitosterol and Palmitic Acid in BALB/c Mice Bearing induced Tumor. *Nutr. Cancer.* **2018,** *70* (4), 650–662.

Boughton, B. A.; Thinagaran, D.; Sarabia, D.; Bacic, A.; Roessner, U. Mass Spectrometry Imaging for Plant Biology: A review. *Phytochem. Rev.* **2016,** *15*, 445–488.

Brown, S. C.; Kruppa, G.; Dasseux, J. L. Metabolomics Applications of FT-ICR Mass Spectrometry. *Mass. Spectrom. Rev.* **2005,** *24*, 223–231.

Cangcang, X.; Huihui, Z.; Lingli, M.; Xiaoping, Y. Artemisinins as Anticancer Drugs: Novel Therapeutic Approaches, Molecular Mechanisms, and Clinical Trials. *Front. Pharmacol.* **2020,** *11*, 529881.

Castro, J.; Pregibon, T.; Chumanov, K.; Markus, R. K. Determination of Catechins and Caffeine in Proposed Green Tea Standard Reference Materials by Liquid

Chromatography-Particle Beam/Elactron Ionization Mass Spectrometry (LC-PB/EIMS). *Talanta.* **2010,** *82*, 1687–1695.

Chawla, G.; Ranjan, C. Principle, Instrumentation, and Applications of UPLC: A Novel Technique of Liquid Chromatography. *Open. Chem. J.* **2016,** *3*, 1–16.

Cheng, L. L.; Lean, C. L.; Bogdanova, A.; Bogdanova, A.; Wright Jr., S. C.; Acherman, J. L.; Brady, T. J.; Garrido, L. Enhanced Resolution of Proton NMR Spectra of Malignant Lymph Nodes using Magic-Angle Spinning. *Magn. Reson. Med.* **2019,** *36* (5), 653–658.

Chong, J.; Soufan, O.; Li, C.; Caraus, I.; Li, S.; Bourque, S.; Wishart, D. S.; Xia, J. MetaboAnalyst 4.0: Towards More Transparent and Integrative Metabolomics Analysis. *Nucleic. Acids Res.* **2018,** *46* (1,2), 486–494.

Clayton, T. A.; Lindon, J. C.; Cloarec, O.; Antti, H.; Charuel, C.; Hanton, C.; Provost, J. P.; Le Net, J. L.; Baker, D.; Walley, R. J.; Everett, J. R.; Nicholson, J. K. Pharmaco-Metabonomic Phenotyping and Personalized Drug Treatment. *Nature.* **2006,** *440* (7087), 1073–1077.

Cloarec, O.; Canpbell, A.; Tseng, L. H.; Braumann, U.; Spraul, M.; Scarfe, G.; Weaver, R.; Nicholson, J. K. Virtual Chromatographic Resolution Enhancement in Cryoflow LC-NMR Experiments Via Statistical Total Correlation Spectroscopy. *Anal. Chem.* **2007,** *79*, 3304–3311.

Crespo-Ortiz, M. P.; Wei, M., Q. Antitumor Activity of Artemisinin and its Derivatives: from a Well-known Antimalarial Agent to a Potential Anticancer Drug. *J. Biomed. Biotechnol.* **2012,** 247597.

Csuk, R.; Barthel, A.; Kluge, R.; Strohl, D.; Kommera, H.; Paschke, R. Synthesis and Biological Evaluation of Antitumour-active Betulin Derivatives. *Bioorg. Med. Chem.* **2010,** *18* (3), 1344–55.

Desai, A. G.; Qazi, G. N.; Ganju, R. K.; El-Tamer, M.; Singh, J.; Saxena, A. K.; Bedi, Y. S.; Taneja, S. C.; Bhat, H. K. Medicinal Plants and Cancer Chemoprevention. *Curr. Drug. Metab.* **2008,** *9* (7), 581–591.

Detour, J.; Bund, C.; Behr, C.; Cebula, H.; Cicek, E. A.; Valenti-Hirsch, M. P.; Lannes, B.; Lhermitte, B.; Nehlig, A.; Kehrli, P.; Proust, F.; Hirsch, E.; Namer, I. J. Metabolomic Characterization of Human Hippocampus from Drug-resistant Epilepsy with Mesial Temporal Seizure. *Epilepsia.* **2018,** *59* (3), 607–616.

Dill, A. L.; Ifa, D. R.; Manicke, N. E.; Ouyang, Z.; Cooks, R. C. Mass Spectrometric Imaging of Lipids using Desorption Electrospray Ionization. *J. Chromatogr. B: Anal. Technol. Biomed. Life Sci.* **2009,** *877*, 2883–2889.

Dinges, S. S.; Vandergrift, L. A.; Wu, S.; Berker, Y.; Habbel, P.; Taupitz, M.; Wu, C. L.; Cheng, L. L. Metabolomic prostate Cancer Fields in HRMAS MRS-profiled Histologically Benign Tissue Vary with Cancer Status and Distance to Cancer. *NMR Biomed.* **2019,** *32* (10), e4038.

Domingo-Almenara, X.; Montenegro-Burke, J. R.; Guijas, C.; Majumder, E. L. W.; Benton, H. P.; Siuzdak, G. Autonomous METLIN-guided in-source Fragment Annotation for Untargeted Metabolomics. *Anal. Chem.* **2019,** *9* (5), 3246–3253.

Dong, H.; Zhang, A.; Sun, H.; Wang, H.; Lu, X.; Wang, M.; Ni, B.; Wang, X. Ingenuity Pathways Analysis of Urine Metabolomics Phenotypes Toxicity of Chuanwu in Wistar Rats by UPLC-Q-TOF-HDMS Coupled with Pattern Recognition Methods. *Mol. BioSys.* **2012,** *8* (4), 1206–1221.

Du, J.-H.; Zhang, H.-D.; Ma, Z.-J.; Ji, K.-M. Artesunate induces Oncosis-like Cell Death in Vitro and has Antitumor Activity Against Pancreatic Cancer Xenografts in Vivo. *Cancer Chemother. Pharmacol.* **2010,** *65*, 895–902.

Duhrkop, K.; Fleischauer, M.; Ludwig, M.; Aksenov, A. A.; Melnik, A. V.; Meusel, M.; Dorrestein, P. C.; Rousu, J.; Bocker, S. SIRIUS 4: A Rapid Tool for Turning Tandem Mass Spectra into Metabolite Structure Information. *Nat. Methods.* **2019,** *16*, 299–302.

Dutta, A.; Shetty, P.; Bhat, S.; Ramachandra, Y.; Hegde, S. A Mass Spectrometric Study for Comparative Analysis and Evaluation of Metabolite Recovery from Plasma by Various Solvent Systems. *J. Biomol. Tech.* **2012,** *23*, 128–135.

Efferth, T. Artemisinins: Their Growing Importance in Medicine. *Trends Pharmacol. Sci.* **2008,** *29* (10), 520–7.

Eiznhamer, D. A.; Xu, Z. Q. Betulinic Acid: A Promising Anticancer Candidate. *IDrugs.* **2004,** *7* (4), 359–73.

Ernst, M.; Silva, D. B.; Silva, R. R.; Vencio, R. Z. N.; Lopes, N. P. Mass Spectrometry in Plant Metabolomics Strategies: From Analytical Platforms to Data Acquisition and Processing. *Nat. Prod. Rep.* **2014,** *31*, 784–806.

Fan, T. W. M.; Lane, A. N. NMR-based Stable Isotope Resolved Metabolomics in Systems Biochemistry. *J. Biomol. NMR.* **2011,** *49*, 267–280.

Farag, M. A.; Porzel, A.; Wessjohan, L. A. Comparative Metabolite Profiling and Fingerprinting of Medicinal Licorice Roots Using a Multiplex Approach of GC-MS, LC-MS and 1D NMR techniques. *Phytochem.* **2012,** *76*, 60–72.

Fardoun, M.; Al-Shehabi, T.; El-Yazbi, A.; Issa, K.; Zouein, F.; Maaliki, D.; Iratni, R.; Eid, A. H. *Ziziphus Nummularia* Inhibits Inflammation-induced Atherogenic Phenotype of Human Aortic Smooth Muscle Cells. *Oxid. Med. Cell Longev.* **2017,** 4134093.

Fernald, K.; Kurokawa, M. Evading Apoptosis in Cancer. *Trends Cell Biol.* **2013,** *23*, 620–633.

Forseth, R. R.; Schroeder, F. C. NMR-Spectroscopic Analysis of Mixtures: from Structure to Function. *Curr. Opin. Chem. Biol.* **2011,** *15*, 38–47.

Fuchs, B.; Sub, R.; Nimptsch, A.; Schiller, J. Application of MALDI-TOF Mass Spectrometry in Lipidomics. *Eur. J. Lipid Sci. Technol.* **2009,** *111*, 83–98.

Fulda, S.; Debatin, K. M. Sensitization for Anticancer Drug-induced Apoptosis by Betulinic Acid. *Neoplasia.* **2005,** *7* (2), 162–70.

Gabelica, V.; Matklund, E. Fundamentals of Ion Mobility Spectrometry. *Curr. Opin. Chem. Biol.* **2018,** *43*, 51–59.

Galhena, A. S.; Harris, G. A.; Nyadong, L.; Murray, K. K.; Fernandez, F. M. Small Molecule Ambient Mass Spectrometry Imaging by Infrared Ablation Metastable-induced Chemical Ionization. *Anal. Chem.* **2010,** *82*, 2178–2181.

Garcia-Oliveira, P.; Otero, P.; Pereira, A. G.; Chamorro, F.; Carpena, M.; Echave, J.; Fraga-Corral, M.; Simal-Gandara, J.; Prieto, M. A. Status and Challenges of Plant-Anticancer Compounds in Cancer Treatment. *Pharmaceuticals.* **2021,** *14*, 157. https://doi.org/10.3390/ph14020157.

Garza, D. R.; Verk, M. C.; Huynen, M. A.; Dutilh, B. E. Towards Predicting the Environmental Metabolome from Metagenomics with a Mechanistic Model. *Nat. Microbiol.* **2018,** *3*, 456–460.

Gogiashvili, M.; Nowacki, J.; Hergenroder, R.; Hengstler, J. G.; Lambert, J.; Edlund, K. HR-MAS NMR Based Quantitative Metabolomics in Breast Cancer. *Metabolites.* **2019,** *9* (2), 19.

Gomez-Casati, D. F.; Zanor, M. I.; Busi, M. V. Metabolomics in Plants and Humans: Applications in the Prevention and Diagnosis of Diseases. *Biomed. Res. Int.* **2013,** Article ID 792527.

Gowda N. G. A.; Raftery D. Advances in NMR-based Metabolomics. *In compr. Anal. Chem. Elvesier B.V.* 2014, 187–211.

Guijas, C.; Montenegro-Burke, J. R.; Domingo-Almenara, X.; Palermo, A.; Warth, B.; Hermann, G.; Koellensperger, G.; Huan, T.; Uritboonthai, W.; Aisporna, A. E.; Wolan, D. W.; Spilker, M. E.; Benton, H. P.; Siuzdak, G. METLIN: A Technology Platform for Identifying Knowns and Unknowns. *Anal. Chem.* **2018b,** *90* (5), 3156–3164.

Guijas, C.; Montenegro-Burke, J. R.; Warth, B.; Spilker, M. E.; Siuzdak, G. Metabolomics Activity Screening for Identifying Metabolites that Modulate Phenotype. *Nat. Biotechnol.* **2018a,** *36*, 316–320.

Haddad, R.; Sparrapan, R.; Eberlin, M. N. Desorption Sonic Spray Ionization for (high) Voltage-free Ambient Mass Spectrometry. *Rapid Commun. Mass Spectrom.* **2006,** *20*, 2901–2905.

Hagel, J. M.; Facchini, P. J. Plant Metabolomics: Analytical Platforms and Integration with Functional Genomics. *Phytochem. Rev.* **2008,** *7*, 479–497.

Hansen, A.; Henderson, S.; Lagos, D.; Nikitenko, L.; Coulter, E.; Roberts, S.; Gratrix, F.; Plaisance, K.; Renne, R.; Bower, M. KSHV-encoded miRNAs Target MAF to induce Endothelial Cell Reprogramming. *Genes Dev.* **2010,** *24*, 195–205.

Harada, T.; Yuba-Kubo, A.; Sugiura, Y.; Zaima, N.; Hayasaka, T.; Goto-Inoue, N.; Wakui, M.; Suematsu, M.; Takeshita, K.; Ogawa, K.; Yoshida, Y.; Setou, M. Visualization of Volatile Substances in Different Organelles with an Atmospheric-pressure Mass Microscope. *Anal. Chem.* **2009,** *81*, 9153–9157.

Harikrishnan, H.; Jantan, I.; Haque, M. A.; Kumolosasi, E. Anti-inflammatory Effects of *Phyllanthus amarus* Schum. & Thonn. through Inhibition of NF-κB, MAPK, and PI3K-Akt Signaling Pathways in LPS-Induced Human Macrophages. *BMC Complement. Altern. Med.* **2018,** *18*(1), 224.

Harris, G. A.; Galhena, A. S.; Fern, F. M. Ambient Sampling/ionization Mass Spectrometry: Applications and Current Trends. *Anal. Chem.* **2011,** *83*, 4508–4538.

Heyman, H. M.; Dubery, I. A. The Potential of Mass Spectrometry Imaging in Plant Metabolomics: A Review. *Phytochem. Rev.* **2016,** *15*, 297–316.

Hou, S.; Zhu, J.; Ding, M.; Lv, G. Simultaneous Determination of Gibberellic Acid, Indole-3-acetic Acid and Abscisic Acid in Wheat Extracts by Solid-phase Extraction and Liquid Chromatography-electrospray Tandem Mass Spectrometry. *Talanta.* **2008,** *76*, 798–802.

Hussin, F.; Eshkoor, S. A.; Rahmat, A.; Othman, F.; Akim, A. The *Centella Asiatica* Juice Effects on DNA Damage, Apoptosis and Gene Expression in Hepatocellular Carcinoma (HCC). *BMC Complement Altern. Med.* **2014,** *14*:32.

Jantan, I. Y.; Ilangkovan, M.; Husain, K.; Chan, K. M. Inhibitory Effects of Compounds from *Phyllanthus Amarus* on Nitric Oxide Production, Lymphocyte Proliferation, and Cytokine Release from Phagocytes. *Drug Des. Devel. Ther.* **2016,** *10*, 1935–45.

Jaroszewski, J. W. Hyphenated NMR Methods in Natural Products Research, Part 1: Direct hyphenation. *Planta Med.* **2005a,** *71*, 691–700.

Jaroszewski, J. W. Hyphenated NMR Methods in Natural Products Research, Part 2: HPLC-SPE-NMR and Other New Trends in NMR hyphenation. *Planta Med.* **2005b,** *71*, 795–802.

Jeong, D. A.; Song, H. J.; Lim, S.; Lee, S. J.; Lim, J. E.; Nam, D-H.; Joo, K. M.; Jeong, B. C.; Jeon, S. S.; Choi, H. Y.; Lee, H. W. Repurposing the Anti-malarial Drug Artesunate as a Novel Therapeutic agent for Metastatic Renal Cell Carcinoma due to its Attenuation of Tumor Growth, Metastasis, and Angiogenesis. *Oncotarget.* **2015,** *6*, 33046–33064.

Jo, K. J.; Cha, M. R.; Lee, M. R.; Yoon, M. Y.; Park, H. R. Methanolic Extracts of *Uncaria rhynchophylla* Induce Cytotoxicity and Apoptosis in HT-29 Human Colon Carcinoma Cells. *Plant Food. Hum. Nutr.* **2008,** *63* (2), 77–82

Kachlicki, P.; Piasecka, A.; Stobiecki, M.; Marczak, L. Structural Characterization of Flavonoid Glycoconjugates and their Derivatives with Mass Spectrometric Techniques. *Molecules.* **2016,** *21*, 1494.

Kessler, N.; Walter, F.; Persicke, M.; Albaum, S. P.; Kalinowski, J.; Goesmann, A. Allocator: An Interactive Web Platform for the Analysis of Metabolomic LC-ESI-MS datasets, Enabling Semi-Automated, User-Revised Compound Annotation and Mass Isotopomer Ratio Analysis. *PLoS One.* **2014,** *9*, e113909.

Khan, T.; Ali, M.; Khan, A.; Nisar, P.; Jan, S. A.; Afridi, S.; Shinwari, Z. K. Anticancer Plants: A Review of the Active Phytochemicals, Applications in Animal Models, and Regulatory Aspects. *Biomol.* **2020,** *10* (1), 47.

Kim, H. K.; Choi, Y. H.; Verpoorte, R. NMR-based Plant Metabolomics: Where Do We Stand, Where Do We Go? *Trends Biotechnol.* **2011,** *29*, 267–275.

Kind, T.; Fiehn, O. Metabolomic Database Annotations via Query of Elemental Compositions: Mass Accuracy is Insufficient Even at Less than 1 ppm. *BMC Bioinform.* **2006,** *7*, 234.

Kind, T.; Tsugawa, H.; Cajka, T.; Ma, Y.; Lai, Z.; Mehta, S. S.; Wohlgemuth, G.; Barupal, D. K.; Showalter, M. R.; Arita, M.; Fiehn, O. Identification of Small Molecules Using Accurate Mass MS/MS Search. *Mass Spectrom. Rev.* **2017,** *9999*, 1–20.

Krishna, S.; Bustamante, L.; Haynes, R. K.; Staines, H. M. Artemisinins: their Growing Importance in Medicine. *Trends Pharmacol. Sci.* **2008,** *29* (10), 520–527.

Kumar, R.; Bohra, A.; Pandey, A. K.; Pandey, M. K.; Kumar, A. Metabolomics for Plant Improvement: Status and Prospects. *Front. Plant Sci.* **2017,** *8*, 1302.

Lalli, P. M.; Sandivo, G. B.; Garcia, J. S.; Haddad, R.; Cosso, R. G.; MAia, D. R. J.; Zacca, J. J.; Maldanerc, A. O.; Eberlin, M. N. Fingerprinting and aging of Ink by Easy Ambient Sonic-spray Ionization Mass Spectrometry. *Analyst.* **2010,** *135*, 745–750.

Lane, A. N.; Fan, T. W. NMR-Based Stable Isotope Resolved Metabolomics in Systems Biochemistry. *Arch. Biochem. Biophys.* **2017,** *628*, 123–131.

Lang, S. J.; Schmiech, M.; Hafner, S.; Paetz, C.; Steinborn, C.; Huber, R.; Gaafary, M. E.; Werner, K.; Schmidt, C. Q.; Syrovets, T.; Simmet, T. Antitumor activity of an *Artemisia Annua* Herbal Preparation and Identification of Active Ingredients. *Phytomedicine.* **2019,** *62*, 152962.

Larive, C. K.; Barding Jr, G. A.; Dinges, M. M. NMR Spectroscopy for Metabolomics and Metabolic Profiling. *Anal. Chem.* **2015,** *87* (1), 133–146.

Leite, D. F.; Kassuya, C. A.; Mazzuco, T. L.; Silvestre, A.; de Melo, L. V.; Rehder, V. L.; Rumjanek, V. M.; Calixto, J. B. The Cytotoxic Effect and the Multidrug Resistance

Reversing Action of Lignans from *Phyllanthus Amarus*. *Planta Med.* **2006,** *72* (15), 1353-8.

Li, Y.; Gu, J. F.; Zou, X.; Wu, J.; Zhang, M. H.; Jiang, J.; Qin, D.; Zhou, J. Y.; Liu, B. X.; Zhu, Y. T.; Jia, X. B.; Feng, L.; Wang, R. P. The Anti-lung Cancer Activities of Steroidal Saponins of *P. polyphylla Smith* var. *chinensis* (Franch.) Hara through Enhanced Immune-stimulation in Experimental Lewis Tumor-bearing C57BL/6 Mice and Induction of Apoptosis in the A549 cell line. *Molecules*. **2013,** *18* (10), 12916-36.

Liu, X.; Zhao, M.; Wu, K.; Chai, X.; Yu, H.; Tao, Z.; Wang, J. Immunomodulatory and Anticancer Activities of Phenolics from Emblica Fruit (*Phyllanthus emblica* L.). *Food Chem.* **2012,** *131* (2), 685-690.

Ljung, K.; Sandberg, G.; Moritz, T. Methods of plant hormone analysis. In *Plant Hormones: Biosynthesis, Signal Transduction, Action;* **2010,** 717-740.

Lommen, A.; van der Kamp, H. J.; Kools, H. J.; van der Lee, M. K.; van der Weg, G.; Mol, H. G. metAlignID: A High-throughput Software Tool Set for Automated Detection of Trace Level Contaminants in Comprehensive LECO Two-dimensional Gas Chromatography Time-of-flight Mass Spectrometry Data. *J. Chromatogr. A* **2012,** *1263*, 169-178.

Lopes, A. S.; Santa Cruz, E. C.; Sussulini, A.; Klassen, A. Metabolomic Strategies Involving Mass Spectrometry Combined With Liquid and gas chromatography. *In*: Metabolomics: From Fundamentals to Clinical Applications. Sussulini A. (ed.). Springer International Publishing: New York City, 2017, 77-98.

Ludwig, C.; Viant, M. R. Two-dimensional J-resolved NMR Spectroscopy: Review of a Key Methodology in the Metabolomics Toolbox. *Phytochem. Anal.* **2010,** *21*, 22-23.

Ma, P.; Zhang, Z.; Zhou, X.; Yun, Y.; Liang, Y.; Lu, H. Feature Extraction from Resolution Perspective for Gas Chromatography-mass Spectrometry Datasets. *RSC Adv.* **2016,** *6*, 113997-114004.

Ma, Z.; Ge, L.; Lee, A. S. Y.; Yong, J. W. H.; Tan, S. N.; Ong, E. S. Simultaneous Analysis of Different Classes of Phytohormones in Coconut (*Cocos nucifera* L.) Water Using High-performance Liquid Chromatography and Liquid Chromatography-tandem Mass Spectrometry after solid-phase extraction. *Anal. Chiml. Acta.* **2008,** *610*, 274–281.

Mahata, S.; Pandey, A.; Shukla, S.; Tyagi, A.; Husain, S. A.; Das, B. C.; Bharti, A. C. Anticancer Activity of *Phyllanthus Emblica* Linn. (Indian gooseberry): Inhibition of Transcription Factor AP-1 and HPV gene expression in cervical cancer cells. *Nutr. Cancer.* **2013,** *65* (1), 88-97.

Mandal, M. K.; Chen, L. C.; Hashimoto, Y.; Yu, Z.; Hiraoka, K. Detection of Biomolecules from Solutions with High Concentration of Salts using Probe Electrosparay and Nano-electrospray Ionization Mass Spectrometry. *Anal. Methods.* **2010,** *2*, 1905–1912.

Manjamalai, A.; Berlin Grace, V. M. Antioxidant Activity of Essential Oils from *Wedelia chinensis* (Osbeck) in Vitro and in Vivo Lung Cancer Bearing C57BL/6 Mice. *Asian Pac. J. Cancer Prev.* **2012,** *13* (7), 3065–71.

Martin, D.; Gutkind, J. S. Human Tumor-Associated Viruses and New Insights into the Molecular Mechanisms of Cancer. *Oncogene.* **2008,** *27*, S31–S42.

Marx, D.; Metzger, J.; Pejchinovski, M.; Gil, R. B.; Frantzi, M.; Latosinska, A.; Belczacka, I.; Heinzmann, S. S.; Husi, H.; Zoidakis, J.; Herget-Rosenthal, M. K. M. Proteomics and Metabolomics for AKI Diagnosis. *Semin. Nephrol.* **2018,** *38* (1), 63–87.

Mirsaleh-Kohan, N.; Robertson, W. D.; Compton, R. N. Electron Ionization Time-of-flight Mass Spectrometry: History Review and Current Applications. *Mass spectrom. Rev.* **2008,** *27*, 237–285.

Mishra, R.; Kaur, G. Aqueous Ethanolic Extract of *Tinospora Cordifolia* as a Potential Candidate for Differentiation based Therapy of Glioblastomas. *PLoS One.* **2013,** *8* (10), e78764.

Mishra, R.; Kaur, G. *Tinospora Cordifolia* Induces Differentiation and Senescence Pathways in Neuroblastoma Cells. *Mol. Neurobiol.* **2015,** *52* (1), 719–33.

Misra, B. B. van der Hooft, J. J. Updates in Metabolomics Tools and Resources: 2014–2015. *Electrophoresis.* **2016,** *37*, 86–110.

Miura, D.; Fujimura, Y.; Wariishi, H. Insitu Metabolomic Mass Spectrometry Imaging: Recent Advances and Difficulties. *J. Proteomics.* **2012,** *25*, 5052–5060.

Mohamed, S. I. A.; Jantan, I.; Nafiah, M. A.; Seyed, M. A.; Chan, K. M. Lignans and Polyphenols of *Phyllanthus Amarus* Schumach and Thonn Induce Apoptosis in HCT116 Human Colon Cancer Cells through Caspases-Dependent Pathway. *Curr. Pharm. Biotechnol.* **2021,** *22*(2), 262–273.

Motta, A.; Paris, D.; Melck, D. Monitoring Real-time Metabolism of Living Cells by Fast Two-dimensional NMR Spectroscopy. *Anal. Chem.* **2010,** *82*, 2405–2411.

Munson, B. Chemical Ionization Mass Spectrometry: Theory and Applications. In *Encycl. Anal. Chem.* 2000, 1–22.

Naidoo, D. B.; Chuturgoon, A. A.; Phulukdaree, A.; Guruprasad, K. P.; Satyamoorthy, K.; Sewram, V. *Centella Asiatica* Modulates Cancer Cachexia Associated Inflammatory Cytokines and Cell Death in Leukaemic THP-1 Cells and Peripheral Blood Mononuclear Cells (PBMC's). *BMC Complement Altern Med.* **2017,** *17* (1), 377.

Nakabayashi, R.; Saito, K. Metabolomics for Unknown Plant Metabolites. *Anal. Bioanal. Chem.* **2013,** *405* (15), 5005–5011.

Narayanan, D. L.; Saladi, R. N.; Fox, J. L. Ultraviolet Radiation and Skin Cancer. *Int. J. Dermatol.* **2010,** *49*, 978–986.

Nyadong, L.; Galhena, A. S.; Fernandez, F. M. Desorption Electrospray/metastable-Induced Ionization: a Flexible Multimode Ambient Ion Generation Technique. *Anal. Chem.* **2009,** *81*, 7788–7794.

Padalia, H.; Chanda, S. Characterization, Antifungal and Cytotoxic Evaluation of Green Synthesized Zinc Oxide Nanoparticles using *Ziziphus Nummularia* Leaf Extract. *Artif Cells Nanomed Biotechnol.* **2017,** *45* (8), 1751–1761.

Panda, A.; Parida, A. K.; Rangani, J. Advancement of Metabolomics Techniques and their Applications in Plant Science. *In* Plant Metabolites and Regulation under Environmental Stress. Ahmad P, Ahanger MA, Singh VP, Tripathi DK, Alam P and Alyemeni MN (Eds.). Academic Press: UK & US 2018, 1–36.

Pareek, A.; Godavarthi, A.; Issarani, R.; Nagori, B. P. Antioxidant and Hepatoprotective Activity of *Fagonia Schweinfurthii* (Hadidi) Hadidi Extract in Carbon Tetrachloride Induced Hepatotoxicity in HepG2 Cell line and Rats. *J Ethnopharmacol.* **2013,** *150* (3), 973–81.

Passarelli, M. K.; Winograd, N. Lipid Imaging with Time-of-Flight Secondary Ion Mass Spectrometry (TOF-SIMS). *Biochimica et Biophysica Acta - Molecular and cell Biology of Lipids.* **2011,** *1811*, 976–990.

Pegasus, H. T. ChromaTOF Software Instruction Manual, Version 3.3. **2003**. Available at: http://www.scielo.br/scielo.php?script=sci_nlinks&ref=000133&pid=S0100-40422011000600009000032&lng=en.

Piasecka, A.; Kachlicki, P.; Stobiecki, M. Analytical Methods for Detection of Plant Metabolomes Changes in Response to Biotic and Abiotic Stresses. *Int. J. Mol. Sci.* **2019,** *20* (2), 379.

Porcari, A. M.; Fernandes, G. D.; Barrera-Arellano, D.; Eberlin, M. N.; Alberici, R. M. Food Quality and Authenticity Screening Via Easy Ambient Sonic-spray Ionization Mass Spectrometry. *Anal.* **2016,** *141*, 1172–1184.

Portoles, T.; Sancho, J. V.; Hernandez, F.; Newton, A.; Hancock, P. Potential of Atmospheric Pressure Chemical Ionization Source in GC-QTOF MS for Peaticide Residue Analysis. *J. Mass Spectrom.* **2010,** *45*, 926–936. (SPELLING)

Prinsloo, G.; Vervoort, J. Identifying anti-HSV Compounds from Unrelated Plants using NMR and LC-MS Metabolomic Analysis. *Metabolomics.* **2018,** *18* (14), 134.

Raina, P.; Hall, P. Comparison of Gass Chromatography-mass Spectrometry and Gas Chromatography-Tandem Mass Spectrometry with Electron Ionization and Negative-ion Chemical Ionization for Analyses of Pesticides at Trace Levels in Atmospheric Samples. *Anal. Chem. Insights.* **2008,** 111–125.

Ralston-Hooper, K.; Hopf, A.; Oh, C.; Zhang, X.; Adamec, J.; Sepulveda, M. S. Development of GCxGC/TOF-MS Metabolomics for Use in Ecotoxicological Studies with Invertebrates. *Aquat. Toxicol.* **2008,** *88*, 48–52.

Ramautar, R.; de Jong, G. J. Recent Developments in Liquid Phase Separation Techniques for Metabolomics. *Bioanal.* **2014,** *6*, 1011–1026.

Rassias, D. J.; Weathers, P. J. Dried Leaf *Artemisia Annua* Efficacy Against Non-small Cell Lung Cancer. *Phytomedicine.* **2019,** *52*, 247–253.

Reo, N. V. NMR-based Metabolomics. *Drug Chem. Toxicology.* **2002,** *25*, 375–382.

Reuter, S.; Gupta, S. C.; Chaturvedi, M. M.; Aggarwal, B. B. Oxidative Stress, Inflammation, and Cancer: How are they linked? *Free Radic. Biol. Med* **2010,** *49*, 1603–1616.

Ruhland, E.; Bund, C.; Outilaft, H.; Piotto, M.; Namer, I. J. A Metabolic Database for Biomedical Studies of Biopsy Specimens by High-Resolution Magic Angle Spinning Nuclear MR: a Qualitative and Quantitative Tool. *Magn. Reson. Med.* **2019,** *82* (1), 62–83.

Sato, D.; Kondo, S.; Yazawa, K.; Mukudai, Y.; Li, C.; Kamatani, T.; Katsuta, H.; Yoshihama, Y.; Shirota, T.; Shintani, S. The Potential Anticancer Activity of Extracts Derived from the Roots of *Scutellaria Baicalensis* on Human Oral Squamous Cell Carcinoma Cells. *Mol. Clin. Oncol.* **2013,** *1* (1), 105–111.

Scheubert, K.; Hufsky, F.; Petras, D.; Wang, M.; Nothias, L. F.; Duhrkop, K.; Bandeira, N.; Dorrestein, P. C.; Bocker, S. Significance Estimation for Large Scale Metabolomics Annotations by Spectral Matching. *Nat. Commun.* **2017,** *8*, 1494.

Schrader, W.; Klein, H. W. Liquid Chromatography/Fourier Transform Ion Cyclotron Resonance Mass Spectrometry (LC-FTICR MS): An Early Overview. *Anal. Bioanal. Chem.* **2004,** *379* 1013–1024.

Segers, K.; Declerck, S.; Mangelings, D.; Heyden, Y. V.; Eeckhaut. Analytical Techniques for Metabolomic Studies: A Review. *Bioanal.* **2019,** *11* (24), 2297–2318.

Sharma, A.; Saggu, S. K.; Mishra, R.; Kaur, G. Anti-brain Cancer Activity of Chloroform and Hexane Extracts of *Tinospora cordifolia* Miers: an in Vitro Perspective. *Ann. Neurosci.* **2019,** *26* (1), 10–20.

Shen, H.; Tao, S.; Liu, J.; Huang, Y.; Chen, H.; Li, W.; Zhang, Y.; Chen, Y.; Su, S.; Lin, N. Global Lung Cancer Risk from PAH Exposure Highly Depends on Emission Sources and Individual Susceptibility. *Sci. Rep.* **2014,** *4*, 1–8.

Shen, X.; Wang, R.; Xiong, X.; Yin, Y.; Cai, Y.; Ma, Z.; Liu, N.; Zhu, Z. J. Metabolic Reaction Network-based Recursive Metabolite Annotation for Untargeted Metabolomics. *Nat. Commun.* **2019,** *10*, 1516.

Singh, A. Tools for Metabolomics. *Nat. Methods.* **2020,** *17* (1), 24.

Slezakova, S.; Ruda-Kucerova, J. Anticancer Activity of Artemisinin and its Derivatives. *Anticancer Res.* **2017,** *37*, 5995–6003.

Song, P.; Wu, L.; Guan, W. Dietary Nitrates, Nitrites, and Nitrosamines Intake and The Risk of Gastric Cancer: A meta-analysis. *Nutrients.* **2015,** *7*, 9872.

Stewart, B. W.; Wild, C. P. *World Cancer Report 2014*; WHO Press; World Health Organization: Geneva, Switzerland 2014, ISBN 978–92-832–0443-5.

Sumner, L. W.; Lei, Z.; Nikolou, B. J.; Saito, K. Modern Plant Metabolomics: Advanced Natural Product gene Discoveries, Improved Technologies, and Future Prospects. *Nat. Prod. Rep.* **2015,** *32*, 212–229.

Sun, H.; Li, X.; Zhang, A.; Zhang, K.; Yan, G.; Han, Y.; Wu, F.; Wang, X. Exploring Potential Biomarkers of Coronary Heart Disease Treated by Jing Zhi Guan Xin Pian Using High-throughput Metabolomics. *RSV Adv.* **2019,** *9* (20), 11420–11432.

Sun, H.; Wang, M.; Zhang, A.; Ni, B.; Dong, H.; Wang, X. UPLC-Q-TOF-HDMS Analysis of Constituents in the Root of Two Kinds of Aconitum using a Metabolomics Approach. *Phytochem. Anal.* **2013,** *24* (3), 263–276.

Sung, H.; Ferlay, J.; Siegel, R. L.; Laversanne, M.; Soerjomataram, I.; Jemal, A.; Bray, F. Global Cancer Statistics 2020: GLOBOCAN Estimates of Incidence and Mortality Worldwide for 36 Cancers in 185 Countries. *Ca Cancer J. Clin.* **2021,** *71*, 209–249.

Tang, C.; Zhao, C. C.; Yi, H.; Geng, Z. J.; Wu, X. Y.; Zhang, Y.; Liu, Y.; Fan G. Traditional Tibetan Medicine in Cancer Therapy by Targeting Apoptosis Pathways. *Front. Pharmacol.* **2020,** *11*, 976.

Tayyari, F.; Gowda, G. A. N.; Gu, H.; Raftery, D. 15N-Cholamine-a Small Iostope Tag for Combining NMR- and MS-based Metabolite Profiling. *Anal. Chem.* **2013,** *85*, 8715–8721.

Tsugawa, H.; Cajka, T.; Kind, T.; Ma, Y.; Higgins, B.; Ikeda, K.; Kanazawa, M.; Vandergheynst, J.; Fiehn, O.; Arita, M. MS-DIAL: Data-independent MS/MS Deconvolution for Comprehensive Metabolome Analysis. *Nat. Methods.* **2015,** *12*, 523–526.

Tsugawa, H.; Nakabayashi, R.; Mori, T.; Yamada, Y.; Takahashi, M.; Rai, A.; Sugiyama, R.; Yamamoto, H.; Nakaya, T.; Yamazaki, M.; Kooke, R.; Bac-Molenaar, J. A.; Oztolan-Erol, N.; Keurentjes, J. J. B.; Arita, M.; Saito, K. A Cheminformatics Approach to Characterize Metabolomes in Stable-isotope-Labeled Organisms. *Nat. Methods.* **2019,** *16*, 295–298.

Turan, I.; Demir, S.; Kilinc, K.; Burnaz, N. A.; Yaman, S. O.; Akbulut, K.; Mentese, A.; Aliyazicioglu, Y.; Deger, O. Antiproliferative and Apoptotic Effect of *Morus nigra* Extract on Human Prostate Cancer Cells. *Saudi Pharm. J.* **2017,** *25* (2), 241–248.

Turner, M. F.; Heuberger, A. L.; Kirkwood, J. S.; Collins, C. C.; Wolfrum, E. J.; Broeckling, C. D. Non-targeted Metabolomics in Diverse Sorghum Breeding Lines Indicates Primary and Secondary Metabolite Profiles are Associated with Plant Biomass Accumulation and Photosynthesis. *Front. Plant Sci.* **2016,** *7*, 953.

Valent, P.; Bonnet, D.; De Maria, R.; Lapidot, T.; Copland, M.; Melo, J. V.; Chomienne, C.; Ishikawa, F.; Schuringa, J. J.; Stassi, G. Cancer Stem Cell Definitions and Terminology: The Devil is in the Details. *Nat. Rev. Cancer.* **2012,** *12*, 767–775.

Van der Graaf M. *In Vivo* Magnetic Resonance Spectroscopy: Basic Methodology and Clinical Applications. *Eur. Biophys. J.* **2010,** *39* (4), 527–540.

Verhoeven, A.; Giera, M.; Mayboroda, O. A. KIMBLE: A Versatile Visual NMR Metabolomics Workbench in KNIME. *Anal. Chim. Acta.* **2018,** *1044*, 66–76.

Verhoeven, A.; Slagboom, E.; Wuhrer, M.; Giera, M.; Mayboroda, O. A. Automated Quantification of Metabolites in Blood-derived Samples byNMR. *Anal. Chim. Acta.* **2017,** *976*, 52–62.

Vinaixa, M.; Schymanski, E. L.; Neumann, S.; Navarro, M.; Salek, R. M.; Yanes, O. Mass Spectral Databases for LC/MS– and GC/MS-based Metabolomics: State of the Field and Future Prospects. *Trends Anal. Chem.* **2016,** *78*, 23–34.

Vincenti, M. The Renaissance of Desorption Chemical Ionization Mass Spectrometry: Characterization of Large Involatile Molecules and Nonpolar Polymers. *Int. J. Mass Spectrom.* **2001,** *212*, 505–518.

Wang, H.; Sun, W.; Zhang, J.; Yang, X.; Lin, T.; Ding, L. Desorption Corona Beam Ionization Source for Mass Spectrometry. *Analyst.* **2010,** *135*, 688–695.

Wang, Y.; Huang, X.; Han, J.; Zheng, W.; Ma, W. Extract of *Perilla frutescens* Inhibits Tumor Proliferation of HCC via PI3K/AKT Signal Pathway. *Afr. J. Tradit. Complement. Altern. Med.* **2012,** *10* (2), 251–7. eCollection 2013.

WHO Report on the Global Tobacco Epidemic, 2011: Warning About the Dangers of Tobacco, 3rd ed.; World Health Organization: Geneva, Switzerland, 2011.

Wiseman, J. M.; Ifa, D. R.; Song, Q.; Cooks, R. G. Tissue Imaging at Atmospheric Pressure Using Desorption Electrospray Ionization (DESI) Mass Spectrometry. *Angew. Chem. Int. Ed.* **2006,** *45*, 7188–7192.

Wishart, D. S.; Tzur, D.; Knox, C.; Eisner, R.; Guo, A. C.; Young, N.; Cheng, D.; Jewell, K.; Arndt, D.; Sawhney, S.; Fung, C.; Nikolai, L.; Lewis, M.; Coutouly, M. A.; Forsythe, I.; Tang, P.; Shrivastava, S.; Jeroncic, K.; Stothard, P.; Amegbey, G.; Block, D.; Hau, D. D.; Wagner, J.; Miniaci, J.; Clements, M.; Gebremedhin, M.; Guo, N.; Zhang, Y.; Duggan, G. E.; Macinnis, G. D.; Weljie, A. M.; Dowlatabadi, R.; Bamforth, F.; Clive, D.; Greiner, R.; Li, L.; Marrie, T.; Sykes, B. D.; Vogel, H. J.; Querengesser, L. *Nucleic Acids Res.* **2007,** *35*, D521–6.

Wu, T.; Geng, J.; Guo, W.; Gao, J.; Zhu, X. Asiatic Acid Inhibits Lung Cancer Cell Growth in Vitro and in Vivo by Destroying Mitochondria. *Acta Pharm. Sin. B.* **2017,** *7* (1), 65–72.

Xie, L. J.; Chen, Q. F.; Chen, M. X.; Yu, L. J.; Huang, L.; Chen, L.; Wang, F. Z.; Xia, F. N.; Zhu, T. R.; Wu, J. X.; Yin, J.; Liao, B.; Shi, J.; Zhang, J. H.; Aharoni, A.; Nan, Y.; Shu, W.; Xiao, S. Unsaturation of Very-long-chain Ceramides Protects Plant from Hypoxia-induced Damages by Modulating Ethylene Signaling in *Arabidopsis.* **PLoS** Genet. **2015,** *11*, e1005143.

Yang, Q.; Zhang, A.; Miao, J.; Sun, H.; Han, Y.; Yan, G.; Wu, F.; Wang, X. Metabolomics Biotechnology, Applications and Future Trends: A Systemic Review. *RSC Adv.* **2019,** *9*, 37245–37257.

Ye, T.; Zhang, S.; Gowda, N. G. A.; Raftery, D. Nuclear Magnetic Resonance and Statistical Analysis. In Encyclopedia of Analytical Chemist; Meyers RA (Ed.). John Wiley, Eds.; NJ. 2010. https://doi.org/10.1002/9780470027318.a9139

Yu, J. S.; Kim, A. K. *Platycodin D* Induces Apoptosis in MCF-7 Human Breast Cancer Cells. *J. Med. Food.* **2010,** *13* (2), 298–305.

Zhang, A.; Ma, Z.; Sun, H.; Zhang, Y.; Liu, J.; Wu, F.; Wang, X. High-throughput Metabolomics Evaluate the Efficacy of Total Lignans from *Acanthophanax senticosus* Stem against Ovariectomized Osteoporosis Rat. *Front. Pharmacol.* **2019,** *10*, 553.

Zhang, A.; Sun, H.; Wang, P.; Wang, X. Salivary Proteomics in Biomedical Research. *Clin. Chim. Acta.* **2013,** *415*, 261–265.

Zhang, W.; Chang, J.; Lei, Z.; Huhman, D.; Sumner, L. W.; Zhao, P. X. MET-COFEA: A Liquid Chromatography/mass Spectrometry Data Processing Platform for Metabolite Compound Feature Extraction and Annotation. *Anal. Chem.* **2014,** *86* (13), 6245–6253.

Zhang, W.; Lei, Z.; Huhman, D.; Sumner, L. W.; Zhao, P. X. MET-XAlign: a Metabolite Cross-alignment Tool for LC/MS-based Comparative Metabolomics. *Anal. Chem.* **2015,** *87* (18), 9114–9119.

Zhao, H. J.; Liu, T.; Mao, X.; Han, S. X.; Liang, R. X.; Hui, L. Q.; Cao, C. Y.; You, Y.; Zhang, L. Z. *Fructus phyllanthi* Tannin Fraction Induces Apoptosis and Inhibits Migration and Invasion of Human Lung Squamous Carcinoma Cells in Vitro Via MAPK/MMP Pathways. *Acta Pharmacol. Sin.* **2015,** *36* (6), 758–68.

Zhao, L. H.; Liu, X.; Yan, H. X.; Li, W. Y.; Zeng, X.; Yang, Y.; Zhao, J.; Liu, S. P.; Zhuang, X. H.; Lin, C. Genomic and Oncogenic Preference of HBV Integration in Hepatocellular Carcinoma. *Nat. Commun.* **2016,** *7*, 1–10.

Zhao, T.; Sun, Q.; Marques, M.; Witcher, M. Anticancer Properties of *Phyllanthus Emblica* (Indian Gooseberry). *Oxid. Med. Cell Longev.* **2015,** 950890.

Zhao, Y.; Liu, J.; Liu, L. Artesunate Inhibits Lung Cancer Cells via Regulation of Mitochondrial Membrane Potential and Induction of Apoptosis. *Mol. Med. Rep.* **2020,** *22* (4), 3017–3022.

Zhou, X.; Sun, W.-J.; Wang, W.-M.; Chen, K.; Zheng, J.-H.; Lu, M. D.; Li, P.-H.; Zheng, Z.-Q. Artesunate Inhibits the Growth of Gastric Cancer Cells through the Mechanism of Promoting Oncosis both in Vitro and in Vivo. *Anti-cancer Drugs.* **2013,** *24*, 920–927.

Zrodnikov, Y.; Davis, C. E. The Highs and Lows of FAIMS: Predictions and Future Trends for High Field Asymmetric Waveform Ion Mobility Spectrometry. *J. Nanomed. Nanotechnol.* **2012,** *3* (5), 109e.

CHAPTER 9

Computational Approaches Used in Anticancer Plants

FULDEN ULUCAN-KARNAK[1], ZEYNEP YILMAZ-SERCINOGLU[2], ONUR SERCINOGLU[3], and AHMAD ALI[4]

[1]*Ege University, Institute of Health Sciences, Department of Medical Biochemistry, Izmir, Turkey*

[2]*Marmara University, Faculty of Engineering, Department of Bioengineering, Istanbul, Turkey*

[3]*Gebze Technical University, Faculty of Engineering, Department of Bioengineering, Kocaeli, Turkey*

[4]*University Department of Life Sciences, University of Mumbai, Vidyanagari, Mumbai, India*

ABSTRACT

Cancer affects millions of people worldwide. A lot of research is conducted to find effective and low-cost medicine. Plant-derived natural-based products have gained attention over the past decades as novel therapeutic agents. Nature is an enormous source of therapeutic candidate compounds with its chemical diversity. Anticancer plant metabolites are imminent substitutions to chemically synthesized drugs in the progression of drug discovery. Potential anticancer molecules can be identified by bioinformatics-based tools. Computational approaches may thus pave the way for fast and cost-effective identification of potential drug candidates and molecular targets. In this chapter, we provide an overview of the use of herbal resources for cancer treatment, drug design strategies–in, particularly structure-based

Plant-Derived Anticancer Drugs in the OMICS Era: Biosynthesis, Functions, and Applications.
Deepu Pandita, Anu Pandita (Eds.)

drug design, and example applications of drug design for plant-based compounds.

9.1 INTRODUCTION

The plant-derived products have been an irreplaceable part of human civilizations. Besides the food and shelter requirements, they offer immense medicinal benefits for the treatment of simple as well as complex disorders. In fact, all known marketed drugs have derived inspiration from natural compounds exhibiting desirable physicochemical properties (Ali, 2020). However, even with the advances in the field of medicine, we witness numerous disorders that are manageable but currently, there is no cure. Cancer is one such disease that has taken over 10 million lives, globally, in the year 2020 alone (WHO, 2021). In India, over 2.25 million people are estimated to be living with cancer at present(NICPR, 2021). To a large extent, ancient medicinal systems like Unani, Ayurveda, and Chinese medicinal systems have reported the use of various common and rare plants as medicinal agents. Hence, there is definitely hope for finding a cure for cancer and other currently untreatable diseases, given the huge diversity of medicinal plants. Unfortunately, the same diversity of natural products (NPs) extracted from plant origin makes it challenging to explore their potential as medicinal agents (Veeresham, 2012). Also, the available data from ancient records are extremely raw and the mechanism of action of various medicinal preparations as single compounds or concoctions are rarely elucidated till date.

To facilitate drug discovery from plant origin and overcome the above challenges, various computational approaches have been designed to compare huge data sets of available information. In order to discover a novel drug, the desired compound is required to pass through seven phases of testing and standardization. These include targeting of disease and selective mechanisms of action of the desired compound, its identification, optimization of its activity, pre-clinical and clinical testing, and pharmacogenomics optimization (Wong et al., 2016). At times, the potential phytochemicals require slight modification in structure to improve properties like stability and binding of drugs. For this purpose, the computer-aided drug design (CADD) is a well-known study model that can integrate various aspects of basic and applied research, identify specific molecules with the desired potential and generate analogs for designing new drugs based on the available information (Cui et al., 2020). The computer-assisted approaches thus enable us to interpret meaningful data and generate information in simple feasible formats that allow crucial insights into understanding and development of new drugs on the identification of potential phytochemicals.

The cancer cells develop resistance to single target mechanisms after a few rounds of treatment, making them ineffective. The targeted therapy using CADD and other computer-assisted approaches is hence a powerful strategy for cancer treatment since it allows multiple target drug therapies. It also reduces the time and cost of drug design. The importance of these two parameters can be comprehended with the estimated time-scale of 12–14 years and 270–800 million dollars required to develop and market a new drug. Fortunately, a recent study has reported the use of systemic biological approaches along with CADD to develop a new cocktail for drug therapy that treats multiple targets for cancer treatment (Wong et al., 2016; Chan et al., 2019). Considering the scope of plants as medicinal agents and the undeniable importance of CADD and other computer-assisted approaches, this chapter describes their combined scope to develop anticancer drugs in near future.

9.2 ANTICANCER PLANTS

It is reported that over 3000 plant species possessing anticancer properties have been researched since 1950s, and over 60% of them are converted into commercial anticancer agents (Kuruppu et al., 2019). For centuries, plants have been used as medicinal agents to treat several diseases, especially among the Asian and African populations. They remain valuable sources of medical drugs and pharmaceutically active compounds. They include many chemical ingredients which are responsible for their anticancer effects. For instance, polyphenols, flavonoids, brassinosteroids, and taxols are well-known phytochemicals (Greenwell and Rahman, 2015; Sofowora et al., 2013).

9.2.1 TYPES OF ANTICANCER PLANTS

The bioactive compounds, also known as secondary metabolites, are produced by plants during the stationary growth phases. They are not essential for the development of plants. The bioactive compounds can be mainly categorized into four groups such as terpenoids, phenolics, alkaloids, and flavonoids (Seca and Pinto, 2018; Kopustinskiene et al., 2020). Most commonly known and used anticancer agents are alkaloids (vinblastine, vincristine, and camptothecin), terpenoids (lycopene and gamma-tocopherol), polyphenols (etoposide, resveratrol, curcumin, and epigallocatechin gallate) and flavonoids (apigenin, genistein, and kaempferol) (Ramakrishna et al., 2021). Some other examples of chemical compounds inhibiting cancer cell signaling pathways include lignans, saponins, terpenes, taxanes, vitamins, minerals, glycosides, and gums (Iqbal et al., 2017).

Although it is not possible to list all anticancer plants by their class and names, we can categorize them based on activation mechanisms on cancer cells, into six main categories; (i) antimitotics, (ii) topoisomerase inhibitors, (iii) Reactive oxygen species (ROS) inducers, (iv) angiogenesis inhibitors, (v) histone deacetylases inhibitors, and (vi) mitotic kinase inhibitors (Amin et al., 2009).

Plant based anticancer bioactive compounds	Antimitotics
	Topoisomerase inhibitors
	ROS inducers
	Angiogenesis inhibitors
	Histone deacetylases inhibitors
	Mitotic kinase inhibitors

FIGURE 9.1 Categorization of plant-derived bioactive compounds according to activation mechanism (Amin et al., 2009).

In this part, the activation mechanisms of bioactive compounds are summarized. The antimitotic drugs play an important role in the inhibition of the polymerization process of microtubules by activating the spindle assembly checkpoint (SAC) that blocks the transition from metaphase to anaphase. These drug activities can be separated into two groups as microtubule-destabilizing agents (due to the concentration) or microtubule-stabilizing agents (van Vuuren et al., 2015). Colchicine, dolastatin, and vinca alkaloid derivatives such as vinblastine, vincristine, vinorelbine, vindesine, and vinflunine are examples of destabilizing agents. The taxan derivatives such as paclitaxel, doxetaxel, cabazitaxel, and ixabepilone are the few examples of stabilizing agents. Combretastatin A-4 phosphate is also a drug used for disruption of tumor vasculature (Kaul et al., 2019). Podophyllotoxin is an example of a natural antimitotic compound that affects cell growth by inhibiting topoisomerase II. Etoposide, teniposide, and the water-soluble prodrug, etoposide phosphate are examples of Podophyllotoxin (You, 2005; Ardalani et al., 2017).

DNA topoisomerases are nuclear enzymes that play a remarkable role in the catalysis of DNA molecules to prevent topological changes (Binaschi et al., 1995; Skok et al., 2020). DNA replication and transcription lead to conformational changes in DNA helix and results in helical tension in the rest of the DNA molecule. Topoisomerases release this tension with the aid of transient single-stranded (i.e., type I topoisomerases) or double-stranded (i.e., type II topoisomerases) changes in DNA double helix. This is a very important process for the proliferation of cells (Skok et al., 2020). Human topoisomerase family including topoisomerase I and topoisomerase II alpha are known as useful chemotherapeutic agents for many cancer types. To reduce their side effects, combination therapies (DNA repair, epigenetic modifications, signaling modulators, and immunotherapy) can be considered (Wang and Tse-Dinh, 2019). Natural sources of topoisomerase inhibitors can also be obtained from anticancer molecules and thus help in cancer chemotherapy. Etoposide, anthracyclines like doxorubicin (adriamycin or ADR) and daunorubicin, camptothecin derivatives like topotecan and irinotecan, paclitaxel, docetaxel, vincristine, vinblastine, mitomycin C, actinomycin D, bleomycin are the currently recognized chemotherapeutic agents. Lamellarin D, thaspine, erybraedin C, evodiamine, albanol A, and many others are recently identified as novel agents from natural sources (Jain et al., 2016; Pommier, 2006; Scotti et al., 2018).

The ROS inducers increase ROS levels over the cytotoxic threshold and this increase selectively kills cancer cells (Zahra et al., 2021). The ROS level is related to redox homeostasis and increased levels result in cell death (Kim et al., 2019). With increased metabolic rate, gene mutation, and relative hypoxia, ROS are released from tumor cells. When the level of ROS increases, tumor promotion, progression, DNA mutation, and programmed cell death are also induced (Perillo et al., 2020; Paramanya and Ali, 2019).

The ROS involve highly reactive species such as hydroxyl radicals (-OH), alkoxyl radicals, superoxide anion (O_2^-), singlet oxygen ($^1O_2$), and hydrogen peroxide (H_2O_2). The death of cancer cells is induced by ROS because they have higher ROS content compared to normal cells. Anticancer drugs, chemotherapy, and radiotherapy treatments are currently used to kill cancer cells by ROS induction (Perillo et al., 2020; Zou et al., 2017; Krumova and Cosa, 2016; Phaniendra et al., 2015). Induction of ROS can be regarded as a potential therapy for cancer and viral infections among others. ROS inducers affect the RNA replication and DNA repair processes. The quinones are the main class of natural ROS inducers (Nadhan et al., 2021; Calaf et al., 2018). Epigallocatechin-3-gallate (EGCG)-the polyphenolic compound from green tea with antioxidant properties, is another example of a natural ROS inducer (Ouyang et al., 2020).

Angiogenesis is a well-known process of generating new blood vessels. It is a fundamental process of biological development, wound healing as well as the formation of cancer (Otrock et al., 2007). This important process is modulated by activator and inhibitor molecules. The aggressiveness of the tumor cells can be determined by the levels of angiogenic factors. Angiogenesis inhibitors provide a reduction in morbidity and mortality from carcinomas (Nishida et al., 2006). Angiogenesis inhibitors can be divided into direct and indirect inhibitors. Direct ones target endothelial cells and indirect ones target tumor cells and prevent the expression of pro-angiogenic factors. Most angiogenesis inhibitors show clinical benefits when used in combination with other chemotherapeutic/targeted therapies as compared to their use as monotherapy (El-Kenawi and El-Remessy, 2013; Haibe et al., 2020).

Histone deacetylase (HDAC) inhibitors (HDACi) are anticancer agents that affect regulation (DNA methylation or demethylation and/or histone acetylation or deacetylation), cell death induction, apoptosis, and cell cycle in cancer cells (Kim and Bae, 2011). HDAC inhibitors have an important role in inducing cancer cell cycle arrest, differentiation, and cell death. However, its mechanism in cancer cells is not uniform and stable, and differs in cancer types, inhibitor types, and doses (Eckschlager et al., 2017a; Damaskos et al., 2017). Also, they inhibit zinc-containing HDAC enzyme functions (Kroesen et al., 2014). They act as transcriptional repressors by removing acetyl groups from histones, but resistance to HDACi and non-effective therapy in solid tumors can be seen often. Therefore, they can be used as a therapeutic agent with the combination of standard chemotherapeutic drugs in cancer treatment (Suraweera et al., 2018; Hontecillas-Prieto et al., 2020; Thurn et al., 2011). HDACi are becoming a great candidate for therapeutic agents of several diseases such as cancer, autoimmune disease, and neurological damage. This is due to their low toxicity, anticancer properties, and ability to alter various cellular pathways. Therefore, new researches show that HDACi can be used as a single or combination therapeutic agent as immunological modulators in immunotherapy with low or no resistance (Kroesen et al., 2014; Banik et al., 2019; Wang et al., 2020; Bensaid et al., 2018; Jenke et al., 2021).

Mitotic kinases control chromosome transmission accuracy and it is regarded as a key parameter of cancer management. If there is no proper cell cycle and DNA repair mechanism, cancer can occur. Therefore, anti-mitotic agents and inhibitors that regulate the mitotic kinases are important for cancer treatment strategies (Schmit and Ahmad, 2007). Mitotic kinase inhibitors have three main roles in cancer cells including i) targeting cell cycles and minimizing the toxicity on the liver and heart, ii) blocking DNA damage and metastasis, and iii) blocking resistance due to repeated DNA damage. Therefore, they are effective even on chemotherapy-resistant tumors (Yan et al., 2020). The list of mitotic kinases includes CDK (cyclin-dependent kinase; CDK1 and CDK2), Aurora (Aurora-A and Aurora-B) and Plk (Polo-like kinase; Plk1, Plk) families, Bub1, Haspin, and Mps1 among others (Welburn and Jeyaprakash, 2018). Plant-derived inhibitors of mitotic kinase families can be recognized from the literature via docking and computer-based approaches (Jung et al., 2015; de Groot et al., 2015; Shin et al., 2018; Hijjawi et al., 2021; Park et al., 2021).

9.2.2 PLANT-DERIVED DRUGS

Anticancer compounds are extracted from plants and characterized with many advanced techniques. The plant-derived medicinal bioactive extracts can be tested in vitro and in vivo to evaluate their anticancer activities before using them as drugs. After successful in vitro and in vivo studies, it is essential to perform clinical trials. Phase III clinical trials are required for marketing permissions. Based on the regulatory guidelines of The Food and Drug Administration (FDA) and the European Medicines Agency (EMA), all potential drugs must meet the requirements of determining rules and successful phase trial results. This ensures that the potential drug is approved with sufficient data on quality, safety, and efficacy (Fig. 9.2) (Khan et al., 2019; Chanda and Nagani, 2013; Ebrahim et al., 2020; Iqbal et al., 2017).

With the developing technology, it is not possible to screen all plants for their anticancer effects. To plan the time and research cost, in silico design strategies are very useful tools for determining new, effective, and affordable anticancer drugs (Dai et al., 2016; Cui et al., 2020). Also, they are convenient methods to limit animal models with the aid of rational and safe design properties for potential drug candidates and repositioning marketed drugs (Brogi et al., 2020).

9.2.2.1 COMPUTER-AIDED DRUG DISCOVERY AND DESIGN APPROACHES FOR PLANT-BASED NPS

A typical drug discovery and development pipeline starts from the identification of a suitable target molecule, often a protein that plays a significant role in the pathogenesis of a disease of interest, and ends with the successful completion of all clinical trial stages and usage approval of an identified drug candidate by relevant regulatory bodies (Fig. 9.3) (Macalino et al., 2015). The overall workflow seems straightforward, yet

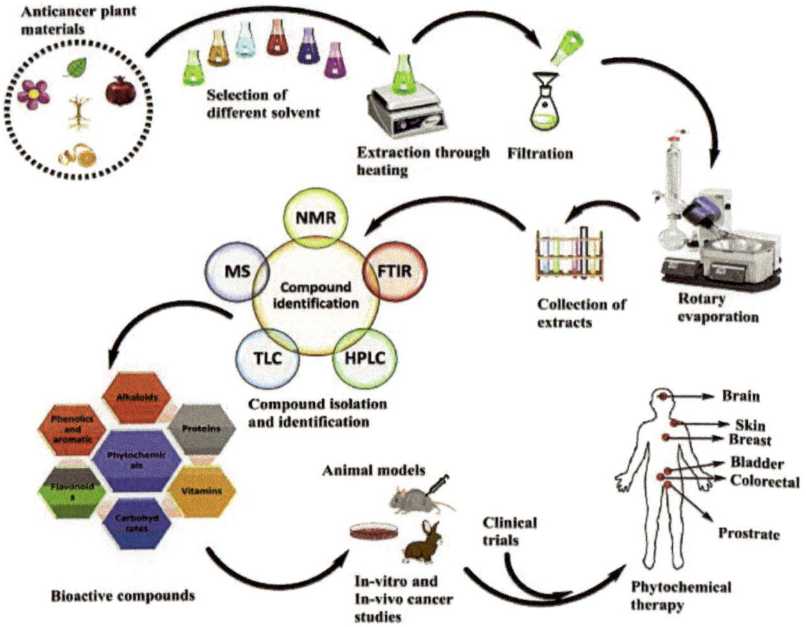

FIGURE 9 2 General strategies of plant based extracts for evaluating their anticancer activity (Iqbal et al., 2017).

Source: Reprinted with permission from Iqbal et al., 2017. © 2017 Hainan Medical University. https://creativecommons.org/licenses/by-nc-sa/4.0/

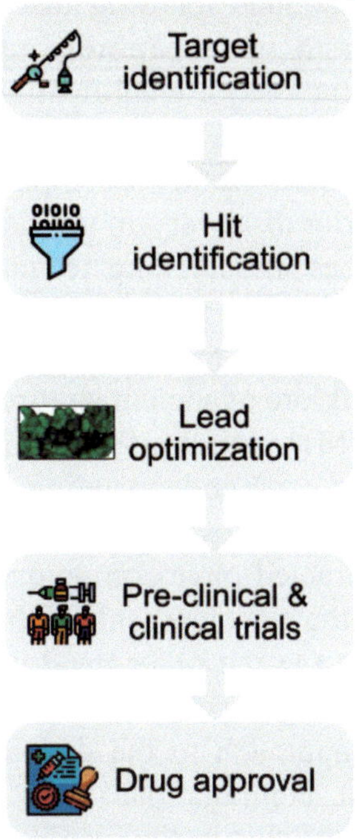

FIGURE 9.3 A typical drug discovery pipeline.

each of the intermediate steps should be carefully planned and executed to increase the chances of a successful drug discovery campaign. Computational approaches have been developed to aid each step of the drug discovery pipeline, however many of the established methods have been most useful in designing and selection of novel drug candidates in pre-clinical stages prior to further developmental steps. In particular, *target identification* (prediction of drug targets for specific disease conditions and/or candidate small molecules) and *hit identification* (identification of small molecule "hits" which likely interact with the identified target) are often performed using computational approaches (Li et al., 2019a).

Plant-based natural compounds have played a major role in the past for the treatment of many diseases, including different types of cancer (Agbarya et al., 2014; Cragg and Pezzuto, 2016; Grothaus et al., 2010; Graham et al., 2000; Huang et al., 2021; Hartwell, 1971; Lamari and Cordopatis, 2008; Rahman and Khan, 2013). Indeed, the large structural and chemical diversity of NPs, in general, provides an advantage over conventional small compounds for drug discovery. On the other hand, difficulties associated with incompatibility of natural product extracts with established screening assays, identification of the actual compounds showing biological activity, and the need to obtain significant amounts of the extract have led pharmaceutical companies to turn to large small-molecule libraries for drug discovery in the past (Atanasov et al., 2021). However, recent advances in screening technologies specific to natural extracts have revived the interest in natural resources for drug discovery.

The discovery of potent phytocompounds to treat diseases including cancer is rooted in the folklore of ancient cultures, for example, Traditional Chinese Medicine (TCM) and Ayurveda-Traditional Indian Medicine (Fridlender et al., 2015). As our understanding of both phytochemistry and human molecular biology improved, the molecular mechanisms behind the activity of many extracted phytocompounds have been elucidated in more detail and led to the development of the field of pharmacognosy (Cahlíková et al., 2020). On the other hand, traditional approaches still require biological screening experiments, which inevitably introduce a "trial-and-error" based approach to the drug discovery process (Zhang et al., 2020). In contrast, computational drug design methodologies are inherently highly "rational," that is, the identification of drug candidates is based on data-driven modeling and prediction of specific small molecule target protein interactions (Ban et al., 2017; Cui et al., 2020; Leelananda and Lindert, 2016; Macalino et al., 2015; Sliwoski et al., 2014). To this end, computational approaches may both provide a rational background to the activity of known bioactive phytocompounds as well as a novel for drug development such as repurposing of known plant-based drugs for the treatment of different cancer types and finding potential targets for previously characterized phytocompounds (Yang et al., 2019; Ho et al., 2018; Koulouridi et al., 2019; Macalino et al., 2015; Rallabandi et al., 2020; Romano and Tatonetti, 2019; Temml and Schuster, 2021).

Approaches used in computer-aided drug design (CADD) and discovery are traditionally classified into two main categories: Structure-based drug design (SBDD) and ligand-based drug design (LBDD) (Macalino et al., 2015). Although the main focus of CADD methods has been primarily based on drug discovery from synthetic small molecule libraries, the same principles apply to the discovery of plant-based natural compounds as well (Singh and Bharadvaja, 2021). On the other hand, the differences between properties of synthetic small molecules, drugs, and natural compounds also warrant careful implementation of CADD methodologies for plant-based natural compounds (Feher and Schmidt, 2003; Huang et al., 2021; Ntie-Kang et al., 2014; Santana et al., 2021). In the following, we focus on SBDD-molecular docking in particular and provide a brief overview while highlighting points to consider when applying SBDD methods for plant-based natural drug discovery without delving into technical details of the introduced methodologies. In addition, we briefly review recent trends and approaches in traditional CADD methodologies, such as molecular dynamics (MD) in drug design, ensemble docking, and drug design targeting the cryptic or allosteric binding pockets.

9.2.2.2 STRUCTURE-BASED DRUG DESIGN

Cancer is a complex disease (de Anda-Jáuregui and Hernández-Lemus, 2020; Knox, 2010). Despite the complexity of underlying molecular mechanisms in different cancer types, different types of OMICs data have consistently pointed toward several "key" proteins, often performing crucial roles in disease development (Abdelmoez et al., 2017; Cohen et al., 2020; de Anda-Jáuregui and Hernández-Lemus, 2020; Ghandi et al., 2019; Menyhárt and Győrffy, 2021; Kummar and Doroshow, 2013). Examples include protein kinases (Klaeger et al., 2017; Qiao et al., 2021; Quan et al., 2017; Roskoski, 2015), G-protein coupled receptors (Bar-Shavit et al., 2016; Jiang et al., 2020; Liu et al., 2016; Schiöth and Lagerström, 2008), P-glycoprotein (Lopes-Rodrigues et al., 2016; Mealey and Fidel, 2015; Pokharel et al., 2017; Waghray and Zhang, 2018), nuclear receptors (Porter et al., 2019) and HDAC (Eckschlager et al., 2017; McClure et al., 2018; Witt et al., 2009; Yoon and Eom, 2016). A rather straightforward strategy for anticancer drug discovery is thus modulating the activity of these key cancer proteins via synthetic or naturally occurring molecules. The molecular mechanism underlying such modulation is often based on a physical interaction between the drug candidate (such as a plant-derived compound) and the target protein. If the three-dimensional structure of the target protein is available, then this can be exploited for discovering possible physical interactions using SBDD approaches.

The availability of the target (receptor) protein structure is thus a prerequisite for SBDD (Van Montfort and Workman, 2017). Protein Data Bank (PDB) is a central public database storing experimental structural information on many different proteins (Berman et al., 2003; Berman et al., 2000; Burley et al., 2021). As of July 2021, this database stores more than 1,80,000 macromolecular protein structures, which correspond to around 70,000 unique protein sequences. Due to their high importance, multiple structures of many cancer-related proteins have been deposited at PDB as well. For example, more than 90 experimental structures of the androgen receptor ligand-binding domain are available from the PDB (Sakkiah et al., 2016).

X-ray crystallography (Maveyraud and Mourey, 2020), Nuclear Magnetic Resonance (Emwas et al., 2020), and more recently cryo-EM (Renaud et al., 2018) are widely used protein structure determination methods. Even though these methods have been successfully used in the past to determine structures of many biologically relevant proteins, their implementation at a proteome-scale is still not feasible due to difficulties associated with obtaining enough sample for purification, sample preparation, and other factors such as the presence of transmembrane regions and high conformational flexibility of some proteins. For this reason, computational protein structure determination has been an active area of research, and a variety of molecular modeling methods have been developed over the last decade (Deng et al., 2018). To this end, homology modeling has been a popular structure prediction method, which is often successful in predicting structures of proteins based on their sequence similarity and/or homology to related proteins with known experimental 3D structures (Deng et al., 2018; Haddad et al., 2020; Muhammed and Aki-Yalcin, 2019).

9.2.2.3 MOLECULAR DOCKING

Molecular docking is an essential method used in SBDD (Liu et al., 2018). The aim of a molecular docking simulation is to find an optimal structural fit between a given (small) molecule (the *ligand*) and a macromolecule (often a protein, the *receptor*). Depending on whether the flexibilities of ligands and/or receptors are considered, molecular docking simulations can be categorized as rigid or flexible. Pioneering works on molecular docking simulations were conducted using the rigid docking approach, in which conformations of both the ligand and the receptor are kept fixed, and the search for the "optimal fit" is performed based on a "lock-and-key" principle. As computational capacities of common computer hardware have increased with the development of faster and cheaper processing units, it has become standard practice to generate many possible ligand conformation, and use this "conformer library" instead of a single ligand conformation in molecular docking. This way, ligand flexibility is considered. Nevertheless, even this is an over-simplification of a real-world ligand binding process, which is a dynamic process where receptor flexibility also plays a role. However, the degrees of freedom associated with protein structures are still so large that it is often not feasible to generate alternative protein conformations without performing resource-demanding atomistic MD simulations (Hospital et al., 2015), although the increasing availability of high-performance computing resources for researchers is currently driving a paradigm shift toward "dynamic docking" (Gioia et al., 2017; Pinzi and Rastelli, 2019).

A typical molecular docking simulation consists of two major steps: (1) conformational space search and (2) scoring (Bitencourt-Ferreira and de Azevedo, 2019). In conformational space search, different conformations of the putative ligand molecule are generated by modifying the dihedral (torsional) angles within the molecule as well as rotational and translational degrees of freedom within a pre-determined binding site/area, often defined by a "grid." The binding site usually consists of a pocket or cleft on the protein surface. Yet, depending on the function of the protein, it may also rest deeper within the protein. If there are already native ligand(s) identified along with the protein structure, the respective binding site may be chosen after removing the ligand from the structure file. If no information on the binding site is available, binding pocket detection/prediction tools may be used, or "blind docking" may be performed, where the used program detects suitable binding sites prior to molecular docking simulation (Agoni et al., 2020; Volkamer et al., 2012).

Conformational search can be performed either systematically or stochastically. In a systematic search, ligand conformations are generated in a gradual manner, where the energy of the generated conformer is evaluated toward obtaining a conformer with the minimum energy, representing the most probable binding mode of the ligand. In contrast, stochastic search generates ligand conformations randomly. Hence, a larger variety of alternative ligand conformations are tested than those in systematic search strategies, albeit at a higher computational cost.

Once the conformational space search is complete, the resulting ligand conformations within the binding site are evaluated to select the "best" binding pose of the ligand having favorable interactions with the receptor binding site residues. This is usually performed using a scoring function (Huang, 2014; Huang et al., 2010; Li et al., 2019b). Scoring functions used in molecular docking may be classified into four main categories: (1) physics-based, (2) knowledge-based, (3) empirical, and (4) machine learning-based scoring functions (Liu and Wang, 2015).

9.2.2.4 STRUCTURE-BASED VIRTUAL SCREENING (SBVS) VIA MOLECULAR DOCKING

If the interactions between a limited number of ligands and a target receptor protein are investigated, repeating the docking simulation multiple times for each ligand, and manually checking scoring results in terms of consistency as well as performing a visual inspection may be a reasonable approach (Lill et al., 2021). However, molecular docking is more often used in a "virtual screening" (VS) context, where a database of potential ligand molecules is screened against a selected target via molecular docking simulations to filter out non-binders from binders and select those molecules with strong affinity for the target protein (Fig. 9.4) (Klebe, 2006; Macalino et al., 2015; Maia et al., 2020). Such SBDD VS (SBVS) approaches are now established procedures for drug discovery in academic as well as industrial settings (Phillips et al., 2018). For anti-cancer plant-based drug discovery, relevant database(s) and target protein structures may be used in such SBVS campaigns.

Since large molecule databases are often used in SBVS, the computational efficiency of the docking protocol is of utmost importance to make the most of the time and resource-saving aspects of a CADD approach. Increasing the efficiency of search and scoring steps is thus a major focus of molecular docking software development, in addition to integration with high-performance computing infrastructures (Dolezal et al., 2015; Dong et al., 2018; Jaghoori et al., 2016; Trager et al., 2016; Zhang et al., 2013). Moreover, a typical SBVS campaign also involves a filtering step in which a sub-group of molecules for the actual docking-based screen is selected. This selection is usually based on molecular properties describing the drug-likeness of a given compound (Agoni et al., 2020; Tian et al., 2015).

A key criterion to consider a molecule as a drug is a favorable ADME/T (adsorption, distribution, metabolism, excretion, and toxicity) profile (Ferreira and Andricopulo, 2019; Norinder and Bergström, 2006;

Kar and Leszczynski, 2020). In other words, a molecule with a good ADME/T profile should pass through the intestinal wall, enter blood circulation, travel to the intended site, bind to its target with high affinity to perform its intended function, and finally get eliminated from the body to prevent toxicity build-up. Several drug-likeness criteria have been developed in the past to select potential drug candidates from large databases (Mignani et al., 2018), including the widely used Lipinski's Rule of Five (Ro5), which is mainly related to oral bioavailability (Lipinski et al., 2001). The Ro5 consists of four criteria describing the drug-likeness of a given molecule: Molecular weight less than 500 Da, octanol/water partition coefficient (clogP) less than 5, number of hydrogen bond acceptors less than 10, and number of hydrogen bond donors less than 5 (the name Ro5 comes from the fact that all the numbers in the criteria are multiples of 5).

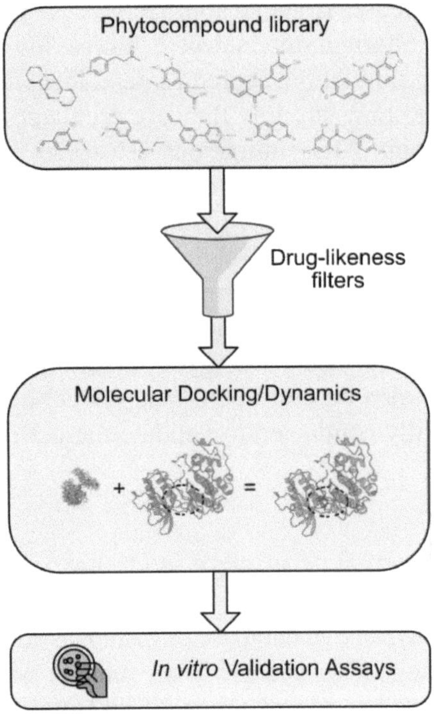

FIGURE 9.4 A typical SBVS workflow.

On the other hand, when drug-likeness criteria are applied in a VS study on NPs, such as those extracted from medicinal plants, the differences between the properties of synthetic molecules obtained by combinatorial synthesis and NPs should be considered as well. It is well-known that NPs are characterized by complex scaffolds, higher molecular mass, chiral centers, and a higher number of oxygen atoms and aromatic groups, compared to the average properties of small-molecule drugs (Grabowski and Schneider, 2012; Ntie-Kang et al., 2019). As a result, they tend to show weaker bioavailability and poor ADME/T profiles. The NPs are considered an important source of oral drugs, and do not necessarily conform fully to the Ro5 (Doak et al., 2014). For example, a previous study showed that a majority of previously identified NP-based anticancer drugs showed violations of the Ro5 (Ntie-Kang et al., 2014); nevertheless, most of the NPs showed only two Ro5 violations. Thus, a more "relaxed" filtering step, allowing for up to two Ro5 violations during drug-likeness filtering step, may be a reasonable approach for NPs.

Following the filtering step, selected molecules are subjected to the molecular docking simulation, scored as described above, and eventually ranked according to how strongly they are predicted to bind to the target protein. At this point, MD simulations (Hospital et al., 2015) may be performed to "validate" the obtained poses of top-scoring ligands. The purpose of MD simulations here is to check whether the predicted interactions between the ligand and the protein remain stable when both the ligand and receptor flexibility are considered. Moreover, more accurate binding free energy calculations, for example, by using the Molecular Mechanics/Poisson Boltzmann Surface Area (MM/PBSA) method (Genheden and Ryde, 2015), may also be performed using MD simulations. Finally, in vitro tests are usually conducted to validate the biological activity of the selected molecule(s).

9.2.2.5 TARGET FISHING (INVERSE VS) VIA MOLECULAR DOCKING

In a regular VS study, a large database of ligands is screened for binding to a single target protein. The increase in the number of structures available from the PDB as well as recent advances in protein structure prediction allows an opposite approach for VS as well, in which a large database of proteins is screened for binding of a single ligand molecule. This reverse/

inverse screening approach is called target fishing (Xu et al., 2018). Target fishing is particularly relevant for NPs, as the details of the molecular mechanism behind the biological activity of a plant extract are often unknown, and in most cases based on interaction with multiple target proteins (Temml and Schuster, 2021b).

9.2.2.6 BEST PRACTICES AND GENERAL CONSIDERATIONS FOR MOLECULAR DOCKING APPLICATIONS

Molecular docking is now considered an established and proven method for SBDD. However, despite years of research experience in the scientific community, discriminating binders of a target protein from non-binders via molecular docking simulations is still a challenging task (Chen, 2015; Plewczynski et al., 2011). This is largely due to the inherent limitations of the method itself. To this end, inaccuracies of scoring functions, limitations in the conformational sampling of ligands, and in particular, the lack of receptor flexibility in the standard docking approach are major limiting factors (Antunes et al., 2015). As a result, there is not a single well-established "gold standard" protocol, but rather a set of "best practices" that can be applied to reduce the uncertainty and increase confidence in molecular docking results (Neves et al., 2021; Torres et al., 2019). Here, we give a brief overview of approaches used to tackle scoring function (in) accuracy and conformational sampling limitations. Incorporating receptor flexibility can usually be achieved via MD simulations, which are reviewed in the next section.

As the number of software alternatives for molecular docking has increased over years, researchers were naturally interested in comparing the performance of these software in terms of their accuracy in predicting the correct pose of the ligand within the binding site of the target protein and/or selecting true binders from a pool of molecules in a VS context. This can be ideally done prospectively by testing the accuracy of docking predictions via experimental validations of ligand binding. However, these experiments are very costly and accessing the required high-throughput screening data, often the intellectual property of pharmaceutical companies is cumbersome. For this purpose, benchmarking datasets were assembled (Lagarde et al., 2015).

Benchmarking datasets have been prepared specifically to test accuracies in either pose/binding affinity (or sampling/scoring power, respectively) or VS. For pose prediction, the dataset includes curated sets of target structures with ligands in their experimentally observed binding poses. A typical benchmarking dataset for VS consists of two types of compounds for each target including active and inactivate compounds. Active compounds are those with documented, experimental binding activity on the selected protein target. Consequently, inactivate compounds are those that are not detected to bind to the selected target. However, due to the bias toward reporting only active molecules in the literature, datasets including "decoy" compounds (compounds that are assumed not to bind to the target protein) are used instead.

Assessing the quality of molecular docking protocols with appropriate benchmark datasets is a common practice today, and state-of-the-art docking software is indeed developed with the help of these datasets. On the other hand, a common misconception among researchers employing docking strategies in their studies is that if a particular docking protocol/software has been validated against a certain dataset, it may be used in an R and D context to design/screen drugs for any protein target. Carefully designed comparative evaluations of docking software indicated that even when the correct binding pose is often generated successfully by the docking program, it is not always ranked among the top-scorers due to possible limitations of the scoring function used (Bhattacharyya and Vishveshwara, 2011), indicating that there is no "one-fits-all" approach in molecular docking.

In light of such considerable levels of variance and uncertainty with respect to the output of molecular docking software, establishing a reliable computational workflow through a rigorous selection and, if necessary, a validation procedure is key to increase the chances of success and speedy drug discovery. First, good literature research is essential, and evaluation may be based on several key questions such as "which benchmarking dataset was used to validate the software?," "is there any information available on the performance of a specific docking program on the selected target protein (or protein class)?", "is there any target-specific scoring function available?." For natural sources, another key aspect is "whether the used benchmarking dataset included NPs."

Literature information often yields useful information that may guide the selection of a docking protocol for a specific protein target (Acharya et al., 2019; Boittier et al., 2020; Glaab, 2016; Serçinoğlu et al., 2021). However, conducting an internal molecular docking validation study is still a better and more reliable strategy (Kontoyianni, 2017; Neves et al., 2021; Scior et al., 2012; Temml and Schuster, 2021b). This is performed basically by first compiling a dataset specific to the selected target protein, and then by checking the performance of the docking protocol as described previously. To this end, three approaches may be used, depending on how much structural data is available. If at least a crystal structure, including the target protein and a small molecule ligand bound to the same target binding site is available, a "re-docking" study may be conducted, in which the ligand is removed from the binding site, and docked again to test whether the workflow is able to reproduce the experimentally observed binding pose. Root Mean Square Deviation (RMSD) from the experimentally observed pose is a popular metric used as a measure of accuracy in this context (Lohning et al., 2017). If multiple crystal structures including different ligands bound to the same target protein are available, a more advanced procedure called cross-docking may be performed. In cross-docking, ligands from different crystal structures are docked onto the binding site on other structures. This way, possible binding site variations can be considered. Finally, if no crystal structure is available for any ligands of the selected target protein, previous knowledge of ligand activity on the target may still be used. In this case, a training-test dataset (in the same spirit as the VS benchmarking sets described above) may be prepared, including active and inactive ligands, and the docking protocol may be validated based on its ability to distinguish binders from non-binders. In all these approaches, the selection of ligands of similar size to NPs is an important consideration.

Finally, consensus approaches may also be used to establish reliable docking workflows. In such approaches, validation is conducted based on multiple docking workflow alternatives (e.g., different software or scoring functions) (Charifson et al., 1999; Poli and Tuccinardi, 2018; Torres et al., 2019). Consensus approaches are based on the idea that if the same output is generated by alternative workflows, the reliability of the docking results is increased.

9.3 MOLECULAR DYNAMICS IN STRUCTURE-BASED DRUG DESIGN

The importance of MD in protein science has long been recognized, as all proteins are involved in energy exchange with their surroundings to perform their functions (Henzler-Wildman and Kern, 2007). Indeed, members from various protein families have been found to evolve to conserve or regulate their function and stability (Abriata et al., 2015; Echave and Wilke, 2017; Serçinoğlu and Ozbek, 2020; Sikosek and Chan, 2014) as well as their dynamics (Saldaño et al., 2016; Tiwari and Reuter, 2018).

The most important contribution of MD simulation to CADD has been the incorporation of protein flexibility into the computational drug discovery workflows (Antunes et al., 2015; Feixas et al., 2014; Salo-Ahen et al., 2020). In this regard, combining molecular docking with MD simulations in SBDD has become popular in recent years (Santos et al., 2019). MD simulations in this regard may be used as part of several computational approaches including ensemble docking (Amaro et al., 2018), cryptic binding pocket identification (Vajda et al., 2018), binding free energy calculations, MD-based allosteric drug design (Chatzigoulas and Cournia, 2021) and dynamic docking (Gioia et al., 2017). Ensemble docking is based on the idea that performing MD simulations of the ligand-free receptor protein structure prior to SBVS and using multiple receptor conformations instead of a single-often crystal-structure in the screening workflow will eventually lead to more accurate results (Amaro et al., 2018). Conducting MD simulations prior to SBVS may also be used to scan for possible, alternative binding sites which are not observed in static crystal structures and therefore termed "cryptic" (Durrant and McCammon, 2011; Hollingsworth et al., 2019). Allosteric drug design is another hot area of research that is highly advantageous for finding novels drug candidates acting on key molecular targets, as these pockets are often formed by non-conserved residues and may therefore offer a chance for increased selectivity (Chatzigoulas and Cournia, 2021; Perricone et al., 2018).

9.4 SUCCESSFUL APPLICATIONS OF DRUG DISCOVERY

The CDK2 is an important member of serine/threonine protein kinase family which plays a critical role during the cellular division of eukaryotic cells. CDK2 over-expression is unfortunately related to broad types of cancers. Medicinal plants are being used for centuries to treat many diseases including cancer. Inhibitors of CDK2 are an important field of research around the world. In 2007, 20 of 21 CDK2 inhibitors were in clinical trials (Khan et al., 2017). Phytochemicals are therapeutic compounds with anticancer properties and are extracted from plants. Khan and colleagues investigated the inhibition CDK2 by phytochemicals. They selected 10 of 2300 phytochemicals depending on low S-score. Next, 4 of these 10 selected phytochemicals were further analyzed as anticancer agents depending on the docking score. Neocalyxins A, Remangiflavanone B, Kushenol T, and Elenoside were found to strongly bind to the CDK2 binding site (Khan et al., 2017).

Aurora kinases are also a member of serine/threonine kinases and their overexpression is related to many cancers such as urogenital, breast, and colon cancer (Hijjawi et al., 2020; Jung et al., 2015). Experimental studies showed that mitosis is disturbed and results in cell death when aurora kinases are inhibited. This information is valuable to assess the aurora kinases as an important target to be inhibited to cure cancer. In the study Jung, 28 flavones were examined for their inhibitory action of Aurora B (aurB). According to in vitro experiments of 28 flavones, quercetagetin, and fisetin were found to have the highest pIC50 values. To elucidate the information on pharmacophores, molecular docking analysis was conducted with a selective aurora kinase inhibitor of aurB (VX-680). Quercetagetin binding energies were comparable to VX-680, revealing good binding to aurB (Jung et al., 2015).

Isothymusin is a flavone that is not investigated thoroughly as an anticancer agent. Singh and colleagues conducted molecular docking studies with isothymusin (Singh et al., 2021). Proliferation markers such as hyaluronidase and dihydrofolate reductase were found to be inhibited by isothymusin together with enzymes, for example, cycloxygenase-2 (COX-2) associated with the second stage of cancer. Anti-proliferative properties of isothymusin may pave the way for the synthesis of analogs to treat leukemia, lung, colon, skin, kidney, hepatic, and genital cancers.

As mentioned before, angiogenesis is a pivotal process to supply energy to the tumorigenic tissue or cell to sustain cancer proliferation. Therefore, vascular endothelial growth factor (VEGF) is an essential target molecule to treat cancer, together with matrix metalloproteinases (MMP) and tyrosine kinase (TK). Phytochemicals extracted from *Caesalpinia bonduc* were used to elucidate their interaction with TK, VEGF, and MMP, in silico. 7,4′-dihydroxy-3,11-dehydrohomoisoflavanone (74DH), 7-hydroxy-4′-methoxy-3,11-dehydrohomoisoflavanone (7H4M), kaempferol-3-O-β-d-xylopyranoside (K3βd), kaempferol-3-O-α-l-rhamnopyranosyl-(1 → 2)-β-D-xylopyranoside (K3αl), 4,4′-dihydroxy-2’-methoxy-chalcone (44DH), quercetin-3-methyl and luteolin were investigated through molecular docking analysis. Drug-likeness of these seven compounds was investigated with Lipinski rule of 5 (RO5), Ghose filter, Veber rule, Egan rule, and Muegge rule. Five of seven compounds (7H4M, 74DH, 44DH, K3βd, quercetin-3-methyl and luteolin) showed good pharmacokinetic properties and they were further investigated with molecular docking. The binding affinity and docking score of these seven compounds were found to be lower than that of commercial analogs, which means stronger binding to the target. All compounds were weakly inhibiting the human ether-a-go-go-related gene (hERG) and did not show significant toxicity to humans. However, 7H4M and 74DH are highly toxic to honey bees. These results may be beneficial for the development of new anticancer drugs (Iheagwam et al., 2019).

Bulbine frutescens (*B. frutescens*) is a medicinal plant used for the treatment of burns and skin wounds in South Africa. It was reported to be an inhibitor of HIV-1 protease, and have anti-proliferative activity. Isofuranonapthoquinone 1 extracted from *B. frutescens* has an inhibitory effect on glutathione transferase P1-1 protein, which plays a role in detoxification-mediated drug resistance of anticancer drugs. Moreover, an extract of *B. frutescens* is found to have an inhibitory effect on Notch signaling in breast cancer. In the study of Kushwaha and colleagues, the inhibitory effect of Knipholone compounds on ABC transporter protein is first reported. In this study, 23 phytochemicals are screened for their binding characteristics to ATP-binding cassette (ABC) transporter. Of the 23 phytochemicals selected, 4'-Demethylknipholone 2'-β-D-glucopyranoside (4DMK) was found to have a minimum binding score compared to the diltiazem which is the standard ABC transporter inhibitor. In addition, 4DMK has higher activity at a lower concentration (15.08 μM) compared to felodipine which has the same effect at a concentration of 127.3 μM. They stated that 4DMK has satisfactory results in RMSD (Kushwaha et al., 2021).

The TCM has an esteemed collection of compounds to be investigated for the treatment of cancer. In 2016, Dai and friends investigated TCM Database@Taiwan to predict possible anticancer compounds. The first screening of 21,334 compounds revealed 5278 possible anticancer agents. They used the method they developed and named it CDRUG. The CDRUG integrates relative-weighted fingerprinting and measurement of similarity between the known compounds and the compound of interest. In their study, 346 of 5278 compounds were similar to the compounds proven to be effective on 60 cancer cell lines. Moreover, according to anticancer activity enrichment analysis (ACEA), 57 plants were identified to possibly contain anticancer compounds. Among these, 24 plants were not studied thoroughly, which means they may have a hidden potential as anticancer agents (Dai et al., 2016).

In 2019, a large-extent investigation of Brazilian biodiversity for potential anticancer NPs were conducted for the first time. During the study, 331 of 2221 compounds, taken from Nuclei of Bioassays, Ecophysiology, and Biosynthesis of NPs Database (NuBBEDB), were found to possess anticancer properties after their analysis with CDRUG. In their study, methyl 6,7,8-trimethoxydihydrocinnamate and 3,4,5-trimethoxydihydrocinnamic acid were the compounds mentioned as potential anticancer agents for the first time in the literature. MD simulations of pedalitin (a tetrahydroxy-monohydroxy-flavone) and 5,6,7,3′,4′,5′-hexamethoxyflavone were stable and these molecules had comparable interaction with reference inhibitors. Dihydrokavain is one of the kavalactones extracted from kava plant with an anxiolytic property. This compound was found interesting and recommended to be explored as anticancer drug in this study (Galúcio et al., 2019). However, it was already stated that crude extracts of kava has an inhibitory effect on osteosarcoma cells in 2015 (Dai et al., 2015) and on leukemia cancer cell lines and ovarian tumors earlier in 2005 (Tabudravu and Jaspars, 2005). A recent study was conducted to show the effect of kavain constitutes on oral squamous cell carcinoma cells in vitro (Celentano et al., 2020).

In 2018, anti-inflammatory plants, used for centuries in Indian medicine, were investigated to assess their potential as an anticancer drug. These plants were used by Indian tribes for centuries in different regions. Prediction of Activity Spectra for Substances (PASS) assessed 23 phytochemicals derived from 20 plants. PASS is a widely used tool to analyze the relationship between structure and activity. Those predicted plants were used by tribes to cure tumors. Selected compounds were further investigated with CLC-Pred tool to assess their cytotoxicity against different cancer cell lines and tissues in relation with tumor type. CLC-Pred tool uses the PASS training sets. As a result of CLC-Pred tool, selected compounds were found to be most effective on, but not limited to, carcinoma, and adenocarcinoma cells.

According to the result of admetSAR, Diospyrin from *Diospyros montana* Roxb. and Friedelin from *Mallotus philippensis* (Lam.) Müll. Arg. were found to have high absorption and metabolism and low toxicity; while Aristolochic acid from *Aristolochia bracteolata* Lam. was found to have high toxicity together with good absorption and metabolism in the human body. The admetSAR is therefore an important tool to predict ADME/T profile of the phytochemicals. Of course, the investigations were not limited to diospyrin, friedelin, and aristolochic acid. Since it was an extensive study, readers were kindly directed to read the above study for more information about the ancient medicinal wisdom of Ayurveda (Pavithra and Arumugam, 2018).

In a recent study, 21 phytochemicals from the phenolic group were investigated for their interaction with 1118 cancer stem cell genes. Resveratrol, epigallocatechin gallate, curcumin, quercetin, and genistein were the top five phenolics and were further evaluated for their potential as anticancer molecules against cancer stem cells. Oral bioavailability and drug-likeness of the phenolics were also investigated. Moreover, associated disease networks related to cancer stem cells (CSC) genes were also investigated. The presence of more than three aromatic rings is regarded as a sign that the drug cannot be developed further. Based on this fact, all of the studied phenolics were identified as potential drugs since they had three or fewer aromatic rings (Ritchie and Macdonald, 2009). Epigallocatechin gallate was the only phenolic compound violating the Lipinski rule of five and had low Caco-2 permeability. According to ADME profile of selected phenolics, none of them was found to be hepatoxic and skin sensitive (Mandal et al., 2020).

9.5 CONCLUSIONS

The discovery of novel drugs is extremely crucial for the treatment of currently untreatable diseases like cancer. However, the standard protocols for drug discovery require over a decade of analysis, testing, and clinical trials. Moreover, several million dollars are invested during the whole process of drug discovery. Many times, the novel compounds identified as potential anticancer agents pass the initial tests but fail clinical trials during to factors like toxicity, time of activity, target non-specificity, side effects, and many more. Hence it is necessary to develop programs and strategies to speed up the drug discovery processes cost-effectively. This is largely achieved with the help of CADD and similar approaches that combines artificial intelligence with biological information to constructively generate drug scaffolds, analyze protein interactions and accurately predict drug binding affinity and toxicity of molecules. These predictions walk us halfway through the drug-designing protocols of traditionally used approaches that lead to the validation of experimental procedures in a short time. With further improvement in artificial intelligence leading to superior CADD software and related programs, combined with valuable literature on plant-based compounds, an effective treatment for cancer is possible in near future.

ACKNOWLEDGMENTS

Figures 9.3 and 9.4 were designed using resources from Flaticon.com.

KEYWORDS

- **anticancer**
- **cancer**
- **computational biology**
- **computer-aided drug design**
- **plant secondary metabolites**

REFERENCES

Abdelmoez, A.; Coraça-Huber, D. C.; Thurner, G. C.; Debbage, P.; Lukas, P.; Skvortsov, S.; Skvortsova, I. I. Screening and İdentification of Molecular Targets for Cancer Therapy. *Cancer Lett.* **2017,** *387*, 3–9.

Abriata, L. A.; Palzkill, T.; Dal Peraro, M. How Structural and Physicochemical Determinants Shape Sequence Constraints in a Functional Enzyme. *PLoS One* **2015,** *10*, e0118684.

Acharya, R.; Chacko, S.; Bose, P.; Lapenna, A.; Pattanayak, S. P. Structure Based Multitargeted Molecular Docking Analysis of Selected Furanocoumarins against Breast Cancer. *Sci. Rep.* **2019,** *9*, 1–13.

Agbarya, A.; Ruimi, N.; Epelbaum, R.; Ben-Arye, E.; Mahajna, J. Natural Products as Potential Cancer Therapy Enhancers: A Preclinical Update. *SAGE Open Med.* **2014,** *2*, 2050312114546 92.

Agoni, C.; Olotu, F. A.; Ramharack, P.; Soliman, M. E. Druggability and Drug-likeness Concepts in Drug Design: Are Biomodelling and Predictive Tools Having their Say? *J. Mol. Model* **2020,** *26*, 1–11.

Ali, A. Herbs that Heal: The Philanthropic Behavior of Nature. *Ann. Phytomed.* **2020,** 9(1), 7–17.

Amaro, R. E.; Baudry, J.; Chodera, J.; Demir, Ö.; McCammon, J. A.; Miao, Y.; Smith, J. C. Ensemble Docking in Drug Discovery. *Biophys. J.* **2018,** *114*, 2271–2278.

Amin, A.; Gali-Muhtasib, H.; Ocker, M.; Schneider-Stock, R. Overview of Major Classes of Plant-Derived Anticancer Drugs. *Int. J. Biomed. Sci.* **2009,** *5*, 1–11.

Antunes, D. A.; Devaurs, D.; Kavraki, L. E. Understanding the Challenges of Protein Flexibility in Drug Design. *Expert Opin. Drug Discovery* **2015,** *10*, 1301–1313.

Ardalani, H.; Avan, A.; Ghayour-Mobarhan, M. Podophyllotoxin: A Novel Potential Natural Anticancer Agent. *Avicenna J. Phytomed.* **2017,** *7*, 285–294.

Atanasov, A. G.; Zotchev, S. B.; Dirsch, V. M.; Orhan, I. E.; Banach, M.; Rollinger, J. M.; Barreca, D.; Weckwerth, W.; Bauer, R.; Bayer, E. A.; Majeed, M.; Bishayee, A.; Bochkov, V.; Bonn, G. K.; Braidy, N.; Bucar, F.; Cifuentes, A.; D'Onofrio, G.; Bodkin, M.; Supuran, C. T. Natural Products in Drug Discovery: Advances and Opportunities. *Nat. Rev. Drug Discovery* **2021,** *20*, 200–216.

Ban, F.; Dalal, K.; Li, H.; LeBlanc, E.; Rennie, P. S.; Cherkasov, A. Best Practices of Computer-Aided Drug Discovery: Lessons Learned from the Development of a Preclinical Candidate for Prostate Cancer with a New Mechanism of Action. *J. Chem. Inform. Model* **2017,** *57*, 1018–1028.

Banik, D.; Moufarrij, S.; Villagra, A. Immunoepigenetics Combination Therapies: An Overview of the Role of HDACs in Cancer Immunotherapy. *Int. J. Mol. Sci.* **2019,** *20*, 2241.

Bar-Shavit, R.; Maoz, M.; Kancharla, A.; Nag, J. K.; Agranovich, D.; Grisaru-Granovsky, S.; Uziely, B. G Protein-coupled Receptors in Cancer. *Int. J. Mol. Sci.* **2016,** *17*, 1320.

Bensaid, D.; Blondy, T.; Deshayes, S.; Dehame, V.; Bertrand, P.; Grégoire, M.; Errami, M.; Blanquart, C. Assessment of new HDAC İnhibitors for İmmunotherapy of Malignant Pleural Mesothelioma. *Clin. Epigenetics* **2018,** *10*, 79.

Berman, H. M.; Westbrook, J.; Feng, Z.; Gilliland, G.; Bhat, T. N.; Weissig, H.; Shindyalov, I. N.; Bourne, P. E. The Protein Data Bank. *Nucleic Acids Res.* **2000,** *28*, 235–242.

Berman, H.; Henrick, K.; Nakamura, H. Announcing the Worldwide Protein Data Bank. *Nat. Struct. Biol.* **2003,** *10*, 980.

Bhattacharyya, M.; Vishveshwara, S. Probing the Allosteric Mechanism in Pyrrolysyl-tRNA Synthetase using Energy-Weighted Network Formalism. *Biochem.* **2011,** *50*, 6225–6236.

Binaschi, M.; Zunino, F.; Capranico, G.; Mechanism of Action of DNA Topoisomerase İnhibitors. *Stem Cells* **1995,** 13, 369–379.

Bitencourt-Ferreira, G.; de Azevedo, W. F. How Docking Programs Work. *Methods Mol. Biol.* **2019,** *2053*, 35–50.

Boittier, E. D.; Tang, Y. Y.; Buckley, M. E.; Schuurs, Z. P.; Richard, D. J.; Gandhi, N. S. Assessing Molecular Docking Tools to Guide Targeted Drug Discovery of cd38 İnhibitors. *Int. J. Mol. Sci.* **2020,** *21*, 1–19.

Brogi, S.; Ramalho, T. C.; Kuca, K.; Medina-Franco, J. L.; Valko, M. In silico Methods for Drug Design and Discovery. *Front. Chem.* **2020,** *8*, 612.

Burley, S. K.; Bhikadiya, C.; Bi, C.; Bittrich, S.; Chen, L.; Crichlow, G. V.; Christie, C. H.; Dalenberg, K.; Di Costanzo, L.; Duarte, J. M.; Dutta, S.; Feng, Z.; Ganesan, S.; Goodsell, D. S.; Ghosh, S.; Green, R. K.; Guranovic, V.; Guzenko, D.; Hudson, B. P.; Zhuravleva, M. RCSB Protein Data Bank: Powerful New Tools for Exploring 3D Structures of Biological Macromolecules for Basic and Applied Research and Education in Fundamental Biology, Biomedicine, Biotechnology, Bioengineering and Energy Sciences. *Nucleic Acids Res*. **2021,** *49*, D437–D451.

Cahlíková, L.; Šafratová, M.; Hošťálková, A.; Chlebek, J.; Hulcová, D.; Breiterová, K.; Opletal, L. Pharmacognosy and its Role in the System of Profile Disciplines in Pharmacy: *Nat. Prod. Commun*. **2020,** *15*, 1–7.

Calaf, G. M.; Urzua, U.; Termini, L.; Aguayo, F. Oxidative Stress in Female Cancers. *Oncotarget*. **2018,** *9*, 23824–23842.

Celentano, A.; Yiannis, C.; Paolini, R.; Zhang, P.; Farah, C. S.; Cirillo, N.; Yap, T.; McCullough, M. Kava Constituents Exert Selective Anticancer Effects in Oral Squamous Cell Carcinoma Cells in Vitro. *Sci. Rep*. **2020,** *10*, 1–11.

Chan, H. C. S.; Shan, H.; Dahoun, T.; Vogel, H.; Yuan, S. Advancing Drug Discovery via *Artificial Intelligence. Trends Pharmacol. Sci.* **2019,** *40*, 592–604.

Chanda, S.; Nagani, K. In vitro and in vivo Methods for Anticancer Activity Evaluation and Some Indian Medicinal Plants Possessing Anticancer Properties : An Overview. *J. Pharmacogn. Phytochem*. **2013,** *2*, 140–152.

Charifson, P. S.; Corkery, J. J.; Murcko, M. A.; Walters, W. P. Consensus Scoring: A Method for Obtaining İmproved Hit Rates from Docking Databases of Three-Dimensional Structures into Proteins. *J. Med. Chem.* **1999,** *42*, 5100–5109.

Chatzigoulas, A.; Cournia, Z. Rational Design of Allosteric Modulators: Challenges and Successes. *Comput. Mol. Sci*. **2021**, e1529.

Chen, Y. C. Beware of Docking! *Trends Pharmacol. Sci.* **2015,** *36*, 78–95.

Cohen, R.; Pudlarz, T.; Delattre, J. F.; Colle, R.; André, T. Molecular Targets for the Treatment of Metastatic Colorectal Cancer. *Cancers*. **2020,** *12*, 2350.

Cragg, G. M.; Pezzuto, J. M. Natural Products as a Vital Source for the Discovery of Cancer Chemotherapeutic and Chemopreventive Agents. Med. *Princ. Pract.* **2016,** *25*, 41–59.

Cui, W.; Aouidate, A.; Wang, S.; Yu, Q.; Li, Y.; Yuan, S. Discovering Anti-Cancer Drugs via Computational Methods. *Front. Pharmacol*. **2020,** *11*, 733.

Cui, W.; Aouidate, A.; Wang, S.; Yu, Q.; Li, Y.; Yuan, S. Discovering Anti-Cancer Drugs via Computational Methods. *Front. Pharmacol*. **2020,** *11*, 733.

Dai, Jun-Qi, Yi-Gang Huang, and Ai-Na He. Dihydromethysticin Kavalactone Induces Apoptosis in Osteosarcoma Cells through Modulation of PI3K/Akt Pathway, Disruption of Mitochondrial Membrane Potential and Inducing Cell Cycle Arrest. *Int. J. Clin. Exp. Pathol.* **2015,** *8*(5): 4356.

Dai, S. X.; Li, W. X.; Han, F. F.; Guo, Y. C.; Zheng, J. J.; Liu, J. Q.; Wang, Q.; Gao, Y. D.; Li, G. H.; Huang, J. F. In Silico İdentification of Anti-Cancer Compounds and Plants from Traditional Chinese Medicine Database. *Sci. Rep*. **2016,** *6*, 25462.

Damaskos, C.; Valsami, S.; Kontos, M.; Spartalis, E.; Kalampokas, T.; Kalampokas, E.; Athanasiou, A.; Moris, D.; Daskalopoulou, A.; Davakis, S.; Tsourouflis, G.; Kontzoglou, K.; Perrea, D.; Nikiteas, N.; Dimitroulis, D. Histone Deacetylase İnhibitors: An Attractive Therapeutic Strategy Against Breast Cancer. *Anticancer. Res.* **2017,** *37*, 35–46.

de Anda-Jáuregui, G.; Hernández-Lemus, E. Computational Oncology in the Multi-Omics Era: State of the Art. *Front. Oncol*. **2020,** *10*, 423.

de Groot, C. O.; Hsia, J. E.; Anzola, J. V.; Motamedi, A.; Yoon, M.; Wong, Y. L.; Jenkins, D.; Lee, H. J.; Martinez, M. B.; Davis, R. L.; Gahman, T. C.; Desai, A.; Shiau, A. K. A Cell Biologist's Field Guide to Aurora Kinase Inhibitors. *Front. Oncol*. **2015,** *5*, 285.

Deng, H.; Jia, Y.; Zhang, Y. Protein Structure Prediction. *Int. J. Mod. Phys. B.* **2018,** *32*. https://doi.org/10.1142/S021797921840009X

Doak, B. C.; Over, B.; Giordanetto, F.; Kihlberg, J. Oral Druggable Space Beyond the Rule of 5: İnsights from Drugs and Clinical Candidates. *Chem. Biol.* **2014,** *21*, 1115–1142.

Dolezal, R.; Ramalho, T. C.; França, T. C. C.; Kuca, K. Parallel Flexible Molecular Docking in Computational Chemistry on High Performance Computing Clusters. *Lect. Notes Comput. Sci.* **2015,** 9330, 418–427.

Dong, D.; Xu, Z.; Zhong, W.; Peng, S. Parallelization of Molecular Docking: A Review. *Curr. Top. Med. Chem.* **2018,** *18*, 1015–1028.

Durrant, J. D.; McCammon, J. A. Molecular Dynamics Simulations and Drug Discovery. *BMC Biol.* **2011,** *9*, 71.

Ebrahim, H. Y.; Osman, S. A.; Haffez, H. R.; Hassan, Z. A. In-Vıtro Screenıng of Some Plant Extracts for theır Potentıal Antıcancer Actıvıty. *African J. Tradit. Complement. Altern. Med.* **2020,** *17*, 1–8.

Echave, J.; Wilke, C. O. Biophysical Models of Protein Evolution: Understanding the Patterns of Evolutionary Sequence Divergence. *Annual Rev. Biophys.* **2017,** *46*, 85–103.

Eckschlager, T.; Plch, J.; Stiborova, M.; Hrabeta, J. Histone Deacetylase Inhibitors as Anticancer Drugs. *Int. J. Mol. Sci.* **2017,** *18*, 1414.

El-Kenawi, A. E.; El-Remessy, A. B. Angiogenesis İnhibitors in Cancer Therapy: Mechanistic Perspective on Classification and Treatment Rationales. *Br. J. Pharmacol.* **2013,** *170*, 712–729.

Emwas, A. H.; Szczepski, K.; Poulson, B. G.; Chandra, K.; McKay, R. T.; Dhahri, M.; Alahmari, F.; Jaremko, L.; Lachowicz, J. I.; Jaremko, M. NMR as a "Gold Standard" Method in Drug Design and Discovery. *Molecules* **2020,** *25*, 4597.

Feher, M.; Schmidt, J. M. Property distributions: Differences Between Drugs, Natural Products, and Molecules from Combinatorial Chemistry. *J. Chem. Inf. Comput. Sci.* **2003,** *43,* 218–227.

Feixas, F.; Lindert, S.; Sinko, W.; McCammon, J. A. Exploring the Role of Receptor Flexibility in Structure-Based Drug Discovery. *Biophys. Chem.* **2014,** *186*, 31–45.

Ferreira, L. L. G.; Andricopulo, A. D. ADMET Modeling Approaches in Drug Discovery. *Drug Discov. Today* **2019,** *24*, 1157–1165.

Fridlender, M.; Kapulnik, Y.; Koltai, H. Plant Derived Substances with Anti-Cancer Activity: From Folklore to Practice. *Front. Plant Sci.* **2015,** 6, 1–9.

Galúcio, J. M.; Monteiro, E. F.; de Jesus, D. A.; Costa, C. H.; Siqueira, R. C.; Dos Santos, G. B.; Lameira, J.; da Costa, K. S. In Silico Identification of Natural Products with Anticancer Activity Using a Chemo-Structural Database of Brazilian Biodiversity. *Comput. Biol. Chem.* **2019,** 107102.

Genheden, S.; and Ryde, U. The MM/PBSA and MM/GBSA Methods to Estimate Ligand-Binding Affinities. *Expert Opin. Drug Discov.* **2015,** *10*, 449–461.

Ghandi, M.; Huang, F. W.; Jané-Valbuena, J.; Kryukov, G. V.; Lo, C. C.; McDonald, E. R.; Barretina, J.; Gelfand, E. T.; Bielski, C. M.; Li, H.; Hu, K.; Andreev-Drakhlin, A. Y.; Kim, J.; Hess, J. M.; Haas, B. J.; Aguet, F.; Weir, B. A.; Rothberg, M. V.; Paolella, B. R.; Sellers, W. R. Next-generation Characterization of the Cancer Cell Line Encyclopedia. *Nature* **2019,** *569*, 503–508.

Gioia, D.; Bertazzo, M.; Recanatini, M.; Masetti, M.; Cavalli, A. Dynamic docking: A Paradigm Shift in Computational Drug Discovery. *Molecules* **2017,** *22*, 2029.

Glaab, E. Building a Virtual Ligand Screening Pipeline Using Free Software: A survey. *Brief. Bioinform.* **2016,** *17*, 352–366.

Grabowski, K.; Schneider, G. Properties and Architecture of Drugs and Natural Products Revisited. *Curr. Chem. Biol.* **2012,** *1*, 115–127.

Graham, J. G.; Quinn, M. L.; Fabricant, D. S.; Farnsworth, N. R. Plants Used Against Cancer - An Extension of the Work of Jonathan Hartwell. *J. Ethnopharmacol.* **2000,** *73*, 347–377.

Greenwell, M.; Rahman P. K. S. M. Medicinal Plants: Their Use in Anticancer Treatment. *Int. J. Pharm. Sci. Res.* **2015,** *6*, 4103–4112.

Grothaus, P. G.; Cragg, G. M.; Newman, D. J. Plant Natural Products in Anticancer Drug Discovery. *Curr. Org. Chem.* **2010,** *14*, 1781–1791.

Haddad, Y.; Adam, V.; Heger, Z. Ten Quick Tips for Homology Modeling of High-Resolution Protein 3D Structures. In F. Ouellette (Ed.), *PLoS Comput. Biol.* 2020, *16*, e1007449.

Haibe, Y.; Kreidieh, M.; El Hajj, H.; Khalifeh, I.; Mukherji, D.; Temraz, S.; Shamseddin, A. Resistance Mechanisms to Anti-angiogenic Therapies in Cancer. *Front. Oncol.* **2020,** *10*.

Hartwell, J. L. Plants used Against Cancer. A Survey. *Lloydia.* **1971,** *34*, 103–160.

Henzler-Wildman, K.; Kern, D. Dynamic Personalities of Proteins. *Nature.* **2007,** *450*, 964–972.

Hijjawi, M. S.; Reem, F. A.; Mutasem, O. T. Structure-Based Discovery and Bioactivity Evaluation of Novel Aurora-A Kinase Inhibitors as Anticancer Agents via Docking-Based Comparative Intermolecular Contacts Analysis (DbCICA). *Molecules* **2021,** *25*, 6003.

Ho, T. T.; Tran, Q. T.; Chai, C. L. The Polypharmacology of Natural Products. *Future Med. Chem.* **2018,** *10*, 1361–1368.

Hollingsworth, S. A.; Kelly, B.; Valant, C.; Michaelis, J. A.; Mastromihalis, O.; Thompson, G.; Venkatakrishnan, A. J.; Hertig, S.; Scammells, P. J.; Sexton, P. M.; Felder, C. C.; Christopoulos, A.; Dror, R. O. Cryptic Pocket Formation Underlies Allosteric Modulator Selectivity at Muscarinic GPCRs. *Nat. Commun.* **2019,** *10*, 3289.

Hontecillas-Prieto, L.; Flores-Campos, R.; Silver, A.; de Álava, E.; Hajji, N.; García-Domínguez, D. J. Synergistic Enhancement of Cancer Therapy Using HDAC Inhibitors: Opportunity for Clinical Trials. *Front. Genet.* **2020,** *11*.

Hospital, A.; Goni, J. R.; Orozco, M.; Gelpi, J. L. Molecular Dynamics Simulations: Advances and Applications. *Adv. Appl. Bioinform. Chem.* **2015,** *8*, 37–47.

Huang, M.; Lu, J.J.; Ding, J. Natural Products in Cancer Therapy: Past, Present and Future. *Nat. Prod. Bioprospect.* **2021,** *11*, 5–13.

Huang, S. Y.; Grinter, S. Z.; Zou, X. Scoring Functions and their Evaluation Methods for Protein-Ligand Docking: Recent Advances and Future Directions. *Phys Chem. Chem. Phys.* **2010,** *12*, 12899–12908.

Huang, S.Y. Search Strategies and Evaluation in Protein-Protein Docking: Principles, Advances and Challenges. *Drug Discov. Today* **2014**, *19*, 1081–1096.

Iheagwam, F. N.; Ogunlana, O. O.; Ogunlana, O.E.; Isewon, I.; Oyelade, J. Potential Anti-Cancer Flavonoids Isolated From Caesalpinia Bonduc Young Twigs and Leaves: Molecular Docking and In Silico Studies. *Bioinform. Biol. Insights* **2019**.

Iqbal, J.; Abbasi, B. A.; Mahmood, T.; Kanwal, S.; Ali, B.; Shah, S. A.; Khalil, A. T. Plant-Derived Anticancer Agents: A Green Anticancer Approach. *Asian Pac. J. Trop. Biomed.* **2017**, *7*, 1129–1150.

Jaghoori, M. M.; Bleijlevens, B.; Olabarriaga, S. D. 1001 Ways to run AutoDock Vina for virtual screening. *J. Comput-Aided Mol. Des.* **2016,** *30*, 237–249.

Jain, C.; Majumder, H.; Roychoudhury, S. Natural Compounds as Anticancer Agents Targeting DNA Topoisomerases. *Curr. Genomics* **2016,** *18*, 75–92.

Jenke, R.; Reßing, N.; Hansen, F. K.; Aigner, A.; Büch, T. Anticancer Therapy with HDAC Inhibitors: Mechanism-Based Combination Strategies and Future Perspectives. *Cancers (Basel)* **2021**, *13*, 634.

Jiang, Y.; Zhuo, X.; Mao, C. G Protein-coupled Receptors in Cancer Stem Cells. *Curr. Pharm. Des.* **2020,** *26*, 1952–1963. https://doi.org/10.2174/13816128266620030 5130009

Jun Qi, D.; Huang, Y. G.; He, A. N. Dihydromethysticin Kavalactone Induces Apoptosis in Osteosarcoma Cells through Modulation of PI3K/Akt Pathway, Disruption of Mitochondrial Membrane Potential and Inducing Cell Cycle Arrest. *Int. J. Clin. Exp. Pathol.* **2015,** *8*, 4356.

Jung, Y.; Shin, S. Y.; Yong, Y.; Jung, H.; Ahn, S.; Lee, Y. H.; Lim, Y. Plant-Derived Flavones as Inhibitors of Aurora B Kinase and Their Quantitative Structure-Activity Relationships. *Chem. Biol. Drug Des.* **2015,** *85*, 574–585.

Kar, S.; Leszczynski, L. Open Access in Silico Tools to Predict the ADMET Profiling of Drug Candidates. *Expert Opin. Drug Discov*. **2020,** *15*, 1473–1487.

Kaul, R.; Risinger, A. L.; Mooberry, S. L. Microtubule-Targeting Drugs: More than Antimitotics. *J. Nat. Prod.* **2019,** *82*, 680–685.

Khan, T.; Ali, M.; Khan, A.; Nisar, P.; Jan, S. A.; Afridi, S.; Shinwari, N. Anticancer Plants: A Review of the Active Phytochemicals, Applications in Animal Models, and Regulatory Aspects. *Biomolecules* **2019,** *10*, 47.

Khan, W.; Ashfaq, W. A.; Aslam, S.; Saif, S.; Aslam, T.; Tusleem, K.; Maryam, A.; Qamar, M. T. Anticancer Screening of Medicinal Plant Phytochemicals against Cyclin-Dependent Kinase-2 (CDK2): An in-Silico Approach. *Adv. Life Sci.* **2017,** *4*, 113–119.

Kim, H. J.; Bae, S. C. Histone Deacetylase İnhibitors: Molecular Mechanisms of Action and Clinical Trials as Anti-Cancer Drugs. *Am. J. Transl. Res.* **2011,** *3*, 166–179.

Kim, S. J.; Kim, H. S.; Seo, Y. R. Understanding of ROS-Inducing Strategy in Anticancer Therapy. *Oxid. Med. Cell Longev.* **2019,** 1–12.

Klaeger, S.; Heinzlmeir, S.; Wilhelm, M.; Polzer, H.; Vick, B.; Koenig, P. A.; Reinecke, M.; Ruprecht, B.; Petzoldt, S.; Meng, C.; Zecha, J.; Reiter, K.; Qiao, H.; Helm, D.; Koch, H.; Schoof, M.; Canevari, G.; Casale, E.; Re Depaolini, S.; Kuster, B. The Target Landscape of Clinical Kinase Drugs. *Sci.* **2017,** *358*, 6367.

Klebe, G. Virtual Ligand Screening: Strategies, Perspectives and Limitations. *Drug Discov. Today* **2006,** *11*, 580–594.

Knox, S. S. From "omics" to Complex Disease: A Systems Biology Approach to Gene-Environment İnteractions in Cancer. *Cancer Cell Int.* **2010,** *10*, 1–13.

Kontoyianni, M. Docking and Virtual Screening in Drug Discovery. *Methods Mol. Biol.* **2017,** *1647*, 255–266.

Kopustinskiene, D. M.; Jakstas, V.; Savickas, A.; Bernatoniene, J. Flavonoids as Anticancer Agents. *Nutrients* **2020,** *12*, 457.

Koulouridi, E.; Valli, M.; Ntie-Kang, F.; Bolzani, V. D. S. A Primer on Natural Product-Based Virtual Screening. *Phys. Sci. Rev.* **2019,** *4*.

Kroesen, M.; Gielen, P. R.; Brok, I. C.; Armandari, I.; Hoogerbrugge, P. M.; Adema, G. J. HDAC İnhibitors and İmmunotherapy; a Double Edged Sword? *Oncotarget.* **2014,** *5*, 6558–6572.

Krumova, K.; Cosa, G. Overview of Reactive Oxygen Species. *In: Singlet Oxygen: Applications in Biosciences and Nanosciences* 2016, 1–21.

Kummar, S.; Doroshow, J. H. Molecular Targets in Cancer Therapy. *Expert Rev. Anticancer Ther.* **2013,** *13*, 267–269.

Kuruppu, A. I.; Paranagama, P.; Goonasekara, C. L. Medicinal Plants Commonly used Against Cancer in Traditional Medicine Formulae in Sri Lanka. *Saudi Pharm. J.* **2019,** *27*, 565–573.

Kushwaha, P. P.; Maurya, S. K.; Singh, A.; Prajapati, K. S.; Singh, A.T.; Shuaib, M.; Kumar, S. Bulbine Frutescens Phytochemicals as Novel ABC-Transporter Inhibitor: A Molecular Docking and Molecular Dynamics Simulation Study. *J. Cancer Metastatis Treat.* **2021,** *7*, 2.

Lagarde, N.; Zagury, J. F.; Montes, M. Benchmarking Data Sets for the Evaluation of Virtual Ligand Screening Methods: Review and Perspectives. *J. Chem. Inf. Model* **2015,** *55*, 1297–1307.

Lamari, F. N.; Cordopatis, P. Exploring the Potential of Natural Products in Cancer Treatment. *Anticancer Ther.* **2008,** 1–16.

Leelananda, S. P.; Lindert, S. Computational Methods in Drug Discovery. *Beilstein J. Org. Chem.* **2016,** *12*, 2694–2718.

Li, J.; Fu, A.; Zhang, L. An Overview of Scoring Functions Used for Protein-Ligand Interactions in Molecular Docking. *Interdiscip. Sci. Comput. Life Sci.* **2019a,** *11*, 320–328.

Li, K.; Du, Y.; Li, L.; Wei, D. Q. Bioinformatics Approaches for Anti-cancer Drug Discovery. *Curr. Drug Targets* **2019b,** *21*, 3–17.

Lill, M. A.; Fischer, A.; Smiesko, M.; Sellner, M. Decision Making in Structure-Based Drug Discovery: Visual İnspection of Docking Results. *J. Med. Chem.* **2021,** *64*, 2489–2500.

Lipinski, C. A.; Lombardo, F.; Dominy, B. W.; Feeney, P. J. Experimental and Computational Approaches to Estimate Solubility and Permeability in Drug Discovery and Development Settings. *Adv. Drug Del. Rev.* **2001,** *46*, 3–26.

Liu, J.; Wang, R. Classification of Current Scoring Functions. *J. Chem. Inf. Model* **2015,** *55*, 475–482.

Liu, X.; Shi, D.; Zhou, S.; Liu, H.; Liu, H.; Yao, X. Molecular Dynamics Simulations and Novel Drug Discovery. *Expert Opin. Drug Discov.* **2018,** *13*, 23–37.

Liu, Y.; An, S.; Ward, R.; Yang, Y.; Guo, X. X.; Li, W.; Xu, T. R. G Protein-Coupled Receptors as Promising Cancer Targets. *Cancer Lett.* **2016,** *376*, 226–239.

Lohning, A. E.; Levonis, S. M.; Williams-Noonan, B.; Schweiker, S. S. A Practical Guide to Molecular Docking and Homology Modelling for Medicinal Chemists. *Curr. Topics Med. Chem.* **2017,** *17*, 2023–2040.

Lopes-Rodrigues, V.; Sousa, E.; Vasconcelos, M. H. Curcumin as a modulator of P-glycoprotein in cancer: Challenges and perspectives. *Pharmaceuticals* **2016,** *9*, 71.

Macalino, S. J. Y.; Gosu, V.; Hong, S.; Choi, S. Role of computer-aided drug design in modern drug discovery. *Arch. Pharma. Res.* **2015,** *38*, 1686–1701.

Maia, E. H. B.; Assis, L. C.; de Oliveira, T. A.; da Silva, A. M.; Taranto, A. G. Structure-Based Virtual Screening: From Classical to Artificial Intelligence. *Front. Chem.* **2020,** *8*, 343.

Mandal, M.; Sahoo, S. K.; Patra, P.; Mallik, S.; Zhao, Z. In Silico Ranking of Phenolics for Therapeutic Effectiveness on Cancer Stem Cells. *BMC Bioinform.* **2020,** *21*, 1–17.

Maveyraud, L.; Mourey, L. Protein X-ray Crystallography and Drug Discovery. *Molecules* **2020,** *25*, 1030.

McClure, J. J.; Li, X.; Chou, C. J. Advances and Challenges of HDAC Inhibitors in Cancer Therapeutics. *Adv. Cancer Res.* **2018,** *138*, 183–211.

Mealey, K. L.; Fidel, J. P-Glycoprotein Mediated Drug Interactions in Animals and Humans with Cancer. *J. Vet. Intern. Med.* **2015,** *29*, 1–6.

Menyhárt, O.; Győrffy, B. Multi-omics Approaches in Cancer Research with Applications in Tumor Subtyping, Prognosis, and Diagnosis. *Comput. Struct. Biotechnol. J.* **2021,** *19*, 949–960.

Mignani, S.; Rodrigues, J.; Tomas, H.; Jalal, R.; Singh, P. P.; Majoral, J. P.; Vishwakarma, R. A. Present Drug-Likeness Filters in Medicinal Chemistry During the Hit and Lead Optimization Process: How Far Can They be Simplified? *Drug Discov. Today* **2018,** *23*, 605–615.

Muhammed, M. T.; Aki-Yalcin, E. Homology Modeling in Drug Discovery: Overview, Current Applications, and Future Perspectives. *Chem. Biol. Drug Design* **2019,** *93*, 12–20.

Nadhan, R.; Patra, D.; Krishnan, N.; Rajan, A.; Gopala, S.; Ravi, D.; Srinivas, P. Perspectives on Mechanistic İmplications of ROS İnducers for Targeting Viral İnfections. *Eur. J. Pharmacol.* **2021,** *890*, 173621.

National Institute of Cancer Prevention and Research (NICPR) report, 2021. Available at http://cancerindia.org.in/cancer-statistics/(Accessed 26th September 2021).

Neves, B. J.; Mottin, M.; Moreira-Filho, J. T.; Sousa, B. K. de P.; Mendonca, S. S.; Andrade, C. H. Best Practices for Docking-Based Virtual Screening. Mol. Dock. *Comp. Aided Drug Design.* **2021,** 75–98.

Nishida, N.; Yano, H.; Nishida, T.; Kamura, T.; Kojiro, M. Angiogenesis in Cancer. *Vasc. Health Risk Manag.* **2006,** *2*, 213–219.

Norinder, U.; Bergström, C. A. S. Prediction of ADMET Properties. *Chem. Med. Chem.* **2006,** *1*, 920–937.

Ntie-Kang, F.; Lifongo, L. L.; Judson, P. N.; Sippl, W.; Efange, S. M. N. How "Drug-Like" are Naturally Occurring Anti-Cancer Compounds? *J. Mol. Model* **2014,** *20*, 1–13.

Ntie-Kang, F.; Nyongbela, K. D.; Ayimele, G. A.; Shekfeh, S. Drug-likeness" Properties of Natural Compounds. *Phys. Sci. Rev*. **2019,** *4*.

Otrock, Z.; Mahfouz, R.; Makarem, J.; Shamseddıne, A. Understanding the Biology of Angiogenesis: Review of the Most İmportant Molecular Mechanisms. *Blood Cells Mol. Dis.* **2007,** *39*, 212–220.

Ouyang, J.; Zhu, K.; Liu, Z.; Huang, J. Prooxidant Effects of Epigallocatechin-3-Gallate in Health Benefits and Potential Adverse Effect. *Oxid. Med. Cell Longev.* **2020,** 1–14.

Paramanya, A.; Ali, A. Role of Oxidative Stress in Biological Systems. *Middle East J. Sci.* **2019,** 5(2), 155–162.

Park, H.; Jeon, J.; Kim, K.; Choi, S.; Hong, S. Structure-Based Virtual Screening and de Novo Design of PIM1 İnhibitors with Anticancer Activity from Natural Products. *Pharmaceuticals* **2021,** *14*, 275.

Pavithra, C.; Arumugam, R. In Silico Prediction of Anticarcinogenic Bioactivities of Traditional Anti-Inflammatory Plants Used by Tribal Healers in Sathyamangalam Wildlife Sanctuary, India. *Egypt. J. Basic Appl. Sci.* **2018,** *5*, 265–279.

Perillo, B.; Di Donato, M.; Pezone, A.; Di Zazzo, E.; Giovannelli, P.; Galasso, G.; Castoria, G., Miggliaccio, A. ROS in Cancer Therapy: the Bright Side of the Moon. *Exp. Mol. Med.* **2020,** *52*, 192–203.

Perricone, U.; Gulotta, M. R.; Lombino, J.; Parrino, B.; Cascioferro, S.; Diana, P.; Cirrincione, G.; Padova, A. An Overview of Recent Molecular Dynamics Applications as Medicinal Chemistry Tools for the Undruggable Site Challenge. Med. *Chem. Comm.* **2018,** *9*, 920–936.

Phaniendra, A.; Jestadi, D. B.; Periyasamy, L. Free Radicals: Properties, Sources, Targets, and Their Implication in Various Diseases. *Indian J. Clin. Biochem.* **2015,** *30*, 11–26.

Phillips, M. A.; Stewart, M. A.; Woodling, D. L.; Xie, Z. R. Has Molecular Docking Ever Brought us a Medicine? *Mol. Dock.* **2018**.

Pinzi, L.; Rastelli, G. Molecular Docking: Shifting Paradigms in Drug Discovery. *Int. J. Mol. Sci.* **2019**, *20*, 4331.

Plewczynski, D.; Łaźniewski, M.; Augustyniak, R.; Ginalski, K. Can We Trust Docking Results? Evaluation of Seven Commonly Used Programs on PDBbind Database. *J. Computat. Chem.* **2011,** *32*, 742–755.

Pokharel, D.; Roseblade, A.; Oenarto, V.; Lu, J.; Bebawy, M. Proteins Regulating the İntercellular Transfer and Function of P-glycoprotein in Multidrug-Resistant Cancer. *E Cancer Med. Sci.* **2017,** 11.

Poli, G.; Tuccinardi, T. Consensus Docking in Drug Discovery. *Cur.Bioact. Comp.* **2018,** *16*, 182–190.

Pommier, Y. Topoisomerase I İnhibitors: Camptothecins and Beyond. Nat. Rev. *Cancer* **2006,** *6*, 789–802.

Porter, B. A.; Ortiz, M. A.; Bratslavsky, G.; Kotula, L. Structure and Function of the Nuclear Receptor Superfamily and Current Targeted Therapies of Prostate Cancer. *Cancers* **2019,** *11*, 1852.

Qiao, G.; Bi, K.; Liu, J.; Cao, S.; Liu, M.; Pešić, M.; Lin, X. Protein Kinases as Targets for Developing Anticancer Agents from Marine Organisms. *Biochim. Biophys. Acta Gen. Subj.* **2021,** *1865*, 129759.

Quan, C.; Xiao, J.; Liu, L.; Duan, Q.; Yuan, P.; Zhu, F. Protein Kinases as Tumor Biomarkers and Therapeutic Targets. *Curr. Pharm. Design* **2017,** *23*, 17.

Rahman, M. M.; Khan, M. A. Anti-Cancer Potential of South Asian Plants. *Nat. Prod. Bioprospect.* **2013,** *3*, 74–88.

Rallabandi, H. R.; Mekapogu, M.; Natesan, K.; Saindane, M.; Dhupal, M.; Swamy, M. K.; Vasamsetti, B. M. K. Computational Methods Used in Phytocompound-Based Drug Discovery. In: *Plant-derived Bioactives: Chemistry and Mode of Action* 2020, pp. 549–573.

Ramakrishna, W.; Kumari, A.; Rahman, N.; Mandave, P. Anticancer Activities of Plant Secondary Metabolites: Rice Callus Suspension Culture as a New Paradigm. *Rice Sci.* **2021,** *28*, 13–30.

Renaud, J. P.; Chari, A.; Ciferri, C.; Liu, W. T.; Rémigy, H. W.; Stark, H.; Wiesmann, C. Cryo-EM in Drug Discovery: Achievements, Limitations and Prospects. *Nat. Rev. Drug Discov.* **2018,** *17*, 471–492.

Ritchie, T. J.; Macdonald, S. J. F. The Impact of Aromatic Ring Count on Compound Developability – Are Too Many Aromatic Rings a Liability in Drug Design? *Drug Discov. Today* **2009,** *14*, 1011–1020.

Romano, J. D.; Tatonetti, N. P. Informatics and Computational Methods in Natural Product Drug Discovery: A Review and Perspectives. *Front. Genetics* **2019,** *10*, 368.

Roskoski, R. A Historical Overview of Protein Kinases and their Targeted Small Molecule İnhibitors. *Pharmacol. Res.* **2015,** *100*, 1–23.

Sakkiah, S.; Ng, H. W.; Tong, W.; Hong, H. Structures of Androgen Receptor Bound with Ligands: Advancing Understanding of Biological Functions and Drug Discovery. *Expert Opin. Ther. Targets* **2016,** *20*, 1267–1282.

Saldaño, T. E.; Monzon, A. M.; Parisi, G.; Fernandez-Alberti, S. Evolutionary Conserved Positions Define Protein Conformational Diversity. *PLoS Computat. Biol.* **2016,** *12*, e1004775.

Salo-Ahen, O. M. H.; Alanko, I.; Bhadane, R.; Bonvin, A. M. J. J.; Honorato, R. V.; Hossain, S.; Juffer, A. H.; Kabedev, A.; Lahtela-Kakkonen, M.; Larsen, A. S.; Lescrinier, E.; Marimuthu, P.; Mirza, M. U.; Mustafa, G.; Nunes-Alves, A.; Pantsar, T.; Saadabadi, A.; Singaravelu, K.; Vanmeert, M. Molecular Dynamics Simulations in Drug Discovery and Pharmaceutical Development. *Processes* **2020,** *9,* 71.

Santana, K.; do Nascimento, L. D.; Lima e Lima, A.; Damasceno, V.; Nahum, C.; Braga, R. C.; and Lameira, J. Applications of Virtual Screening in Bioprospecting: Facts, Shifts, and Perspectives to Explore the Chemo-Structural Diversity of Natural Products. *Front. Chem.* **2021,** *9*, 662688.

Santos, L. H. S.; Ferreira, R. S.; Caffarena, E. R. Integrating Molecular Docking and Molecular Dynamics Simulations. *Methods Mol. Biol.* **2019,** *2053*, 13–34.

Schiöth, H. B.; Lagerström, M. C. Structural diversity of G Protein Coupled Receptors and Significance for Drug Discovery. *Nat. Rev. Drug Discov.* **2008,** *7*, 339–357.

Schmit, T. L.; Ahmad, N. Regulation of Mitosis via Mitotic Kinases: New Opportunities for Cancer Management. *Mol. Cancer Ther.* **2007,** *6*, 1920–1931.

Scior, T.; Bender, A.; Tresadern, G.; Medina-Franco, J. L.; Martínez-Mayorga, K.; Langer, T.; Cuanalo-Contreras, K.; Agrafiotis, D. K. Recognizing Pitfalls in Virtual Screening: A Critical Review. *J. Chem. Inform. Model* **2012,** *52*, 867–881.

Scotti, L.; Bezerra Mendonca, F. J.; Ribeiro, F. F.; Tavares, J. F.; da Silva, M. S.; Barbosa Filho, J. M.; Scotti, M. T. Natural Product Inhibitors of Topoisomerases: Review and Docking Study. *Curr. Protein Pept. Sci.* **2018,** *19*, 275–296.

Seca, A.; Pinto, D. Plant Secondary Metabolites as Anticancer Agents: Successes in Clinical Trials and Therapeutic Application. *Int. J. Mol. Sci.* **2018,** *19*, 263.

Serçinoğlu, O.; Ozbek, P. Sequence Structure Function Relationships in Class i MHC: A Local Frustration Perspective. *PLoS One* **2020,** *15*, e0232849.

Serçinoğlu, O.; Bereketoglu, C.; Olsson, P.-E.; Pradhan, A. In Silico and in Vitro Assessment of Androgen Receptor Antagonists. *Comput. Biol. Chem.* **2021,** *92*, 107490.

Shin, S.; Lee, Y.; Kim, B.; Lee, J.; Ahn, S.; Koh, D.; Lim, Y.; Lee, Y. H. Inhibitory Effect of Synthetic Flavone Derivatives on Pan-Aurora Kinases: Induction of G2/M Cell-Cycle Arrest and Apoptosis in HCT116 Human Colon Cancer Cells. *Int. J. Mol. Sci.* **2018,** 19, 4086.

Sikosek, T.; Chan, H. S. Biophysics of Protein Evolution and Evolutionary Protein Biophysics. *J. Royal Soc. Interface* **2014,** *11*, 20140419.

Singh, H.; Bharadvaja, N. Treasuring the Computational Approach in Medicinal Plant Research. *Progress Biophysics Mol. Biol.* **2021,** *164*, 19–32.

Singh, S.; Kumari, P.; Hussain, Y.; Luqman, S.; Meena, A.; Kanaojia, D. Isothymusin, a Potential Inhibitor of Cancer Cell Proliferation: An In Silico and In Vitro Investigation. *Curr. Topics Med. Chem.* **2021,** *20*, 1898–1909.

Skok, Ž.; Zidar, N.; Kikelj, D.; Ilaš, J. Dual Inhibitors of Human DNA Topoisomerase II and Other Cancer-Related Targets. *J. Med. Chem.* **2020,** *63*, 884–904.

Sliwoski, G.; Kothiwale, S.; Meiler, J.; Lowe, E. W. Computational Methods in Drug Discovery. *Pharmacol. Rev.* **2014,** *66*, 334–395.

Sofowora, A.; Ogunbodede, E.; Onayade, A. The Role and Place of Medicinal Plants in the Strategies for Disease Prevention. *African J. Tradit. Complement. Altern. Med.* **2013,** *10*, 210–229.

Suraweera, A.; O'Byrne, K. J.; Richard, D. J. Combination Therapy with Histone Deacetylase Inhibitors (HDACi) for the Treatment of Cancer: Achieving the Full Therapeutic Potential of HDACi. *Front. Oncol.* **2018,** *8*.

Tabudravu, J N.; Jaspars, M. Anticancer Activities of Constituents of Kava (Piper methysticum). *South Pac. J. Nat. Appl. Sci.* **2005,** *23*, 26–29.

Temml, V.; Schuster, D. Molecular Docking for Natural Product Investigations: Pitfalls and Ways to Overcome Them. *Mol. Dock. Comput. Aided Drug Design* **2021,** 391–405.

Thurn, K. T.; Thomas, S.; Moore, A.; Munster, P. N. Rational Therapeutic Combinations with Histone Deacetylase İnhibitors for the Treatment of Cancer. *Futur. Oncol.* **2011,** *7*, 263–283.

Tian, S.; Wang, J.; Li, Y.; Li, D.; Xu, L.; Hou, T. The Application of İn Silico Drug-Likeness Predictions in Pharmaceutical Research. *Adv. Drug Del. Rev.* **2015,** *86*, 2–10.

Tiwari, S. P.; Reuter, N. Conservation of İntrinsic Dynamics in Proteins — What Have Computational Models Taught us? *Current Opin. Struct. Biol.* **2018,** *50*, 75–81.

Torres, P. H. M.; Sodero, A. C. R.; Jofily, P.; Silva Jr, F. P. Key Topics in Molecular Docking for Drug Design. *Int. J. Mol. Sci.* **2019,** *20*, 4574.

Trager, R. E.; Giblock, P.; Soltani, S.; Upadhyay, A. A.; Rekapalli, B.; Peterson, Y. K. Docking Optimization, Variance and Promiscuity for Large-Scale Drug-Like Chemical Space Using High Performance Computing Architectures. *Drug Discov. Today* **2016,** *21*, 1672–1680.

Vajda, S.; Beglov, D.; Wakefield, A. E.; Egbert, M.; and Whitty, A. Cryptic Binding Sites on Proteins: Definition, Detection, and Druggability. *Curr. Opin. Chem. Biol.* **2018,** *44*, 1–8.

Van Montfort, R. L. M.; Workman, P. Structure-Based Drug Design: Aiming for a Perfect Fit. *Essays in Biochem.* **2017,** *61*, 431–437.

van Vuuren, R. J.; Visagie, M. H.; Theron, A. E.; Joubert, A. M. Antimitotic Drugs in the Treatment of Cancer. *Cancer Chemother. Pharmacol.* **2015,** *76*, 1101–1112.

Veeresham, C. Natural Products Derived from Plants as a Source of Drugs. *J. Adv. Pharm. Technol. Res.* **2012,** *3*(4): 200–201.

Volkamer, A.; Kuhn, D.; Rippmann, F.; Rarey, M. Dogsitescorer: A Web Server for Automatic Binding Site Prediction, Analysis and Druggability Assessment. *Bioinformatics* **2012,** *28*, 2074–2075.

Waghray, D.; Zhang, Q. Inhibit or Evade Multidrug Resistance P-Glycoprotein in Cancer Treatment. *J. Med. Chem.* **2018,** *61*, 5108–5121.

Wang, W.; Tse-Dinh, Y. C. Recent Advances in Use of Topoisomerase Inhibitors in Combination Cancer Therapy. *Curr. Top. Med. Chem.* **2019,** *19*, 730–740.

Wang, X.; Waschke, B. C.; Woolaver, R. A.; Chen, S. M. Y.; Chen, Z.; Wang, J. H. HDAC İnhibitors Overcome İmmunotherapy Resistance in B-cell Lymphoma. *Protein Cell* **2020,** *11*, 472–482.

Welburn, J. P. I.; Jeyaprakash, A. A. Mechanisms of Mitotic Kinase Regulation: A Structural Perspective. *Front Cell. Dev. Biol.* **2018,** *6*.

Witt, O.; Deubzer, H. E.; Milde, T.; Oehme, I. HDAC family: What are the Cancer Relevant Targets? *Cancer Lett.* **2009,** *277*, 8–21.

Wong, Y. H.; Chiu, C. C.; Lin, C. L.; Chen, T. S.; Jheng, B. R.; Lee, Y. C.; Chen, J.; Chen, B. S. A New Era for Cancer Target Therapies: Applying Systems Biology and Computer-Aided Drug Design to Cancer Therapies. *Curr. Pharm. Biotechnol.* **2016,** *17*(14), 1246–1267.

World Health Organisation (WHO) Factsheet, 2021. Available at https://www.who.int/news-room/fact-sheets/detail/cancer (Accessed 26th September 2021).

Xu, X.; Huang, M.; Zou, X. Docking-Based İnverse Virtual Screening: Methods, Applications, and Challenges. *Biophys. Rep.* **2018,** *4*, 1–16.

Yan, V. C.; Butterfield, H. E.; Poral, A. H.; Yan, M. J.; Yang, K. L.; Pham, C. D.; Muller, F.L. Why Great Mitotic Inhibitors Make Poor Cancer Drugs. *Trends Cancer* **2020,** *6*, 924–941.

Yang, B.; Mao, J.; Gao, B.; Lu, X. Computer-Assisted Drug Virtual Screening Based on the Natural Product Databases. *Curr. Pharm. Biotechnol.* **2019,** *20*, 293–301.

Yoon, S.; and Eom, G. H. HDAC and HDAC Inhibitor: From Cancer to Cardiovascular Diseases. *Chonnam Med. J.* **2016,** *52*, 1.

You, Y. Podophyllotoxin Derivatives: Current Synthetic Approaches for New Anticancer Agents. *Curr. Pharm. Des.* **2005,** *11*, 1695–1717.

Zahra, K. F.; Lefter, R.; Ali, A.; Abdellah, E.; Trus, C.; Ciobica, A.; Timofte, D. The Involvement of the Oxidative Stress Status in Cancer Pathology: A Double View on the Role of the Antioxidants. *Oxid. Med. Cell. Long.* **2021,** 9965916.

Zhang, L.; Song, J.; Kong, L.; Yuan, T.; Li, W.; Zhang, W.; Hou, B.; Lu, Y.; and Du, G. The Strategies and Techniques of Drug Discovery from Natural Products. *Pharmacol. Therap.* **2020,** *216*, 107686.

Zhang, X.; Wong, S. E.; Lightstone, F. C. Message Passing İnterface and Multithreading Hybrid for Parallel Molecular Docking of Large Databases on Petascale High Performance Computing Machines. *J. Computat. Chem.* **2013,** *34*, 915–927.

Zou, Z.; Chang, H.; Li, H.; Wang, S. Induction of Reactive Oxygen Species: an Emerging Approach for Cancer Therapy. *Apoptosis* **2017,** *22*, 1321–1335.

CHAPTER 10

CRISPR/Cas-Mediated Editing of Anticancer Plants

MUHAMMAD SHAN, ZULQURNAIN KHAN, and MUHAMMAD ARSLAN AKHTAR

Institute of Plant Breeding and Biotechnology, MNS University of Agriculture Multan, Multan, Pakistan

ABSTRACT

Cancer is a disease that has a severe impact on the human population worldwide. Newer therapies to treat and prevent this life-threatening disease are continually required. Scientists and researchers are curious about naturally derived secondary metabolites as they are less poisonous to treatments such as chemotherapy. Since the dawn of human existence, plants are being used for medical purposes and provide modern medicine's backbone. Most therapeutic agents for cancer treatments are plants or their derivates, which are secluded and recognized molecules. Traditional biotechnology and new generation sequence (NGS) techniques have been effectively implemented to enhance plant products of biomedical importance. The Cas9 endonuclease and clustered regular short palindrome repeats (CRISPR) are site-driven productive and reliable mutagenesis approaches for specific RNA-driven genome editing. The CRISPR/Cas9 uses the designed RNAs guide to determine the sequence of three base-pair adjacent protospacer adjoining motif (PAM) patterns downstream of the target gene. But, due to the unavailability of the entire genome and mRNA sequences and the lack of adequate transformation and regeneration strategies, a few medical plants have been modified utilizing the CRISPR/Cas tool. Recently, several secondary metabolites of the plants have

Plant-Derived Anticancer Drugs in the OMICS Era: Biosynthesis, Functions, and Applications. Deepu Pandita, Anu Pandita (Eds.)

been designed for CRISPR/Cas editing employing knock-out, knock-in, point-mutation, gene expression fine-tailing, and target-mutagenesis (e.g., alkaloid, terpenoid, flavonoid, phenolic, saponin, etc.). In this chapter, secondary metabolites of anticancer plants will be discussed, along with CRISPR-mediated metabolic engineering and the prospect of CRISPR/Cas in medicinal plants.

10.1 ANTICANCER PLANTS AND SECONDARY METABOLITES

Cancer is the primary source of death after cardiovascular issues (White et al., 2014). Malignant growth is an intrinsic or stochastic confounded heritable illness because of genes' various expressions (Wishart, 2015). The exhibition levels of asbestos, tobacco, medications, radiation, and tumorigenic infection are numerous components responsible for the cell adjustment, coming full circle in a variety in the cell's genetic profile. Malignant cell uncovers polymorphisms and chromosomal anomalies diminish the intersection between cell breaches and normal cells. They have intrinsic development signals, which make them impervious to development concealment signals. They show protection from apoptosis, a modified cell passing vital for sustaining the balance in both cell growth and cell demise in the organism (Fulda, 2009). Such features of a disordered cell are prospective targets for medication improvement, halting cell growth, infiltration, and mobility.

Many medicines are designated and employed to either forestall or correct cancer (Cragg et al., 2016). Nonetheless, terrible fundamental adverse effects for patients, the rapid evolution of pharmaceutical opposition, and the more substantial price of therapy are a portion of the disadvantages rendering them unable in general, malignant growth the management. With the advancement of manufactured oncogenic drugs, malignancy patients are progressively reliant upon elective medications for treatment because of their well-being, accessibility, reasonableness, negligible antagonistic impacts, and less shot at creating an obstruction. Plants are the main wellspring of medication in antiquated occasions (Pan et al., 2014; Petrovska, 2012). Shockingly, they stay a considerable wellspring of medicine till now, prevalently in agricultural nations because of their benefits over business-manufactured medications. World Health Organization (WHO) has announced that approximately 80% of the total populace depends on the natural treatment method than traditional engineered drugs (WHO, 2014–2023).

Malignant growth analysts have concentrated more on regular items as an elective wellspring of disease control and repair. Indian outmoded Atharva Veda and ayurvedic medicine, traditional Chinese treatment, and Egypt Papyrus give rich documentation of plant-based prevention and healing techniques for illnesses and infections (Lemonnier et al., 2017). A few plants such as stalks, leaves, stem bark, roots, seeds' extracts are utilized as natural medicines (Li and Weng, 2017). Almost 60% of the recommended remedies used for anticancer treatment are subordinates of phytochemical constituents. Paclitaxel, vincristine, camptothecin, etoposide, and vinblastine Phyto-extract are widely stated plant-determined anticancer products (Fridlender et al., 2015; Howes, 2018). A few extra optimistic botanical standard combos with antitumor action and respective mechanisms are documented (Lichota and Gwozdzinski, 2018).

Bioactive compounds may not be fundamental for the development as well as advancement of plants. However, phytochemicals have significant adornment exercises, for example, aid in guarding phytopathogens, developing hindrance of contending plants, and contagious microbes, and supporting fertilization. They have different calming and counter-oxidant activities (Adebayo et al., 2015). Against oxidants, abilities incorporate the end of free extreme groups and chelate the dynamic metallic particles that trigger lipid oxidative damage. Such characteristics likewise assist in preventive care. Bioactive compounds of plants are gathered into polyphenols, alkaloids, terpenoids, and flavonoids, dependent on their designs (Singh et al., 2016). Major therapeutic alkaloids incorporate camptothecin, vincristine, and vinblastine. Terpenoids comprise gamma-tocopherol and lycopene. Polyphenols consist of curcumin etoposide, epigallocatechin gallate, and resveratrol, while flavonoids include genistein, apigenin, and kaempferol. Such bioactive combinations apply antitumor impacts autonomously or collaboratively with various combinations via regulation of biochemical and flagging mechanisms, restraint of catalysts essential for disease movement, angiogenesis, cytoskeleton mingling, and cycle arrest (Kojima-Yuasa et al., 2015). Throughout the long term, several various plant extracts have been investigated for their antitumor characteristics. A significant number of bioactive compounds show the potential capacity to suppress cancer development and movement (G Grothaus et al., 2010).

Other anticancer plants and their derived metabolites are referenced in Table 10.1.

10.2 INTRODUCTION TO CRISPR FOR PLANT GENETIC IMPROVEMENTS

Clustered regularly interspaced short palindromic repeats (CRISPR) and CRISPR-associated protein (Cas) is a genome-editing tools. It has arisen late but become broadly famous with the mainly well-known is the CRISPR/Cas9. This technique uses the adaptive immune system of archaea and bacteria; the system depends on particular sites in the genome of bacteria known as CRISPR loci. These loci are made out of operons that encode the protein (Cas9) and repeated spacer sequences. The spacers are derivatives of foreign DNA (plasmid or virus) and are short fragments that have become incorporated into bacteria's genome through recombination (Barrangou et al., 2007; Zhang et al., 2014).

It has two significant parts: gRNA (guide RNA) and protein (Cas9). Cas9 protein is an RNA-dependent DNA endonuclease that arranges with the gRNA. The gRNA is based on 20 nucleotides complementary to the targeted sequence and is essential for the recruitment of Cas9 to the targeted location. It is the principal distinction between the CRISPR/Cas9 and all the other genome engineering tools; it requires the interaction of DNA–RNA, rather than DNA-protein, for targeting the nucleotide sequence. Transcription activator-like effector nucleases (TALENs) and zinc-finger nucleases (ZFNs) focus on the specific pattern through the interaction of DNA–protein, expression, and design of two unique domains of DNA binding (amino acids about 500–700 if there should arise an occurrence of TALEN) are necessary per target site. This procedure is somewhat arduous. Then again, in CRISPR/Cas9, which utilizes the interaction of DNA–RNA, an 18–20 bp oligonucleotide design is necessary. That makes it extremely simple for the adaptation of CRISPR/Cas9 for genome-altering purposes. Furthermore, gRNA and Cas9 need to adhere to a particular sequence called protospacer adjoining motif (PAM), which is placed at the 3′ ends of the targeted sequence to work as a genome-altering tool. On account of *Streptococcus pyogenes* Cas9 (SpCas9), the Cas9 usually utilized for modifying a genome, the 5′-NGG-3′ is perceived as the PAM sequence. Except if, in any case, referenced, the genome

TABLE 10.1 List of Anticancer Plants and Their Secondary Metabolites Along with Targeted Cancer Area.

Anticancer plant	Derived compound	Anticancer part	Gene	Target cancer	References
Clausena excavate	Carbazole alkaloid	Seed	petA	Gastric, liver cancer	(Fadhel et al., 2021)
Morus alba	Skimmianine	Stem bark	IDI	Liver cancer	(Li et al., 2021)
Saffron crocus	Saffron	Dry stigma	rbcL	Pancreatic cancer	(Lambrianidou et al., 2020)
Ginkgo biloba	Ginkgetin, ginkgolide	Flower, leaf	LPS	Lung and breast cancer	(Li et al., 2019)
Ammi majus	Caffeic acid, sinapic acid	Leaf	COMT	Glioma, renal, ovary cancer	(Aydogmus ozturk et al., 2019)
Asparagus racemosus	Steroidal saponins	Root	rhaD	Lung cancer	(Biswas et al., 2018)
Zingiber officinale	Gingerol	Zinger	psbA Y17094_001	Ovary, cervix	(Lima et al., 2018)
Peganum harmala	Harmine	Roots	DYRK2	Breast cancer	(Ayoob et al., 2017)
Artemisia annua	Artemisinin	Whole plant	DBR2 AAR	Liver and breast cancer	(Efferth 2017)
Debregeasia saeneb	Tannins	Stem	spy b1743, JW1732	Internal tumor	(Tariq et al., 2017)
Mangifera indica	Mangiferin	Leaf	CGT UGT13	Colon	(Ganogpichayagrai et al., 2017)
Moringa oleifera	*Moringa oleifera* Protease inhibitor (Mopi)	Flower, leaf	psbA	Abdominal cancer	(Vergara-Jimenez et al., 2017)
Gossypium hirsutum	Gossypol	Whole plant	CYP82D109	Breast, stomach, liver	(Sharifi et al., 2017)
Dioscorea colletti	Dioscin	Rhizome	DAG1	Liver and gastric cancer	(Iqbal et al., 2017)
G. biloba	Ginkgetin, ginkgolide A and B	Leave	LPS	Ovary, colon, and liver cancer	(Xiong et al., 2016)

TABLE 10.1 *(Continued)*

Anticancer plant	Derived compound	Anticancer part	Gene	Target cancer	References
Vigna unguiculata	Black-eyed-pea trypsin/chymotrypsin Inhibitor	Seed	PRSS1 TRP1	Human breast cancer (in vitro)	(Mehdad et al., 2016)
Punica granatum	Epicatechingallate, picatechin,	Leaf	UGT84A24	Lung, bladder, bdublst, and skin cancer	(Wu et al., 2016) (Awad et al., 2015)
Curcuma longa	Tannins	Seed	CURS1	Cervical A	(Perone et al., 2018)
Punica granatam	Linoleic acids	Fruit, leaf	FADX FAC	Breast	(Awad et al., 2015)
P. granatam	Quercetin	Leaf	UGT84A23 CDL15_Pgr003363, CRG98_046	Colon cancer	(Awad et al., 2015)
Sylibum marianum	Silymarin	Flower	abc2	Colorectal	(Ozturk et al., 2015)
Tylophora indica	Tylophorine	Bark, fruit	rPB2	Lymphoma	(Kv et al., 2014)
Vitis vinifera	Cyanidin	Fruits, bark	UFGT AlUFGT1	Colon cancer	(Esfahanian et al., 2013)
Plumbago zeylanica	Rolb	Roots	B5TGI3_9CARY	Blood, skin	(Hiradeve et al., 2011)
crocus sativus	Saffron	Flowers	psbD	Ovarian cancer	(Hosseinpour Chermahini et al., 2009)
Viscum album	Viscumin, digallic acid	Sprouts	ML1_VISAL	Breast, cervix, ovary, stomach,colon, kidney, and lung cancer	(Zarkovic et al., 2001)

altering experiments introduced in the present review have been finished utilizing SpCas9 (Fig. 10.1).

A few kinds of CRISPR defensive systems working in cells of different microbes are portrayed exhaustively somewhere else (Gilles and Averof, 2014; Haft et al., 2005). The most "famous" is the CRISPR/Cas type II-A found in the *S. pyogenes* and made out of three genes that encode Cas9 protein, trans-initiating crRNA (tracrRNA), and CRISPR RNA (crRNA). All-inclusive hereditary constructs encoding counterfeit components of CRISPR/Cas "genome editor" have been made (Doudna and Charpentier, 2014). Additionally, a worked-on variant of the system, working as a complex of sgRNA and Cas9, comprising CRISPR tracrRNA and short, mature crRNA, was made. The guided sequence recognizes the DNA site

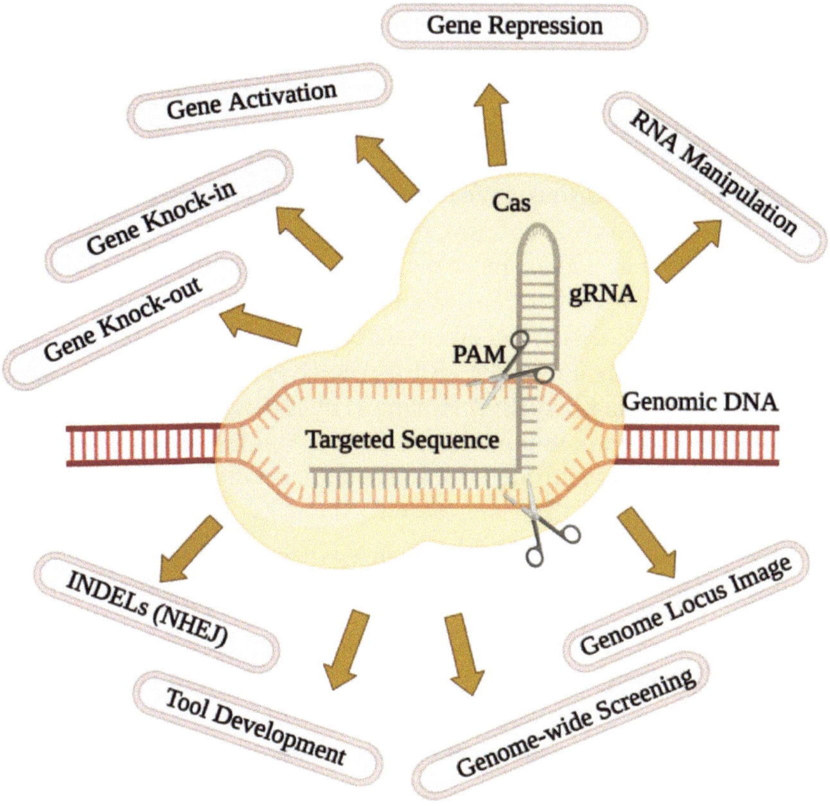

FIGURE 10.1 CRISPR/Cas tool sketch and its probable applications in anticancer plants.

and binds to it, and Cas9 cuts the targeted point of DNA (Graham and Root, 2015). Cas9 recruitment typically brings about DSBs at the targeted site in the DNA; however, the accidental changes known as off-target effects have occasionally been prompted. The development of CRISPR/Cas9 technology has been used for precise genome editing with minor consequences for the genome by improving the explicitness or keeping away from the double strand break (DSB) (Jaganathan et al., 2018; Wang et al., 2016). Besides, once the ideal transgenic plants were produced, the expulsion of the foreign transgenes was assessed conscientiously (Jaganathan et al., 2018). The CRISPR system can be utilized to make hereditarily modified cells grown in living organisms and cultures (Cho et al., 2013). In the primary case, viral vectors, or plasmids that give elevated and stable CRISPR/Cas9 components are brought into cells. In the subsequent case, cultured protoplasts and plasmid coding CRISPR/Cas components are utilized to get hereditarily modified plants (Shan et al., 2013). Another methodology, functional for plants, is the utilization of *Agrobacterium*, a "genetic engineer," that contains a unique plasmid holding onto CRISPR/Cas9 (Lowder et al., 2016; Zhang et al., 2014).

Since CRISPR-Cas technology was effectively designed to alter plant genomes in 2013, various endeavors have been prepared to transform it into an influential tool. As of now, CRISPR-Cas has the capacity of multiplex editing; that is, it alters more than one gene at a time (Donohoue et al., 2018). What's more, CRISPR-Cas can target not just open reading frame (ORF) (Liang et al., 2019) and untranslated region (Mao et al., 2018) of one gene yet additionally non-coding RNAs (ncRNAs), including long ncRNA (Li et al., 2018) and microRNA (Chang et al., 2016), just as regions of the promoter (Seth and communications 2016). Single-base replacements at targets exclusive of requiring DSBs have additionally been achieved (Hess et al., 2017). Now, we portray the CRISPR-Cas optimization regarding the broadened advancement of Cas proteins, the improvement of Cas promoters, and the sgRNAs strengthening with multiplexing ability.

10.3 REQUISITE OF CRISPR/CAS IN ANTICANCER PLANTS

The plant breeding strategies were made before the approach of genetics laws, which have taken advantage of hybrid vigor and grain yield in different harvest plants through novel cytogenetic and hybridization manipulations. The progress further acquired energy by developing novel biotechnological techniques to work with genetic engineering and gene transfer to integrate new traits in plants. Afterward, biofortification of harvests has introduced an intriguing part of present-day plant biotechnology to battle appetite and ailing health (Jauhar, 2006). The foremost transgenic plant was delivered by utilizing TMV (tobacco mosaic virus) to exhibit the idea of CP (coat protein)-interceded cross-protection (Abel et al., 1986).

The plant biotechnology period was begun in the mid-1980s through breaking examination of the *Agrobacterium*-intervened transformed plant (Bevan et al., 1983). Soon, the biomarkers were utilized in harvests to offer high-resolution hereditary maps and exploit the genetic link among plant markers and traits (Paterson et al., 1988). By the mid-1990s, biotechnology was effectively coordinated into crop improvement and plant breeding which was demonstrated in the marketing of several genetically engineered crops (Delannay et al., 1995). Later on, various hereditarily designed harvests were effectively raised to handle abiotic and biotic stress, deliver eatable vaccines, and make healthfully prevalent genotypes (Jauhar, 2006).

Prior, ZFNs and TALENs accounted for protein-based genome-altering techniques at the transcriptional level to control the genome (Chen and Gao, 2015). Both methods use an endonuclease called Fok-I protein for gene knock-out by creating DSBs in the targeted region of DNA (Gaj et al., 2013). Although, the utilization of these strategies in targeting specific sequences of a genome is restricted by the necessity of two distinct protein chimera models that also can detect scarcely accessible areas which flanking the targeted sequence of a DNA (Kim et al., 1996; Li et al., 2011). Likewise, the tools turned out to be less viable because of the event of those sequences alongside the appropriate direction dimerization ability of both proteins with the specified length of spacer (Händel et al., 2009; Urnov et al., 2010). The CRISPR/Cas9 system enjoys the upper hand over ZFN and TALEN for being simple with basic steps of cloning required, high multiplex simplicity, and enormous scale library formation ability (Sharma et al., 2017). The appearance of the CRISPR/Cas9 tool not needing dimerization of protein and intervenes exceptionally proficient genome altering by utilizing designed gRNAs that recognize a three base-pair sequence of a PAM present downstream of the targeted DNA sequence (Cho et al., 2013; Mali et al., 2013). The CRISPR/Cas9 system is a good and accessible substantial part mutagenic tool for genetic modification using gRNA. That identified the few most important benefits: (1) The gene of interest is knocked out though quantity distinction in RNAi creates incomplete knock-down; (2) genomic changes are steady and effectively viable in the offspring introducing massive applications in the breeding of plants (Barrangou et al., 2015; Liu et al., 2016). The capacity of CRISPR/Cas9 intervenes in genome altering to induce specific DSBs inside the genome, which are fixed by either the homology-coordinated fix (HDR) or non-homologous end-joining (NHEJ) mechanism of the cell (Shalem et al., 2015) (Fig. 10.1). On the other hand, NHEJ-interceded irregular deletion (INDELS) or insertion for the most part harms the (ORFs) of the coding sequence of the protein or loses the cis-regulatory components of non-coding sequences such as enhancers, promoters, and so forth (Liu et al., 2016).

Since the immemorial time, plants and their items have been utilized as a productive cause of nutraceuticals, biomaterials, pharmaceuticals, and food for human beings (Dey et al., 2021). Plant-based regular items have filled in as possible leading to drug revelation to improve human morbidity and mortality (Dey et al., 2017b). The adequacy of clinical herbalism in opposition to countless diseases has been examined and approved, employing different preclinical and clinical investigations (Anand et al., 2020; Kaur et al., 2020). Numerous biotechnological mediations have been functional to adapt pathways of secondary metabolites of the plant to elevate the development of significant secondary metabolites of therapeutic and dietary utilization (Dey et al., 2017a).

The NGS strategies approach has shown incredible guarantee in examining medicinal plants' biosynthetic pathways and genetic diversity. Novel breeding techniques based on biotechnology, for example, targeted genome-altering strategies, have been an excellent toolbox for engineering modified medicinal plants with enhanced profiles of secondary metabolite (Niazian, 2019).

10.4 LIMITATION OF CRISPR/CAS IN ANTICANCER PLANTS

10.4.1 OFF-TARGETING

CRISPR/Cas9 nucleases, even though they produce exact and helpful editing in a genome in a broad array of living beings, might likewise cause unfortunate off-targeted mutations taking after the on-target sequence analyses and restricting remedial ramifications of that technique (Kleinstiver et al., 2016). The excellent methods to limit these off-targeted effects (OTEs) to enhance sgRNA to boost the on-targeted impacts and limit off-targeted events by determining the binding of off-targeted encourage secondary structure and sgRNA mismatching. It utilizes artificial change to confine transcription of Cas9 and its translation; protein designing interceded streamlining of exceptionally explicit Cas9 and use of the pair cas9 nickases (Chen et al., 2019; Doench et al., 2016; Kimberland et al., 2018; Shen et al., 2019).

10.4.2 GENOMES INSTABILITY

Cas9 and DSBs are a significant concern for genome instability in numerous organisms, limiting the CRISPR/Cas9 system utilization, particularly in *Streptomyces*. It is measured as a characteristic storage facility of industrial critical natural products and multiple pharmacologically, DSBs basis broad genome rearrangements and deletions in the linear chromosomes (6–12 Mb) (Hoff et al., 2018). Then again, without DSB-free exceptionally change single-nucleotide declaration known as base editing. Deaminase-based DNA base editor and CRISPRi have been considered productive genome-altering toolkits (Eid et al., 2018; Tong et al., 2020).

10.4.3 CAS9 TOXICITY

In green algae and bacteria, the expression of Cas9 regularly prompts poisonousness bringing about weakened development. Cas9 harmfulness can be managed through Cas9 alternatives to diminish the Cas9 level in intracellular by utilizing fragile promoters (constitutive or inducible), controlling the size and Cas9 transient expression or recurrence of edits of the targeted gene, for example, Cas9d 10a and Cas9n (Dow et al., 2015; Ye et al., 2020). One more bright methodology was incorporating anti-Cas9 parts (for example, the anti-CRISPR DNA mimicAcrIIA4 as Cas9-sgRNA-AcrIIA4 complex) to control the expression of Cas9 to diminish poisonousness and OTEs (Shin et al., 2017). In any respect, to present no confirmation of Cas9 harmfulness has been revealed in crops.

10.4.4 NHEJ ERROR-PRONE NATURE

Because of the NHEJ, the prevailing pathways in the DSB recombination, many of the modifications by CRISPR/Cas9 in plants bring about a greater incidence of irregular deletion toward the targeted site (Feng et al., 2013). To avoid stochastic gene interruption, prosperous, just as precise editing at a targeted site is required of great importance for plant breeders. The Frameshift mutation is likewise the different result of the random exactness of the indels range. HDR proficiency is additionally diminished complexly because of challenges with NHEJ, which is as yet predominant (Lu and Zhu, 2017). To stifle the NHEJ pathway or work with HDR pathways, tiny molecules such as L755507, Scr7, and resveratrol have been accounted for to restrain NHEJ essential parts, such as KU80, DNA ligase IV, and KU70 (Li et al., 2017b; Weber et al., 2015).

10.4.5 GENOME EDITING OF POLYPLOID PLANT

The polypoid genomes Complexity has been a significant worry in classical breeding, present-day genome engineering methods, and CRISPR/Cas innovation. In addition, site-directed mutagenesis, the considerable genome size, and large copy numbers interceded the knock-out exceptionally. Homologous genes with the absence of annotated genome for designing appropriate sgRNAs confine the broad guarantee of CRISPR/Cas editing technology in numerous polyploid plants (Vats et al., 2019). In any case, CRISPR/Cas9 altering has many benefits and applications over the orthodox breeding techniques since it can associatively focus the numerous metabolic pathway and genes, not displaying any relationship drag.

10.4.6 TRANSFECTION EFFICIENCY

One of the crucial drawbacks of the CRISPR/Cas9 tool is little transfection proficiency, limiting its wide pertinence. The absence of an effective transfection procedure and choice of appropriate plasmid restrict the utilization of the CRISPR/Cas9 system in numerous organisms. Productive delivery methods of sgRNA and Cas9 utilizing plasmid included using lipid nanoparticle encapsulate with Cas9/sgRNA plasmid (DNA) for effective transfection (Zhang et al., 2017). Additionally, direct nuclear or cytosolic Cas9 delivery with sgRNA via transporter nanoparticles was likewise revealed as a viable transfection system (Mout et al., 2017).

10.4.7 *TRANSFORMATION TECHNIQUES AND REGENERATION PROTOCOLS*

Numerous plants need effective regeneration protocols and transformation (Altpeter et al., 2016). As in multiple cases, the isolated protoplasts have been effectively utilized in more effective modification with strong gene target capability (Zhang et al., 2010). In a tobacco plant, protoplasts have been accounted for as a beautiful explanation for the regeneration of plants utilizing ZFNs and TALENs (Zhang et al., 2013).

10.4.8 *VITAL MOLECULAR ASSETS & TOOLS*

Essential molecular assets like transformation protocols, vectors, score-able markers, and promoters are deficient in numerous higher organisms and plants well-known to deliver usual significant products by the massive cutoff of the appliance and additional advancement of CRISPR/Cas system (Tong et al., 2019).

10.4.9 *LINKING OF PHENOTYPE TO GENOTYPE*

The exact edit recognition step restricts the cost or time viability of the CRISPR/Cas9 system. To interface genotype by phenotype, high data transmission biosensors are utilized effectively in various reports yet with restricted accessibility in numerous applications (Tong et al., 2019). CRISPR, a multi-functional genome-wide technology, is anticipated as late as a high data genotype-phenotype mapping innovation (Lian et al., 2019).

10.4.10 *PRIMORDIAL CRISPR'S ROLE*

In different bacteria and as well as *Streptomyces numerous* native CRISPR/Cas [viz. Type II (Type II-C) or type I-E and numerous more] occurs and offer security against foreign nucleic acids (Sangal et al., 2013). The potential collaborations between the introduced and indigenous CRISPR/

Cas system might be one more energizing yet less undocumented part of the future review (Tong et al., 2019).

10.5 CRISPR-MEDIATED METABOLIC ENGINEERING

Throughout the pre-CRISPR era, different metabolic designing devices effectively exhibited guidelines for auxiliary metabolite mechanisms in plants. For instance, taxadiene (taxol antecedent) creation in *Escherichia coli* was augmented by designing methylerythritol-phosphate (MEP) and terpenoid–framing pathways. That additionally comes about in negligible indole aggregation and P450-intervened 5α-oxidation of taxadiene to taxadien-5α-ol, prompting the creation of taxol (Ajikumar et al., 2010). In *Saccharomyces cerevisiae*, the mevalonate pathway created amorphadiene and dihydroartemisinic corrosive (artemisinin antecedent). It was produced utilizing overexpressing each chemical in the pathway that came about in multiplied artemisinic corrosive and high amorpha-4,11-diene creation (Westfall et al., 2012). Throughout the pre-CRISPR time, heterologous articulation of plant qualities in microbial hosts utilizing pathway remaking filled in as another creation alternative, taking advantage of metabolic designing and manufactured science (Li and Pfeifer, 2014).

NGS procedures have widened the skyline of complete chromosomal and transcriptional information on therapeutic plants. When joined with genomics and proteomics, it can additionally be taken advantage of to make and distinguish anonymous restorative plant-determined regular items (Zhou et al., 2018). Then again, DNA barcoding is a significant device to investigate hereditary variety in therapeutic plants and group them at the species level (Techen et al., 2014).

Restriction site-associated DNA sequencing (RAD-seq) device, utilizing detailed transcriptome describing, might likewise be used for distinguishing proof of qualities and proteins identified with optional metabolite pathways and for fast and exact comprehension of focusing on actuated nearby injuries in genomes (TILLING) populaces (Niazian, 2019). In pre-CRISPR/Cas time, ZFNs, and TALENs protein-based altering techniques for transcriptional level genome control were referred to as a good tool for hereditary just as metabolic designing embroiled to create new characteristics in rejuvenating plants delivering novel metabolites (Pouvreau et al., 2018). What's more, supercombinatorial change of transplastomic beneficiary lines (COSTREL) was accounted for as an inventive hereditary designing methodology to expand the yield of plant secondary metabolites (Fuentes et al., 2016). All manufactured science, NGS, and biotechnological systems have been tried before CRISPR/Cas9 to develop plant attributes and yield further. CRISPR/Cas9 is an essential, exact and effective innovative editing tool that makes it ready for genome changing to clarify the optional metabolic mechanism, enhance quality, and supersize the significant auxiliary metabolites of pharmacological significance. CRISPR/Cas9 framework can intentionally adjust the phytochemical side view in remedial plants as another option and proficient creation technique of business plant-determined items. Table 10.2 presents the therapeutic plants via CRISPR/Cas genome editing to obtain vital secondary metabolites.

10.6 FUTURE PROSPECT OF CRISPR/CAS IN MEDICINAL PLANTS

Efficacious genome editing of medicinal plants that have pharmacological, biomedical, and industrial significance is essential. The metabolic pathways can then be improved by regulating metabolic paths and eliminating level restraint and response hindrance to bioactive compound mechanisms properly. Biomedical industries are constantly expanding, and the CRISPR/Cas genome editing action plan may be a rousing new method for modifying metabolites in therapeutic plants to reveal desired products accurately and adequately. Editing through CRISPR/Cas may not be the preferred procedure for increasing the selected phytochemicals production in creatures with lengthy life expectancy (such as perennial plants) or organisms which have not been altered by transgenes and ribonucleoproteins (RNPs). Bacterial cell factories can be a powerful substitute for secondary metabolic pathway genes that have been heterologously expressed. Genomics tool CRISPR/Cas is an efficient and remarkable innovation that may once again revolutionize plant breeding. Early CRISPR/Cas research focused on modifying single characteristics using error-prone NHEJ. In the past few years, technical advancements have been made in genetic, epigenetic, and transcriptional modulations. The most effective CRISPR/Cas strategies for plants are homologous recombination and disrupting genomic modifications carried by hereditary trait loci through inversions or somatic

TABLE 10.2 List of Anticancer Plants Edited Through CRISPR Genome Edit Tool Along With Consequences

Anticancer plant	Derived compound	Gene	CRISPR method knock-in/ knock-out	Consequence	References
Salvia miltiorrhiza	Tanshinone	(*SmCPS1*)	Knock-out	Antiarrhythmic effects	Varsani et al., 2017
Panax ginseng	Ginseng	SQE1 GSE, SE, SQE	Knockout		Dey 2020
Cameli na sativa (L.) Crantz	Omega-3 Fatty acid, polyunsaturated fatty acid (PUFA)	FAD7 FADD	Knockout	FAD2 genes knock-out increase oleic acid, linolenic acid declined	Lyzenga et al., 2019; Dey 2020
Dendrobium officinale Kimura and Migo	Alkaloids, phenanthrenes, glycosides	MAT	Knockout	Z. C3h, C4h, 4cl, Ccr, and Irx insert, delete, substitution	Zheng et al., 2018
Dioscorea zingiberensis C. H. Wright	Diosgenin	GT4A	Knock-in/ knock-out	Targeted mutagenesis on Dzfps gene	Dey 2020
Nicotiana tabacum L.	Alkaloids, flavonoids	UGT78G1 GT83F	Knock-out	Glycoproteins produce without plant-specific glycans	Gao et al., 2015
Papaver somniferum L	Benzyl quinoline	BEBT1 BPBT	Knock-out	Biosynthesis flux of bias	Alagoz et al., 2016
Salvia miltiorrhiza Bunge	Phenolic acids, diterpenoids	padC pad	Knock-out	Smcps1 knock out. In homozygous mutants, no importanttanshinones viz tanshinone I, tanshinone IIA, and cryptotanshinone observed	Li et al., 2017a; Lambrianidou et al., 2020; Dey 2020
Oryzae	Mortalin-p53 complex	*OsERF922/ Pi21*	Knock-out	Magnaporthe oryzae resistant production	Ahmad et al., 2021

TABLE 10.2 *(Continued)*

Anticancer plant	Derived compound	Gene	CRISPR method knock-in/ knock-out	Consequence	References
P. somniferum	Benzylisoquinoline alkaloids	6OMT PSOMT2	Knock-in	Bias, mainly within the aporphine, bioactive, anticancer, anti-arrhythmic, Anti-HIV, and anti-malarial properties	Courdavault et al., 2020
P. harmala	Harmine	DYRK2	Knock-out	Beta-carboline inhibits the harmine production by CRISPR knock out the beta-carboline gene Knock-out an production of the harmine increase	Gupta et al., 2021
Penicillium chrysogenu	B-Lactam Antibiotics	blr b4409, JW5963	CRISPR–Cas9, recombination	Production of the desired product become increases by CRISPR or recombination technology.	Dey 2020
V. vinifera	Cyanidin	UFGT AIUFGT1	Knock-in	Production of cyanidin become increase	Esfahanian et al., 2013
D. officinale Kimura and Migo	Alkaloids, phenanthrenes, glycosides	MAT	Knock-out	Z. C3h, C4h, 4cl, Ccr, and Irx insert, delete, substitution	Zheng et al., 2018
Z. officinale	Gingerol	psbA Y17094_001	Knock-in	Knockin gingerol gene production of this increase is directly proportional to LTA4H, an inflammatory agent	Lima et al., 2018

cross-overs. The Cas13 system, which breaks down viral mRNA in plants, has also been introduced (Schindele et al., 2020).

The CRISPR/Cas technique is a powerful medium for upgrading plant diversity and bioengineering by inserting transgene into plant genomic sequences. A similar application of the CRISPR/Cas system can carry legume node feature genes into cereals for nitrogen fixation, facilitating the refining of the C4 pathway regulatory elements to intensify carbon fixation proficiency, remarkable attainment of synthetic biology in this field (Chen et al., 2019). A CRISPR–dCas toolkit is already established for genetic engineering to investigate expression patterns, genotyping, chromatin immunoprecipitation, epigenetic engineering, and genome mapping (Xu and Qi, 2019).

Due to cell walls and tissue in plants, species-specific applications require a lengthy and labor-intensive tissue culture step (Chen et al., 2019). These challenges can be overcome by enhancing the transformation through *Agrobacterium* via affecting plant genes and *Agrobacterium* to carry plants' vigorous and faster gene editing (Gelvin, 2010). Novel bacteria as persuasive vectors for the transformation of the plant should be obtained from the natural environment (Rathore and Mullins, 2018). Many evolutionary genes (such as Bbm and Wus2) may also improve transformation efficiency in specific monocots and shorten the plant regeneration time by a significant margin (Hofmann, 2016). The use of transformation through pollens, the shoot top as the target location, and the nanotechnology and virus-like particles as innovative delivery mediators are other innovative transformation strategies. It can be used to attain efficient, fast, and less toxic plant transformation methods (Baskaran et al., 2016; Chen et al., 2019; Kalbande et al., 2016; Kausch et al., 2019; Mohamed and Kumar, 2019; Yang et al., 2017; Zaidi and Mansoor, 2017). The biolistic transformation can deliver and express sgRNA vector into the genome of the plant, but the transformation through *Agrobacterium* remains the most effective and preferred alteration technique (Ma et al., 2016). Regeneration via plant tissue culture may not be necessary within the in-planta transformation strategy (Kalbande et al., 2016). Genome targeting was developed to reduce the need for efficient transformation and regeneration protocols. It relies on simultaneous initiation of the target location mediated by DSB and vector expurgation to activate it in plants. But while NHEJ induction efficiency was lower, CRISPR/Cas12 targeting efficiency was better than that of SaCas9, demonstrating the fitness of

Cas12a in specific for inducing homologous recombination (HR) (Wolter et al., 2019).

CRISPR/Cas as a genome editing tool has enormous potential in metabolic system engineering, cell factory construction, interpreting and influencing bioengineered pathways, and cloning of lengthy genes (Bennett-Baker and Mueller, 2017; Jiang et al., 2015; Liu et al., 2015). Recent advances in cloning strategies and biosynthetic genes allow for a better study of natural byproducts via engineering to obtain bioactive medicinal molecules for industrial purposes. To accomplish that, gene editing of lengthy DNA pieces must be precise and effective.

A dynamic in-vitro CRISPR/Cas9 technique is already successfully used to engineer biosynthetic mechanisms (Liu et al., 2015). Furthermore, Cas9-assisted targeting of chromosome (CATCH) sequences offered an improved model for the precise cloning of lengthy gene sequences in a single attempt. Lengthy bacterial genomes (up to 100 kb) could be sequenced in one step using this strategy (Jiang et al., 2015). A recent proposal is used in CRISPR-mediated isolation of specific mega base-sized regions (CISMR) to isolate contiguous mega base-sized genomic pieces to inspect the DNA and structural variance in various complex genomes (Bennett-Baker and Mueller, 2017).

Knock-out via SpCas9 is one of the many CRISPR/Cas tools that has been extensively studied. In addition, CRISPRi (Bester et al., 2018) and CRISPR activation (CRISPRa) (McInally et al., 2019) can be engineered to control metabolic pathways more effectively than direct gene knock-outs. There was also high efficiency, precision, and multiplexed genome editing with CRISPR-Cas12a/Cpf1 (Yang et al., 2020). Novel Cas9 orthologous proteins with different PAMs and vastly precise Cas9s with reformed PAM characteristics are also studied (Kleinstiver et al., 2015; Song et al., 2019). RNA-guided RNA editing tool CRISPR-Cas13a/C2c2 reprogrammed for knock-down mRNA has been used recently (Cox et al., 2017). By extending sgRNA guide sequences, linking APOBEC1 and Cas9-HF1, and delivering base editors via RNP, new strategies have been developed to improve the specificity of Cas9-linked base editors (Kim et al., 2017; Rees et al., 2017). By influencing metabolic circuits, HDR frequency has been increased, improving the proficiency and efficacy of this procedure (Chen et al., 2019).

The concurrent introduction of many genomic alterations dramatically shortened the plant breeding cycle, resulting in the domestication of many wild plant species in a single generation (Schindele et al., 2020; Wolter et al., 2019). Allele mining can take advantage of the high genetic variance existing in uncommon and semi-domesticated crops and wild relatives and landraces, subsequently expanding the genetic pool of many plants and increasing their yield (Wolter et al., 2019). Aside from that, gene editing using CRISPR/Cas might be used in agriculture as a promising opportunity to combat incursive plant and animal species, which might be influenced to alter pathogens of plants, to instigate unique characteristics, or to form an unwanted weed vulnerable to weedicides or herbicide effectively (Chen et al., 2019).

According to the study, the endoplasmic reticulum (ER) was expanded to increase the yeasts' metabolic ability to produce terpenoids. A CRISPR/Cas9-mediated disruption of PAH1, which encodes the phosphatides acid phosphatase, resulted in the ER expansion. The above strategy can be used without altering metabolic fluxes to have plant triterpenoids and sesquiterpenoids in heterologous hosts (Arendt et al., 2017).

According to recent research, hairy root culture-mediated instigation of artificial polyploidy using CRISPR/Cas9 is an innovative and rousing biotechnological technique to formulate a bioengineering mechanism. It can increase the formation of secondary metabolites in various medicinal plants (Niazian, 2019).

KEYWORDS

- **CRISPR**
- **anticancer plant**
- **secondary metabolites**
- **genome editing**
- **cancer**

REFERENCES

Abel, P. P.; Nelson, R. S.; De, B.; Hoffmann, N.; Rogers, S. G.; Fraley, R. T.; Beachy, R. N. Delay of Disease Development in Transgenic Plants that Express the Tobacco Mosaic Virus Coat Protein Gene. *Sci.* **1986,** *232* (4751), 738–743.

Adebayo, S. A.; Dzoyem, J. P.; Shai, L. J.; Eloff, J. N. The Anti-Inflammatory and Antioxidant Activity of 25 Plant Species Used Traditionally to Treat Pain in Southern African. *BMC Complement Altern. Med.* **2015,** *15* (1), 1–10.

Ahmad, S.; Tang, L.; Shahzad, R.; Mawia, A. M.; Rao, G. S.; Jamil, S.; Wei, C.; Sheng, Z.; Shao, G.; Wei, X. CRISPR-Based Crop Improvements: A Way Forward to Achieve Zero Hunger. *J. Agri. Food Chem.* **2021,** *69* (30), 8307–8323.

Ajikumar, P. K.; Xiao, W.-H.; Tyo, K. E.; Wang, Y.; Simeon, F.; Leonard, E.; Mucha, O.; Phon, T. H.; Pfeifer, B.; Stephanopoulos, G. Isoprenoid Pathway Optimization for Taxol Precursor Overproduction in Escherichia Coli. *Sci.* **2010,** *330* (6000), 70–74.

Alagoz, Y.; Gurkok, T.; Zhang, B.; Unver, T. Manipulating the Biosynthesis of Bioactive Compound Alkaloids for next-Generation Metabolic Engineering in Opium Poppy Using CRISPR-Cas 9 Genome Editing Technology. *Sci. Rep.* **2016,** *6* (1), 1–9.

Albaayit, S. F. A.; Maharjan, R.; Abdullah, R.; Noor, M. H. M. Anti-Enterococcus Faecalis, Cytotoxicity, Phytotoxicity, and Anticancer Studies on Clausena excavata Burum. f.(Rutaceae) Leaves. *Biomed Res. Int* **2021,** *2021.*

Altpeter, F.; Springer, N. M.; Bartley, L. E.; Blechl, A. E.; Brutnell, T. P.; Citovsky, V.; Conrad, L. J.; Gelvin, S. B.; Jackson, D. P.; Kausch, A. P. Advancing Crop Transformation in the Era of Genome Editing. *Plant Cell.* **2016,** *28* (7), 1510–1520.

Anand, U.; Nandy, S.; Mundhra, A.; Das, N.; Pandey, D. K.; Dey, A. A Review on Antimicrobial Botanicals, Phytochemicals and Natural Resistance Modifying Agents From Apocynaceae Family: Possible Therapeutic Approaches against Multidrug Resistance in Pathogenic Microorganisms. *Drug Resist.* **2020,** *51*, 100695.

Arendt, P.; Miettinen, K.; Pollier, J.; De Rycke, R.; Callewaert, N.; Goossens, A. An Endoplasmic Reticulum-Engineered Yeast Platform for Overproduction of Triterpenoids. *Metab. Eng.* **2017,** *40*, 165–175.

Aydoğmuş-Öztürk, F.; Jahan, H.; Beyazit, N.; Günaydın, K.; Choudhary, M. I. The Anticancer Activity of Visnagin, Isolated from Ammi Visnaga L. against the Human Malignant Melanoma Cell Lines, HT 144. *Mol. Biol. Rep.* **2019,** *46* (2), 1709–1714.

Ayoob, I.; Hazari, Y. M.; Lone, S. H.; Khuroo, M. A.; Fazili, K. M.; Bhat, K. A. Phytochemical and Cytotoxic Evaluation of *Peganum harmala*: Structure Activity Relationship Studies of Harmine. *ChemistrySelect.* **2017,** *2* (10), 2965–2968.

Barrangou, R.; Birmingham, A.; Wiemann, S.; Beijersbergen, R. L.; Hornung, V.; Smith, A. v. B. Advances in CRISPR-Cas9 Genome Engineering: Lessons Learned from RNA interference. *Nucleic Acids Res.* **2015,** *43* (7), 3407–3419.

Barrangou, R.; Fremaux, C.; Deveau, H.; Richards, M.; Boyaval, P.; Moineau, S.; Romero, D. A.; Horvath, P. CRISPR Provides Acquired Resistance Against Viruses in Prokaryotes. *Science* **2007,** *315* (5819), 1709–1712.

Baskaran, P.; Soós, V.; Balázs, E.; Van Staden, J. Shoot Apical Meristem Injection: A Novel and Efficient Method to Obtain Transformed Cucumber Plants. *S. Afr. J. Bot.* **2016,** *103*, 210–215.

Bennett-Baker, P. E.; Mueller, J. L. CRISPR-Mediated Isolation of Specific Megabase Segments of Genomic DNA. *Nucleic Acids Res.* **2017.**

Bester, A. C.; Lee, J. D.; Chavez, A.; Lee, Y.-R.; Nachmani, D.; Vora, S.; Victor, J.; Sauvageau, M.; Monteleone, E.; Rinn, J. L. An Integrated Genome-Wide CRISPRa Approach to Functionalize lncRNAs in Drug Resistance. *Cell.* **2018,** *173* (3), 649–664. e20.

Bevan, M. W.; Flavell, R. B.; Chilton, M.-D. A Chimaeric Antibiotic Resistance Gene as a Selectable Marker for Plant Cell Transformation. *Nature.* **1983,** *304* (5922), 184–187.

Biswas, D.; Mathur, M.; Bhargava, S.; Malhotra, H. Anticancer Activity of Root Extracts in Nonsmall Cell Lung Cancer *Asparagus racemosus* A549 cells. *Asian J. Pharm. Pharmacol.* **2018,** *4* (6), 764–70.

Chang, H.; Yi, B.; Ma, R.; Zhang, X.; Zhao, H.; Xi, Y. CRISPR/cas9, A Novel Genomic Tool to Knock Down microRNA in Vitro and in Vivo. *Sci. Rep.* **2016,** *6* (1), 1–12.

Chen, K.; Gao, C. Targeted Gene Mutation in Plants. In *Somatic Genome Manipulation*, Springer: 2015; pp 253–272.

Chen, K.; Wang, Y.; Zhang, R.; Zhang, H.; Gao, C. CRISPR/Cas Genome Editing and Precision Plant Breeding in Agriculture. *Annu. Rev. Plant Biol.* **2019,** *70*, 667–697.

Chermahini, S. H.; Majid, F. A. A.; Sarmidi, M. R.; Taghizadeh, E.; Salehnezhad, S. Impact of Saffron as An Anti-cancer and Anti-tumor Herb. *Afr. J. Pharm. Pharmacol.* **2010,** *4* (11), 834–840.

Cho, S. W.; Kim, S.; Kim, J. M.; Kim, J.-S. Targeted Genome Engineering in Human Cells with the Cas9 RNA-Guided Endonuclease. *Nat. Biotechnol.* **2013,** *31* (3), 230–232.

Courdavault, V.; O'Connor, S. E.; Oudin, A.; Besseau, S.; Papon, N. Towards the Microbial Production of Plant-Derived Anticancer Drugs. *Trends Cancer.* **2020,** *6* (6), 444–448.

Cox, D. B.; Gootenberg, J. S.; Abudayyeh, O. O.; Franklin, B.; Kellner, M. J.; Joung, J.; Zhang, F. RNA Editing with CRISPR-Cas13. *Sci.* **2017,** *358* (6366), 1019–1027.

Cragg, G. M.; Pezzuto, J. M. Natural Products as a Vital Source for The Discovery of Cancer Chemotherapeutic and Chemopreventive Agents. *Med Princ Pract* **2016,** *25* (Suppl. 2), 41–59.

de Lima, R. M. T.; Dos Reis, A. C.; de Menezes, A. A. P. M.; Santos, J. V. d. O.; Filho, J. W. G. d. O.; Ferreira, J. R. d. O.; de Alencar, M. V. O. B.; da Mata, A. M. O. F.; Khan, I. N.; Islam, A. Protective and Therapeutic Potential of Ginger (*Zingiber officinale*) Extract and [6]-Gingerol in Cancer: A Comprehensive Review. *Phytother Res.* **2018,** *32* (10), 1885–1907.

Delannay, X.; Bauman, T.; Beighley, D.; Buettner, M.; Coble, H.; DeFelice, M.; Derting, C.; Diedrick, T.; Griffin, J.; Hagood, E. Yield Evaluation of a Glyphosate-Tolerant Soybean Line After Treatment with Glyphosate. *Crop Sci.* **1995,** *35* (5), 1461–1467.

Dey, A. CRISPR/Cas Genome Editing to Optimize Pharmacologically Active Plant Natural Products. *Pharmacol. Res.***2020,** 105359.

Dey, A.; Bhattacharya, R.; Mukherjee, A.; Pandey, D. K. Natural Products Against Alzheimer's Disease: Pharmaco-Therapeutics and Biotechnological Interventions. *Biotechnol. Adv.* **2017,** *35* (2), 178–216.

Dey, A.; Gorai, P.; Mukherjee, A.; Dhan, R.; Modak, B. K. Ethnobiological Treatments of Neurological Conditions in the Chota Nagpur Plateau, India. *J. Ethnopharmacol.* **2017,** *198*, 33–44.

Dey, A.; Nandy, S.; Mukherjee, A.; Modak, B. K. Sustainable Utilization of Medicinal Plants and Conservation Strategies Practiced by the Aboriginals of Purulia District, India: a Case Study on Therapeutics used Against some Tropical Otorhinolaryngologic and Ophthalmic Disorders. *Environ. Dev. Sustain.* **2021,** *23* (4), 5576–5613.

Doench, J. G.; Fusi, N.; Sullender, M.; Hegde, M.; Vaimberg, E. W.; Donovan, K. F.; Smith, I.; Tothova, Z.; Wilen, C.; Orchard, R. Optimized sgRNA Design to Maximize Activity and Minimize off-Target Effects of CRISPR-Cas9. *Nat. Biotechnol.* **2016,** *34* (2), 184–191.

Donohoue, P. D.; Barrangou, R.; May, A. P. Advances in Industrial Biotechnology using CRISPR-Cas Systems. *Trends Biotechnol.* **2018,** *36* (2), 134–146.
Doudna, J. A.; Charpentier, E. The New Frontier of Genome Engineering with CRISPR-Cas9. *Sci.* **2014,** *346* (6213).
Dow, L. E.; Fisher, J.; O'rourke, K. P.; Muley, A.; Kastenhuber, E. R.; Livshits, G.; Tschaharganeh, D. F.; Socci, N. D.; Lowe, S. W. Inducible in Vivo Genome Editing with CRISPR-Cas9. *Nat.Biotechnol..* **2015,** *33* (4), 390–394.
Efferth, T. In *From Ancient Herb to Modern Drug: Artemisia Annua and Artemisinin for Cancer Therapy*, Seminars in Cancer Biology: Elsevier, 2017; pp 65–83.
Eid, A.; Alshareef, S.; Mahfouz, M. M. CRISPR Base Editors: Genome Editing without Double-Stranded Breaks. *Biochem. J.* **2018,** *475* (11), 1955–1964.
El-Awady, M. A.; Awad, N. S.; El-Tarras, A. E. Evaluation of the Anticancer Activities of Pomegranate (*Punica granatum*) and Harmal (Rhazya stricta) Plants Grown in Saudi Arabia. *Int. J. Curr. Microbiol. App. Sci.* **2015,** *4*, 1158–67.
Esfahanian, Z.; Behbahani, M.; Shanehsaz, M.; Hessami, M. J.; Nejatian, M. A. Evaluation of Anticancer Activity of Fruit and Leave Extracts from Virus Infected and Healthy Cultivars of *Vitis vinifera. Cell J. (Yakhteh).* **2013,** *15* (2), 116.
Feng, Z.; Zhang, B.; Ding, W.; Liu, X.; Yang, D.-L.; Wei, P.; Cao, F.; Zhu, S.; Zhang, F.; Mao, Y. Efficient Genome Editing in Plants Using a CRISPR/Cas System. *Cell Res.* **2013,** *23* (10), 1229–1232.
Fridlender, M.; Kapulnik, Y.; Koltai, H. Plant Derived Substances with Anti-Cancer Activity: from Folklore to Practice. *Front. Plant Sci.* **2015,** *6*, 799.
Fuentes, P.; Zhou, F.; Erban, A.; Karcher, D.; Kopka, J.; Bock, R. A New Synthetic Biology Approach Allows Transfer of An Entire Metabolic Pathway from a Medicinal Plant to a Biomass Crop. *eLife.* **2016,** *5*, e13664.
Fulda, S. Tumor Resistance to Apoptosis. *Int. J. Cancer* **2009,** *124* (3), 511–515.
G Grothaus, P.; M Cragg, G.; J Newman, D. Plant Natural Products in Anticancer Drug Discovery. *Curr Org Chem.* **2010,** *14* (16), 1781–1791.
Gaj, T.; Gersbach, C. A.; Barbas III, C. F. ZFN, TALEN, and CRISPR/Cas-Based Methods for Genome Engineering. *Trends Biotechnol.* **2013,** *31* (7), 397–405.
Ganogpichayagrai, A.; Palanuvej, C.; Ruangrungsi, N. Antidiabetic and Anticancer Activities of *Mangifera indica* cv. Okrong Leaves. *J. Adv. Pharm. Technol. Res.* **2017,** *8* (1), 19.
Gao, J.; Wang, G.; Ma, S.; Xie, X.; Wu, X.; Zhang, X.; Wu, Y.; Zhao, P.; Xia, Q. CRISPR/Cas9-Mediated Targeted Mutagenesis in *Nicotiana tabacum. Plant Mol. Biol.* **2015,** *87* (1–2), 99–110.
Gelvin, S. B. Plant Proteins Involved in *Agrobacterium*-Mediated Genetic Transformation. *Annu. Rev. Phytopathol.* **2010,** *48*, 45–68.
Gilles, A. F.; Averof, M. Functional Genetics for All: Engineered Nucleases, CRISPR and the Gene Editing Revolution. *EvoDevo.* **2014,** *5* (1), 1–13.
Graham, D. B.; Root, D. E. Resources for the Design of CRISPR Gene Editing Experiments. *Genome Biol.* **2015,** *16* (1), 1–21.
Gupta, D.; Sharma, G.; Saraswat, P.; Ranjan, R. Synthetic Biology in Plants, a Boon for Coming Decades. *Mol. Biotechnol.* **2021**, 1–17.

Haft, D. H.; Selengut, J.; Mongodin, E. F.; Nelson, K. E. A Guild of 45 CRISPR-Associated (Cas) Protein Families and Multiple CRISPR/Cas Subtypes Exist in Prokaryotic Genomes. *PLoS Comput. Biol.* **2005,** *1* (6), e60.

Händel, E.-M.; Alwin, S.; Cathomen, T. Expanding or Restricting the Target Site Repertoire of Zinc-Finger Nucleases: the Inter-Domain Linker as a Major Determinant of Target Site Selectivity. *Mol. Ther.* **2009,** *17* (1), 104–111.

Hess, G. T.; Tycko, J.; Yao, D.; Bassik, M. C. Methods and Applications of CRISPR-Mediated Base Editing in Eukaryotic Genomes. *Mol. Cell.* **2017,** *68* (1), 26–43.

Hiradeve, S.; Danao, K.; Kharabe, V.; Mendhe, B. Evaluation of Anticancer Activity of *Plumbago zeylanica* Linn Leaf Extract. *BioMed. Res.* **2010,** *1* (2), 1–9.

Hoff, G.; Bertrand, C.; Piotrowski, E.; Thibessard, A.; Leblond, P. Genome Plasticity is Governed by Double Strand Break DNA Repair in Streptomyces Sci. Rep. **2018,** *8* (1), 1–11.

Hofmann, N. R. A *Breakthrough in Monocot Transformation Methods*. American Society of Plant Biologists: 2016.

Howes, M.-J. R. The Evolution of Anticancer Drug Discovery from Plants. *Lancet Oncol.* **2018,** *19* (3), 293–294.

Iqbal, J.; Abbasi, B. A.; Mahmood, T.; Kanwal, S.; Ali, B.; Shah, S. A.; Khalil, A. T. Plant-Derived Anticancer Agents: A Green Anticancer Approach. *Asian Pac J Trop Biomed.* **2017,** *7* (12), 1129–1150.

Jaganathan, D.; Ramasamy, K.; Sellamuthu, G.; Jayabalan, S.; Venkataraman, G. CRISPR for Crop Improvement: an update Review. *Front. Plant Sci.* **2018,** *9*, 985.

Jauhar, P. P. Modern Biotechnology as an Integral Supplement to Conventional Plant Breeding: the Prospects and Challenges. **2006**.

Jiang, W.; Zhao, X.; Gabrieli, T.; Lou, C.; Ebenstein, Y.; Zhu, T. F. Cas9-Assisted Targeting of Chromosome Segments CATCH Enables One-step Targeted Cloning of Large Gene Clusters. *Nat. Commun.* **2015,** *6*, 8101.

Kalbande, B. B.; Patil, A. S. Plant Tissue Culture Independent *Agrobacterium* Tumefaciens Mediated In-Planta Transformation Strategy for Upland Cotton (*Gossypium hirsutum*). *Journal of Genetic Biotechnol. Tech.* **2016,** *14* (1), 9–18.

Kaur, P.; Gupta, R.; Dey, A.; Malik, T.; Pandey, D. K. Validation and Quantification of Major Biomarkers in "Mahasudarshan Churna"-an Ayurvedic Polyherbal Formulation Through High-performance Thin-layer Chromatography. *BMC complement. med. Ther.* **2020,** *20* (1), 1–11.

Kausch, A. P.; Nelson-Vasilchik, K.; Hague, J.; Mookkan, M.; Quemada, H.; Dellaporta, S.; Fragoso, C.; Zhang, Z. J. Edit at will: Genotype Independent Plant Transformation in the Era of Advanced Genomics and Genome Editing. *Plant Sci.* **2019,** *281*, 186–205.

Kim, D.; Lim, K.; Kim, S.-T.; Yoon, S.-h.; Kim, K.; Ryu, S.-M.; Kim, J.-S. Genome-wide Target Specificities of CRISPR RNA-Guided Programmable Deaminases. *Nat. Biotechnol.* **2017,** *35* (5), 475–480.

Kim, Y.-G.; Cha, J.; Chandrasegaran, S. Hybrid Restriction Enzymes: Zinc Finger Fusions to Fok I Cleavage Domain. *Proc. Natl. Acad. Sci. U. S. A.* **1996,** *93* (3), 1156–1160.

Kimberland, M. L.; Hou, W.; Alfonso-Pecchio, A.; Wilson, S.; Rao, Y.; Zhang, S.; Lu, Q. Strategies for Controlling CRISPR/Cas9 Off-target Effects and Biological Variations in Mammalian Genome Editing Experiments. *J. Biotechnol.* **2018,** *284*, 91–101.

Kleinstiver, B. P.; Pattanayak, V.; Prew, M. S.; Tsai, S. Q.; Nguyen, N. T.; Zheng, Z.; Joung, J. K. High-Fidelity CRISPR–Cas9 Nucleases with no Detectable Genome-wide Off-target Effects. *Nature.* **2016,** *529* (7587), 490–495.

Kleinstiver, B. P.; Prew, M. S.; Tsai, S. Q.; Topkar, V. V.; Nguyen, N. T.; Zheng, Z.; Gonzales, A. P.; Li, Z.; Peterson, R. T.; Yeh, J.-R. J. Engineered CRISPR-Cas9 Nucleases with Altered PAM Specificities. *Nature.* **2015,** *523* (7561), 481–485.

Kojima-Yuasa, A.; Huang, X.; Matsui-Yuasa, I. Synergistic Anticancer Activities of Natural Substances in Human Hepatocellular Carcinoma. *Diseases.* **2015,** *3* (4), 260–281.

Lambrianidou, A.; Koutsougianni, F.; Papapostolou, I.; Dimas, K. Recent Advances on the Anticancer Properties of Saffron (*Crocus sativus* L.) and its Major Constituents. *Molecules* **2021,** *26* (1), 86.

Lemonnier, N.; Zhou, G.-B.; Prasher, B.; Mukerji, M.; Chen, Z.; Brahmachari, S. K.; Noble, D.; Auffray, C.; Sagner, M. Traditional Knowledge-based Medicine: a Review of History, Principles, and Relevance in the Present Context of P4 Systems Medicine. *Prog. Prev. Med.* **2017,** *2* (7), e0011.

Li, B.; Cui, G.; Shen, G.; Zhan, Z.; Huang, L.; Chen, J.; Qi, X. Targeted Mutagenesis in the Medicinal Plant *Salvia miltiorrhiza. Sci. Rep.* **2017,** *7* (1), 1–9.

Li, F.-S.; Weng, J.-K. Demystifying traditional herbal medicine with modern approach. *Nat. Plants.* **2017,** *3* (8), 1–7.

Li, G.; Zhang, X.; Zhong, C.; Mo, J.; Quan, R.; Yang, J.; Liu, D.; Li, Z.; Yang, H.; Wu, Z. Small Molecules Enhance CRISPR/Cas9-Mediated Homology-directed Genome Editing in Primary Cells. *Sci. Rep.* **2017,** *7* (1), 1–11.

Li, M.; Chen, L.; Dai, Y.; Li, J.; Li, F.; Li, Q.; Yu, Z.; Chai, K.; Zhu, Y. Differential Metabolomics and Network Pharmacology Analysis of Silkworm Biotransformation between Mulberry Leaves and Silkworm Droppings. *Evid. based Complement. Altern. Med.* **2021,** *2021.*

Li, M.; Li, B.; Xia, Z.-M.; Tian, Y.; Zhang, D.; Rui, W.-J.; Dong, J.-X.; Xiao, F.-J. Anticancer Effects of Five Biflavonoids from *Ginkgo biloba* L. Male Flowers in Vitro. *Molecules.* **2019,** *24* (8), 1496.

Li, R.; Fu, D.; Zhu, B.; Luo, Y.; Zhu, H. CRISPR/Cas9-Mediated Mutagenesis of lncRNA1459 Alters Tomato Fruit Ripening. *Plant J.* **2018,** *94* (3), 513–524.

Li, T.; Huang, S.; Jiang, W. Z.; Wright, D.; Spalding, M. H.; Weeks, D. P.; Yang, B. TAL Nucleases (TALNs): Hybrid Proteins Composed of TAL Effectors and FokI DNA-Cleavage Domain. *Genome Biol.* **2011,** *39* (1), 359–372.

Li, Y.; Pfeifer, B. A. Heterologous Production of Plant-Derived Isoprenoid Products in Microbes and the Application of Metabolic Engineering and Synthetic Biology. *Curr. Opin. Plant Biol.* **2014,** *19,* 8–13.

Lian, J.; Schultz, C.; Cao, M.; HamediRad, M.; Zhao, H. Multi-Functional Genome-wide CRISPR System for high Throughput Genotype–Phenotype Mapping. *Nat. Commun.* **2019,** *10* (1), 1–10.

Liang, W.; van Wersch, S.; Tong, M.; Li, X. TIR-NB-LRR Immune Receptor SOC 3 Pairs with Truncated TIR-NB Protein CHS 1 or TN 2 to Monitor the Homeostasis of E3 Ligase SAUL 1. *New Phytol.* **2019,** *221* (4), 2054–2066.

Lichota, A.; Gwozdzinski, K. Anticancer Activity of Natural Compounds from Plant and Marine Environment. *Int. J. Mol. Sci.* **2018,** *19* (11), 3533.

Liu, D.; Hu, R.; Palla, K. J.; Tuskan, G. A.; Yang, X. Advances and Perspectives on the use of CRISPR/Cas9 Systems in Plant Genomics Research. *Curr Opin Plant Biol.* **2016,** *30*, 70–77.

Liu, Y.; Tao, W.; Wen, S.; Li, Z.; Yang, A.; Deng, Z.; Sun, Y. In vitro CRISPR/Cas9 System for Efficient Targeted DNA Editing. *MBio.* **2015,** *6* (6), e01714–15.

Lowder, L.; Malzahn, A.; Qi, Y. Rapid Evolution of Manifold CRISPR Systems for Plant Genome Editing. *Front. Plant Sci.* **2016,** *7*, 1683.

Lu, Y.; Zhu, J.-K. Precise Editing of a Target Base in the Rice Genome using a Modified CRISPR/Cas9 System. *Mol. Plant.* **2017,** *10* (3), 523–525.

Lyzenga, W. J.; Harrington, M.; Bekkaoui, D.; Wigness, M.; Hegedus, D. D.; Rozwadowski, K. L. CRISPR/Cas9 Editing of three CRUCIFERIN C Homoeologues Alters the Seed Protein Profile in *Camelina sativa*. *BMC Plant Biol.* **2019,** *19* (1), 1–16.

Ma, X.; Zhu, Q.; Chen, Y.; Liu, Y.-G. CRISPR/Cas9 Platforms for Genome Editing in Plants: Developments and Applications. *Mol. Plant.* **2016,** *9* (7), 961–974.

Mali, P.; Yang, L.; Esvelt, K. M.; Aach, J.; Guell, M.; DiCarlo, J. E.; Norville, J. E.; Church, G. M. RNA-guided Human Genome Engineering via Cas9. *Sci.* **2013,** *339* (6121), 823–826.

Mao, Y.; Yang, X.; Zhou, Y.; Zhang, Z.; Botella, J. R.; Zhu, J.-K. Manipulating plant RNA-silencing Pathways to Improve the Gene Editing Efficiency of CRISPR/Cas9 Systems. *Genome Biol.* **2018,** *19* (1), 1–15.

Mclnally, S. G.; Hagen, K. D.; Nosala, C.; Williams, J.; Nguyen, K.; Booker, J.; Jones, K.; Dawson, S. C. Robust and Stable Transcriptional Repression in GIARDIA using CRISPRi. *Mol. Biol. Cell.* **2019,** *30* (1), 119–130.

Mehdad, A.; Brumana, G.; Souza, A.; Barbosa, J.; Ventura, M.; De Freitas, S. A Bowman–Birk Inhibitor Induces Apoptosis in Human Breast Adenocarcinoma through Mitochondrial Impairment and Oxidative Damage following Proteasome 20S Inhibition. *Cell Death Discov.* **2016,** *2* (1), 1–10.

Mohamed, M. S.; Kumar, D. S. Application of Nanotechnology in Genetic Improvement in Crops. In *Nanoscience for Sustainable Agriculture*, Springer: 2019; pp 3–24.

Mout, R.; Ray, M.; Yesilbag Tonga, G.; Lee, Y.-W.; Tay, T.; Sasaki, K.; Rotello, V. M. Direct Cytosolic Delivery of CRISPR/Cas9-Ribonucleoprotein for Efficient Gene Editing. *ACS Nano.* **2017,** *11* (3), 2452–2458.

Niazian, M. Application of Genetics and Biotechnology for Improving Medicinal Plants. *Planta.* **2019,** *249* (4), 953–973.

Öztürk, B.; Kocaoğlu, E. H.; Durak, Z. E. Effects of Aqueous Extract from *Silybum marianum* on Adenosine Deaminase Activity in Cancerous and Noncancerous Human Gastric and Colon Tissues. *Pharmacogn. Mag.* **2015,** *11* (41), 143.

Pan, S.-Y.; Litscher, G.; Gao, S.-H.; Zhou, S.-F.; Yu, Z.-L.; Chen, H.-Q.; Zhang, S.-F.; Tang, M.-K.; Sun, J.-N.; Ko, K.-M. Historical Perspective of Traditional Indigenous Medical Practices: the Current Renaissance and Conservation of Herbal Resources. *Evid.-based Complement. Altern. Med.* **2014,** *2014*.

Paterson, A. H.; Lander, E. S.; Hewitt, J. D.; Peterson, S.; Lincoln, S. E.; Tanksley, S. D. Resolution of Quantitative Traits into Mendelian Factors by Using a Complete Linkage Map of Restriction Fragment Length Polymorphisms. *Nature.* **1988,** *335* (6192), 721–726.

Petrovska, B. B. Historical Review of Medicinal Plants' Usage. *Phcog Rev.* **2012,** *6* (11), 1.

Pouvreau, B.; Vanhercke, T.; Singh, S. From Plant Metabolic Engineering to Plant Synthetic Biology: the Evolution of the Design/Build/Test/Learn Cycle. *Plant Sci.* **2018,** *273*, 3–12.

Pratheesh, K. V.; Shine, V. J.; Emima, J.; Renju, G. L.; Rajesh, R. Study on the Anti-Cancer activity of *Tylophora indica* leaf extracts on human colorectal cancer cells. *Int. J. Pharmacogn. Phytochem. Res.* **2014,** *6* (2), 355–361.

Perone, S.; Almy, B.; Zelazo, P. D. Toward an Understanding of the Neural Basis of Executive Function Development. In *The Neurobiology of Brain and Behavioral Development*, Elsevier: 2018; pp 291–314.

Rathore, D. S.; Mullins, E. Alternative Non-*Agrobacterium* Based Methods for Plant Transformation. *Annu. Rev. Plant Biol.* **2018**, 891–908.

Rees, H. A.; Komor, A. C.; Yeh, W.-H.; Caetano-Lopes, J.; Warman, M.; Edge, A. S.; Liu, D. R. Improving the DNA Specificity and Applicability of Base Editing Through Protein Engineering and Protein Delivery. *Nat. Commun.* **2017,** *8* (1), 1–10.

Sangal, V.; Fineran, P. C.; Hoskisson, P. A. Novel Configurations of Type I and II CRISPR–Cas Systems in Corynebacterium Diphtheriae. *Microbiology.* **2013,** *159* (Pt_10), 2118–2126.

Schindele, A.; Dorn, A.; Puchta, H. CRISPR/Cas Brings Plant Biology and Breeding into the Fast Lane. *Curr. Opin. Biotechnol.* **2020,** *61*, 7–14.

Seth, K. Current Status of Potential Applications of Repurposed Cas9 for Structural and Functional Genomics of Plants. *Biochem. Biophys. Res. Commun.* **2016,** *480* (4), 499–507.

Shalem, O.; Sanjana, N. E.; Zhang, F. High-throughput Functional Genomics using CRISPR–Cas9. *J. Med. Plant Res.* **2015,** *16* (5), 299–311.

Shan, Q.; Wang, Y.; Li, J.; Zhang, Y.; Chen, K.; Liang, Z.; Zhang, K.; Liu, J.; Xi, J. J.; Qiu, J.-L. Targeted Genome Modification of Crop Plants using a CRISPR-Cas System. *Nat. Biotechnol.* **2013,** *31* (8), 686–688.

Sharifi, F.; Sharififar, F.; Sharifi, I.; Pournamdari, M.; Eslaminejad, T.; Khatami, M. Antioxidant, Anti-proliferation and Cytotoxicity Activities of *Gossypium hirsutum* toward Standard HepG2, A549, MCF-7 and U87 Cancer Cell Lines Compared to HUVEC, 3T3 Normal Cells. *J. Med. Plant Res.* **2017,** 1–10.

Sharma, S.; Kaur, R.; Singh, A. Recent advances in CRISPR/Cas Mediated Genome Editing for Crop Improvement. *Plant Biotechnol. Rep.* **2017,** *11* (4), 193–207.

Shen, C.-C.; Hsu, M.-N.; Chang, C.-W.; Lin, M.-W.; Hwu, J.-R.; Tu, Y.; Hu, Y.-C. Synthetic Switch to Minimize CRISPR Off-target Effects by Self-restricting Cas9 Transcription and Translation. *Nucleic Acids Res. Spec. Publ.* **2019,** *47* (3), e13-e13.

Shin, J.; Jiang, F.; Liu, J.-J.; Bray, N. L.; Rauch, B. J.; Baik, S. H.; Nogales, E.; Bondy-Denomy, J.; Corn, J. E.; Doudna, J. A. Disabling Cas9 by an Anti-CRISPR DNA mimic. *Sci..Adv.* **2017,** *3* (7), e1701620.

Singh, S.; Sharma, B.; Kanwar, S. S.; Kumar, A. Lead Phytochemicals for Anticancer Drug Development. *Front. Plant Sci.***2016,** *7*, 1667.

Song, G.; Zhang, F.; Zhang, X.; Gao, X.; Zhu, X.; Fan, D.; Tian, Y. AcrIIA5 Inhibits a Broad Range of Cas9 Orthologs by Preventing DNA Target Cleavage. *Cell Rep.* **2019,** *29* (9), 2579–2589. e4.

Tariq, A.; Sadia, S.; Pan, K.; Ullah, I.; Mussarat, S.; Sun, F.; Abiodun, O. O.; Batbaatar, A.; Li, Z.; Song, D. A Systematic Review on Ethnomedicines of Anti-cancer Plants. *Phytother. Res.* **2017,** *31* (2), 202–264.

Techen, N.; Parveen, I.; Pan, Z.; Khan, I. A. DNA Barcoding of Medicinal Plant Material for Identification. *Curr. Opin. Biotechnol.* **2014,** *25*, 103–110.

Tong, Y.; Weber, T.; Lee, S. Y. CRISPR/Cas-based Genome Engineering in Natural Product Discovery. *Nat. Prod. Rep.* **2019,** *36* (9), 1262–1280.

Tong, Y.; Whitford, C. M.; Blin, K.; Jørgensen, T. S.; Weber, T.; Lee, S. Y. CRISPR–Cas9, CRISPRi and CRISPR-BEST-Mediated Genetic Manipulation in Streptomycetes. *Nat. Protoc.* **2020,** *15* (8), 2470–2502.

Urnov, F. D.; Rebar, E. J.; Holmes, M. C.; Zhang, H. S.; Gregory, P. D. Genome Editing with Engineered Zinc Finger Nucleases. *Nat. Rev. Genet.* **2010,** *11* (9), 636–646.

Vats, S.; Kumawat, S.; Kumar, V.; Patil, G. B.; Joshi, T.; Sonah, H.; Sharma, T. R.; Deshmukh, R. Genome Editing in Plants: Exploration of Technological Advancements and challenges. *Cells.* **2019,** *8* (11), 1386.

Vergara-Jimenez, M.; Almatrafi, M. M.; Fernandez, M. L. Bioactive Components in *Moringa oleifera* Leaves Protect Against Chronic disease. *Antioxidants.* **2017,** *6* (4), 91.

Wang, H.; La Russa, M.; Qi, L. S. CRISPR/Cas9 in Genome Editing and Beyond. *Annu. Rev. Biochem.* **2016,** *85*, 227–264.

Weber, T.; Wefers, B.; Wurst, W.; Sander, S.; Rajewsky, K.; Kühn, R. Increasing the Efficiency of Homology-Directed Repair for CRISPR-Cas9-induced Precise Gene Editing in Mammalian Cells. *Nat. Biotechnol.* **2015,** *33* (5), 543–548.

Westfall, P. J.; Pitera, D. J.; Lenihan, J. R.; Eng, D.; Woolard, F. X.; Regentin, R.; Horning, T.; Tsuruta, H.; Melis, D. J.; Owens, A. Production of Amorphadiene in Yeast, and its Conversion to Dihydroartemisinic Acid, Precursor to the Antimalarial Agent Artemisinin. *Proc. Natl. Acad. Sci.* **2012,** *109* (3), E111–E118.

White, M. C.; Holman, D. M.; Boehm, J. E.; Peipins, L. A.; Grossman, M.; Henley, S. J. Age and Cancer Risk: a Potentially Modifiable Relationship. *Am. J. Prev. Med.* **2014,** *46* (3), S7-S15.

Wishart, D. S. Is Cancer a Genetic Disease or a Metabolic Disease? *EBioMedicine.* **2015,** *2* (6), 478–479.

Wolter, F.; Puchta, H. In Planta Gene Targeting can be Enhanced by the use of CRISPR/Cas12a. *Plant J.* **2019,** *100* (5), 1083–1094.

Wolter, F.; Schindele, P.; Puchta, H. Plant Breeding at the Speed of Light: the Power of CRISPR/Cas to Generate Directed Genetic Diversity at Multiple sites. *BMC Plant Biol.* **2019,** *19* (1), 1–8.

World Health Organization (WHO). 2014–2023. Traditional, Complementary and Integrative Medicine. http://www.who.int/medicines/areas/traditional/en/.Wu, F.; Zhou, L.; Jin, W.; Yang, W.; Wang, Y.; Yan, B.; Du, W.; Zhang, Q.; Zhang, L.; Guo, Y. Anti-proliferative and Apoptosis-inducing Effect of Theabrownin Against Non-small Cell Lung Adenocarcinoma A549 cells. *Front. pharmacol.* **2016,** *7*, 465.

Xiong, M.; Wang, L.; Yu, H. L.; Han, H.; Mao, D.; Chen, J.; Zeng, Y.; He, N.; Liu, Z. G.; Wang, Z. Y. Ginkgetin Exerts Growth Inhibitory and Apoptotic Effects on Osteosarcoma Cells through Inhibition of STAT3 and Activation of Caspase-3/9. *Oncol. Rep.* **2016,** *35* (2), 1034–1040.

Xu, X.; Qi, L. S. A CRISPR–dCas Toolbox for Genetic Engineering and Synthetic Biology. *J. Mol. Biol.* **2019,** *431* (1), 34–47.

Yang, L.; Cui, G.; Wang, Y.; Hao, Y.; Du, J.; Zhang, H.; Wang, C.; Zhang, H.; Wu, S.-B.; Sun, Y. Expression of Foreign Genes Demonstrates the Effectiveness of Pollen-mediated Transformation in Zea Mays. *Front. Plant Sci.* **2017,** *8*, 383.

Yang, Z.; Edwards, H.; Xu, P. CRISPR-Cas12a/Cpf1-Assisted Precise, Efficient and Multiplexed Genome-editing in Yarrowia Lipolytica. *Metab. Eng. Commun.* **2020,** *10*, e00112.

Ye, S.; Enghiad, B.; Zhao, H.; Takano, E. Fine-tuning the Regulation of Cas9 Expression Levels for Efficient CRISPR-Cas9 Mediated Recombination in Streptomyces. *J. Ind. Microbiol.* **2020,** *47* (4–5), 413–423.

Zaidi, S. S.-e.-A.; Mansoor, S. Viral Vectors for Plant Genome Engineering. *Front. Plant Sci.* **2017,** *8*, 539.

Zarkovic, N.; Vukovic, T.; Loncaric, I.; Miletic, M.; Zarkovic, K.; Borovic, S.; Cipak, A.; Sabolovic, S.; Konitzer, M.; Mang, S. An Overview on Anticancer Activities of the *Viscum album* Extract Isorel®. *Cancer Biother. Radiopharm.* **2001,** *16* (1), 55–62.

Zhang, F.; Maeder, M. L.; Unger-Wallace, E.; Hoshaw, J. P.; Reyon, D.; Christian, M.; Li, X.; Pierick, C. J.; Dobbs, D.; Peterson, T. High Frequency Targeted Mutagenesis in Arabidopsis Thaliana using Zinc Finger Nucleases. *Proc. Natl. Acad. Sci.* **2010,** *107* (26), 12028–12033.

Zhang, F.; Wen, Y.; Guo, X. CRISPR/Cas9 for Genome Editing: Progress, Implications and Challenges. *Hum. Mol. Genet.* **2014,** *23* (R1), R40-R46.

Zhang, L.; Wang, P.; Feng, Q.; Wang, N.; Chen, Z.; Huang, Y.; Zheng, W.; Jiang, X. Lipid Nanoparticle-Mediated Efficient Delivery of CRISPR/Cas9 for Tumor Therapy. *NPG Asia Mater.* **2017,** *9* (10), e441-e441.

Zhang, Y.; Zhang, F.; Li, X.; Baller, J. A.; Qi, Y.; Starker, C. G.; Bogdanove, A. J.; Voytas, D. F. Transcription Activator-like Effector Nucleases Enable Efficient Plant Genome Engineering. *Plant Physiol.* **2013,** *161* (1), 20–27.

Zheng, S.-g.; Hu, Y.-d.; Zhao, R.-x.; Yan, S.; Zhang, X.-q.; Zhao, T.-m.; Chun, Z. Genome-wide Researches and Applications on Dendrobium. *Planta.* **2018,** *248* (4), 769–784.

Zhou, Z.; Tan, H.; Li, Q.; Chen, J.; Gao, S.; Wang, Y.; Chen, W.; Zhang, L. CRISPR/Cas9-Mediated Efficient Targeted Mutagenesis of RAS in *Salvia miltiorrhiza. Phytochemistry.* **2018,** *148*, 63–70.

CHAPTER 11

Zinc Finger Nuclease (ZFNs) and Transcription Activator-like Effector Nucleases (TALENs) Based Genome Editing in Enhancement of Anticancer Activity of Plants

POOJA SARASWAT, AMBIKA CHATURVEDI, and RAJIV RANJAN

Dayalbagh Educational Institute, Department of Botany, Dayalbagh, Agra, India

ABSTRACT

Medicinal plants are often used for different medical purposes. Many anticancer drugs are obtained from plant extracts or derived synthetically. These herb plants were initially used to treat humans because of their highly enriched metabolic compounds involved in various physiological activities. Conventional breeding techniques were applied for medicinal plants. Also, to improve the efficiency and production of such metabolites various methods like next-generation sequencing and classical biotechnology were used previously. But, due to the advance in genome editing approaches, this has become much easier. The synthetic nucleases like Zinc Finger Nucleases (ZFNs), Transcription activator-like endonuclease (TALENs), and clustered regularly interspaced short palindromic repeats (CRISPR) are developed in the past recent years providing great opportunities for plant community. These technologies have enabled the identification of pathways involved in various metabolite formations, then later used in

Plant-Derived Anticancer Drugs in the OMICS Era: Biosynthesis, Functions, and Applications.
Deepu Pandita, Anu Pandita (Eds.)

the improvement, and enhancement of plant metabolites discussed in the chapter.

11.1 INTRODUCTION

Cancer is one of the severe diseases that affect a large number of people globally. The increasing number of cancer cases led to an increase in demand for new and effective therapies to cure that life-threatening disease. Nowadays, naturally derived compound drives the attention of researchers because they are less toxic and with least side effects compared to other harsh treatments or therapies. The naturally occurring plant-derived compound used for research regarding the generation of new effective drugs. Different methods are also used to make this technique more effective such as the use of nanoparticles (Greenwell and Rahman, 2015). Plants have several natural substances such as alkaloids, mistletoe plant extracts, taxanes, combretastatin, colchicine, geniposide, camptothecin, salycine, maytanasin, tapsigargin, ellipticine, roscoyitine, artesunate and many other extracts those have anticancerous properties (Lichota and Gwozdzinski, 2018). Some of the natural compounds obtained from plants with anticancerous properties are listed in Table 11.1. Researchers suggest that the numerous molecules use for chemotherapeutic drugs for cancerous treatment are also extracted from plants. Whole plant extracts of plants such as *Artemesia monosperma, Origanum dayi post,* and *Urtica membranacea* have the capacity to kill the human-derived cancerous cell mass via process of apoptosis. Solowey and colleagues conclude that whole plant extract has a recognizable role against tumor cells (Solowey et al., 2014).

For the unbroken production of these anticancerous plant extracts biotechnological approaches are necessary. To obtain cancerous effective medicine from naturally derived products structural modification and synthesis of the compound are considerable tools. Molecular modification using various approaches namely genomics and biotechnology play a key role to enhance the therapeutic potential (Gordaliza, 2007). The combination of plant-derived taxol and micro-RNA are also proven effective in colorectal cancer (CRC), and the taxol combination with Neferine is proven as a powerful weapon against Nasopharyngeal carcinoma (NPC) (Hejazi et al., 2020; Wang et al., 2020). Different techniques used to enhance the in vitro production of anticancerous compounds such as hairy root culture, cambial meristematic cell line culture, metabolic engineering, suspension culture, heterologous host, and elicitation, etc. (Moon et al., 2015; Benyammi et al., 2016; Batra et al., 2004; Miettinen et al., 2014; Zhou et al., 2014; Venugopalan et al., 2016). Nowadays, various techniques have been launched for the biotechnological production of anticancerous compounds involving metabolic engineering, heterologous expression, and elicitation (Changxing et al., 2020). For the metabolic synthesis of taxol biosenthesis taxadiene synthase (TS) is the first gene of the pathway and another gene is 10-deacetyl baccatin III-10-O-acetyl transferase (DBAT) which controls the whole reaction. The cloning of both genes is considered as an effective approach for enhancing the synthesis of Taxol (Ho et al., 2005). Similarly, taxol production can also be enhanced using heterologous expression in which *Ecoli* is a heterologous host. This technique aims to produce anticancerous compounds without anticancerous compound-producing organisms (Huang et al., 2001). In elicitation number of elicitors such as coronatine, methyl jasmonate (MeJA), and salicylic acid is widely used in which salicylic acid plays a key role to enhance alkaloid production (Pieterse and Van Loon, 1999). Transgenic approaches and genome editing approaches are used to modify the production of plant natural products (Wayne et al., 2019). To optimize the plant-derived medicinal significant product classical biotechnology and emerging next-generation technologies are also effective. Different genome editing approaches involve clustered regularly interspaced short palindromic repeats (CRISPR), zinc finger nucleases (ZFNs), meganucleases, transcription activator-like effector nuclease use to enhance crop quality (Ku and Ha, 2020). Nowadays, protein-based editing techniques ZFNs and transcription activator-like endonucleases (TALENs) are also popular for the manipulation of genome. It has been reported that few medicinal plants are successfully engineered using the CRISPR/Cas-editing technique. For the successful engineering of medicinal crops genome editing require the combination of system biology, functional genomics, and NGS for the effective production of plant-derived natural compound (Dey, 2020). ZFNs, a genome editing technique creates genetic variation using editing or deleting of endogenous gene sequences which led to an increase in the transgenic product that is produced by the transgene incorporation at a specific location within the genome (Davies et al., 2017), whether TALENs work by destroying target loci and consider as a more effective approach for genome editing (Yasumoto et al., 2014).

TABLE 11.1 Some Plant Metabolites Used in Anticancer Activities.

Plant compound	Source	Application
Etoposide, teniposide and etopophos	Semisynthetic derivatives of the cyclolignan podophyllotoxin	Neoplasms, including testicular and small-cell lung cancers, lymphoma, leukemia, Kaposi's sarcoma, etc.
Vincristine	Vinca alkaloids extracted from *Catharantus rosea*	Non-Hodgkin lymphoma, Hodgkin's disease, and pediatric solid tumors t
Vinblastine	Vinca alkaloids extracted from *Catharantus rosea*	Ticular cancer, non-Hodgkin lymphoma, breast cancer, head, and neck cancer, cervico-uterine cancer, and bladder cancer also inhibit the mitosis of cancerous cells.
Paclitaxel	The bark of the Western yew Taxus brevifolia (133-136) Taxus baccata (ref)	Disable the mitotic apparatus by disrupting the normal function of microtubules. They act as microtubulin-stabilizing agents
Docetaxel	A semisynthetic analog of paclitaxel obtained from 10-deacetyl-baccatin III.	the stabilizer of microtubules and is cytotoxic against several human cells. It is used in the treatment of locally advanced metastatic breast cancer and non-small-cell lung cancer
Flavopiridol	Dyboxylumbinectiferum	Suppression of Survivin Phosphorylation on Thr^{34} by Flavopiridol Enhances Tumor Cell Apoptosis
Irinotecan	Camptotheca acuminate	Effective in endothelial and pancreas cancer via enhanced apoptosis
Diallyl sulfide, diallyl disulfide, allyl propyl disulfide	*Allium sativum bulb*	Effective in stomach, breast, liver, and colon cancer

11.2 ZFNS AND TALENS AS A GENOME EDITING TOOL

11.2.1 ZFNS

In the field of biomedical, the use of target genome engineering is very renowned, for instance, for the determination of specific DNA segments or non-coding regions, scientists generally use gene silencing then after phenotypes would determine the whole organism or cell. For the study of gene function small interfering RNA (siRNA) is also used extensively. siRNA gene silencing is not that effective whether the conventional methods of gene silencing such as homologous recombination (HR) have low efficiency. ZFNs are extensively used in the field of biomedical research, and allow effective gene editing, not only in the cultured cell but also in whole plants (Kim and Kim, 2014). ZFNs are generally used to target unique loci within the genome ZFNs are restriction enzymes that are engineered to target a specific set of DNA sequences (Jabalameli et al., 2015). In general, ZFNs can be described as the regents that cleave target DNA, with this property of ZFNs they are considered a gene-targeting tool. The ds break which is induced by the ZFNs is subjected to a DNA repair mechanism by the cell that may result in target mutation or gene replacement (Carroll, 2011).

In the architecture of ZFNs, two functional domains are linked together with the help of peptides. In artificial protein ZFNs, nonspecific nuclease domain fused with zinc finger DNA binding domain. Both the ZFNs domain is made up of two cysteine domains ($Cyst_2$) and two Histidine domains (His_2) (Cys_2His_2-Zinc fingers) (Jamieson et al., 2003; Tupler et al., 2001). The interaction of Zinc fingers with DNA depicts by the crystal structure of Zif268-DNA. The finger of ZFNs works as a modular unit with 3 to 4 pair of DNAs and allow sequence-specific interaction via α-helix with a major groove of the DNA (Pavletich and Pabo, 1991; Klug, 1993) due to this specific property of ZFNs, it allow the engineering of novel DNA binding domain. Research also supports the idea to use ZFP TFs in human therapeutics. Engineering of ZFPs bind to the specific small set of sequences within the promoter of the gene of interest Jamieson and colleagues provide methods in their research to design DNA binding domain and also describe their incorporation in novel transcription factors (Jamieson et al., 2003).

To cut the DNA molecule there is a requirement for dimerization of the FokI cleavage domain due to the weak interface of dimer the designing of two sets of fingers which should be directed to each monomeric cleavage domain (Fig. 11.1). Dimerization and cleavage facilitate by high local concentration which occurs due to the binding of two sets of fingers to their recognition sequence (Bibikova et al., 2001; Handel et al., 2009; Shimizu et al. 2009). With the zinc finger protein, ZFNs combine the non-specific domain (cleavage domain) of FOkI endonuclease, which facilitates the delivery of target-specific ds-break within the genome. The engineered ZFN-mediated gene targeting allows desired permanent modification in plants. This site-specific cleavage by engineered ZFNs depends upon how steady the development of zinc finger proteins occurs so it allows reliable specific recognition of the target site. Development of custom ZFNs molecule with required sequence-specificities the (Cys2His2) ZFPs is considered as best approach (Durai et al., 2005). To design, the versatile artificial DNA-binding protein modular structure and modular recognition of zinc finger motifs and zinc finger domain respectively should be versatile. About 30 amino acids consist of each zinc finger motif and fold into $\beta\beta\alpha$ structure and its stabilization occurs through the process of chelation of zinc ion which occurs via conserved Cys_2His_2 residues. The insertion of α-helix into the major groove of ds-DNA primarily each finger binds to triplet within the genome amino acids present at the positions 1, +1, +2, +3, +4, +5, and +6 positions play an imperative role for the initiation of α-helix for every ZF motifs (Beerli;Barbas, 2002; Pabo et al., 2001; Pavletich, 1991).

For the construction of novel ZFNs number of methods are there in the literature. There is a method called “modular assembly” for the collection of zinc fingers that have known DNA-binding sites the ZFNs DNA binding domain needs to assembled there now are numerous web tools and are available the engineering and assembly can also be facilitated by the arches of zinc finger modules (Cathomen and Joung, 2008; Alwin et al., 2005). Several companies also design ZFNs such as SangamoBioSciences (www.sangamo.com), Sigma-Aldrich1; www.sigmaaldrich.comprovides corresponding DNA that contains vectors. A strategy named “Pool Engineering (OPEN)” deals with the in vivo selection methods as well as zinc finger collection (Madre, et al., 2008). Gabriel and colleagues perform a genome-wide analysis of ZFNs specificity. They showed in their work that non-homologous end-joining captures integrate into the lent viral vector which is defective at double standard breaks (Gabriel et al., 2011). Townsend and colleagues Demonstrate gene targeting stimulated by high-frequency ZFNs in tobacco plant acetoacetate synthase genes namely Surah, SuRB, and ALS. They also introduce mutation via ZFN-mediated gene targeting for resistance to herbicides and these mutations were introduced in SuR loci. They also conclude the possibilities of making efficiently targeted sequence mutations in endogenous plant genes (Townsend et al., 2009). Zeevi and colleagues use the engineered ZFNs combined with homing endonuclease and successfully define the multi-transgenic binary vector assembly. By using the system Zeevi and colleagues engineered a binary vector with a carrying capacity of up to nine genes (Zeevi et al., 2012).

11.2.2 TALENS

Target genome editing is capable to modify genes of interest in various organisms which is based on the synthetic nuclease, protein, and specific gene sequence which binds the nuclease to cleave the gene of interest. The initial work with such a synthetic system was performed using ZFNs. As already discussed in the chapter, ZFNs can be used to alter genes (deletion, point mutations, duplication, etc.) in a wide range of organisms and cells which earlier proved to be an efficient tool for genomic modifications.

Later, TALENs emerged as a better tool than ZFNs and grabbed the attention of researchers toward its easy and rapid designing system and precise genome editing. Similar to ZFNs, TALENs is made up of a synthesis TALE binding domain, and a Fok I cleavage domain. Transcription activator-like effectors (TALEs) are a class of proteins that belongs to plant pathogens which helped in the identification of TALE repeats (DNA-binding domain) (Bogdanove and Voytas, 2011). Based on the simple repeat variable di-residue (RVD)-nucleotide recognition code, the customized TALEs DNA binding domain, could target any sequence given (Bogdanove and Voytas, 2011). The TALE repeats are 33 to 35 amino acids long sequences with amino acids known as RVD which is specific to any of the base pairs (Boch et al., 2009) (Fig. 11.1). The understanding of RVD code resulted in the development of new artificial nucleases specific to any site which further fuses with the two domains of TALE repeats and FokI endonuclease, combinedly known as TALENs (Miller et al., 2011). TALE repeats bind to the target site with an affinity of up to 96% (Miller et al., 2011). TALEs have an advantage over ZFNs in terms of the length of the sequences which can be attached to the desired site. The TALENs can bind to comparatively larger sequences than ZFNs (Guilinger et al., 2014). Also, TALENs can bind to a site with few constraints as it has multiple possibilities for each base pair of a random sequence of DNA (Reyon et al., 2012). TALENs do have limitations because of their large size in comparison to ZFNs. A cDNA of size 3 kb codes for the TALEN whereas a ZFNs is coded by a cDNA approximately 1 kb in length. The larger size makes it difficult to deliver inside the cells such a complexity limits its use in therapeutics (Holkers et al., 2013).

TALENs-based editing has been adopted for its application in various plants so far (Mahfouz et al., 2011; Shan et al., 2013; Zhang et al., 2013). Fok I functioning as a dimer is used to cleave the target site. The resulting DSBs obtained undergo a DNA repair system either by non-homologous end joining (NHEJ) or HR. The NHEJ-based repair allows re-joining of broken DNAs which may lead to indel formation and is used to develop knockout mutants. On the other hand, when DSBs get repaired through the HR mechanism, this creates insertions in the target site.

Targeted gene mutagenesis also known as TGM, brings changes in the gene function or disrupts using NHEJ mechanism of correction. Such genetic manipulations have been seen in the plant including *Arabidopsis*. TGM performed using TALENs is used to insert genes of interest in any part of the genome with HR based approach. This technology can be used to insert various genes at the same locus and is also helpful in the selection of genes with higher expression. Targeted tagging is another method for TGM in which tag or reporter genes are inserted for the labeling of an endogenous gene (Chen et al., 2013). Also, the gene replacement done by TALENs, uses HR DNA repair pathway in which a donor DNA template complementary to the target site is delivered into the cell. Thus, the DSBs obtained from the TALENs are further repaired by the donor templates which ultimately bring changes. It is also known that paired TALENs when introduced in the cells may result in complex target gene mutations like inversion, deletions, etc. (Shan et al., 2013).

11.3 ZFNS AND TALENS MEDIATED GENE EDITING FOR ANTICANCEROUS PLANT DEVELOPMENT

There has been a lot of work done related to the applications of TALEN technology benefiting plants and other organisms. Many of the mutations performed in plants are usually NHEJ-dependent. It is seen that most of the anticancer-related work is done on humans (Ren et al., 2020; Puria et al., 2021). Also, many works have been done on the enhancement of

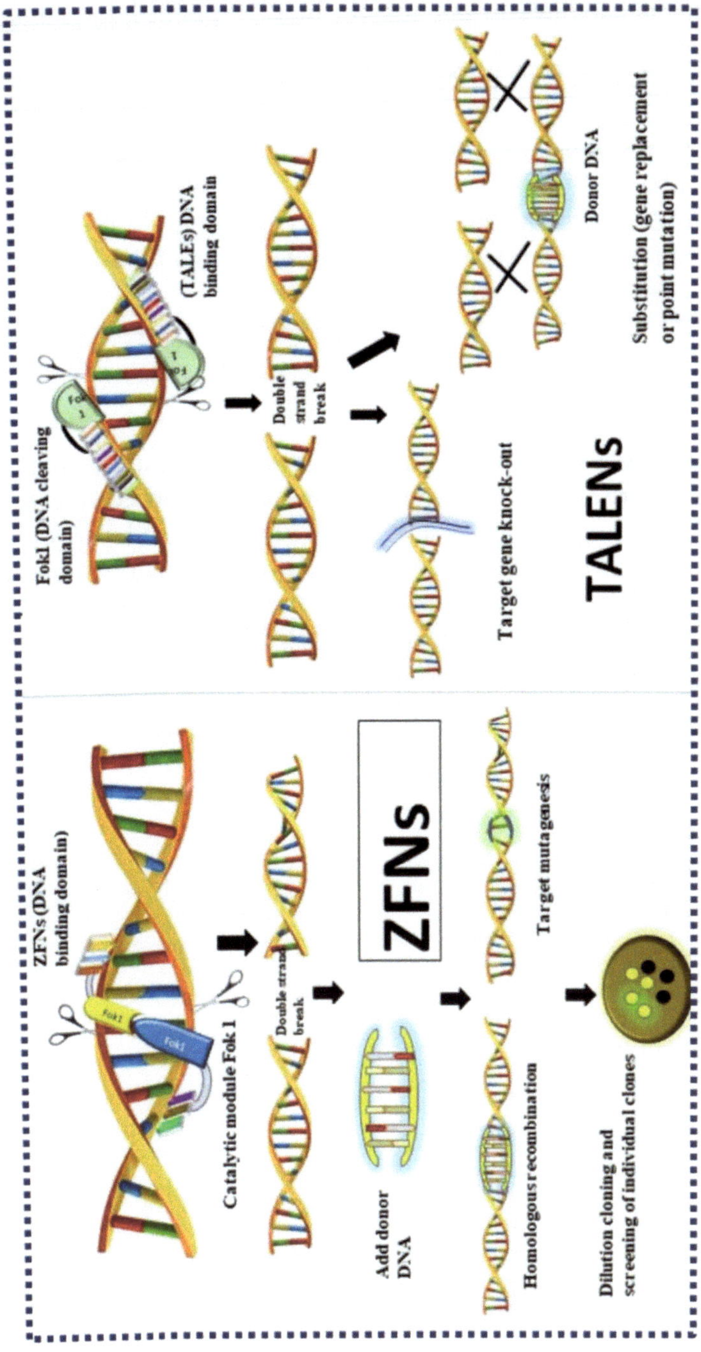

FIGURE 11.1 Structure and functioning of ZFNs and TALENs.

anticancer metabolites in endophytic fungi explained by Ramesha and colleagues (2020). There is less knowledge about the use of ZFNs and TALENs enhancing anticancer activity in plants. Due to the development of CRISPR/Cas system, the applications of ZFNs and TALENs have been reduced to an extent as CRISPR has taken over these two previously developed techniques. The applications of CRISPR have surely enabled the enhancement of anticancerous activity in plants (Li et al., 2017). But still, there is a need to develop other techniques so that they can also be applied to broad-scale applications.

11.4 CONCLUSION

ZFNs and TALEN-mediated mutations are still lagging in many organisms. There are several challenges that need to be addressed so that this method can be used regularly in different organisms and plants. The target specificity has to be increased along with efficient transformation methods. Some advancement in ZFNs and TALENs will surely widen the areas of application in crop plants enhancing various traits.

KEYWORDS

- **ZFNs**
- **TALENs**
- **CRISPR/Cas**
- **anticancer activity**
- **metabolites**

REFERENCES

Alwin, S.; Gere, M. B.; Guhl, E.; Effertz, K.; Barbas III, C. F.; Segal, D. J.; et al. Custom Zinc-finger Nucleases for Use in Human Cells. *Mol. Ther.* **2005,** *12*, 610–617.

Batra, J.; Dutta, A.; Singh, D.; Kumar, S.; Sen, J. Growth and Terpenoid Indole Alkaloid Production in Catharanthus Roseus Hairy Root Clones in Relation to Left-and Right-Termini-Linked Ri T-DNA Gene Integration. *Plant Cell Rep.* **2004,** *23*, 148–154.

Beerli, R. R.;Barbas, C. F. Engineering Polydactyl Zinc-Finger Transcription Factors. *Nat. Biotechnol.* **2002,** *20*, 135–141.

Benyammi, R.; Paris, C.; Khelifi-Slaoui, M.; Zaoui, D.; Belabbassi, O.; Bakiri, N.; et al. Screening and Kinetic Studies of Catharanthine and Ajmalicine Accumulation and their Correlation with Growth Biomass in Catharanthus Roseus Hairy Roots. *Pharmaceut. Biol.* **2016,***54*, 2033–2043.

Bibikova, M.; Carroll, D.; Segal, D. J.; Trautman, J. K.; Smith, J.; Kim, Y. G.; Chandrasegaran, S. Stimulation of Homologous Recombination through Targeted Cleavage by Chimeric Nucleases. *Mol. Cell. Biol.* **2001,** *21*, 289–297.

Boch, J.; Scholze, H.; Schornack, S.; Landgraf, A.; Hahn, S.; Kay, S.; et al. Breaking the Code of DNA Binding Specificity of TAL-type III Effectors. *Sci.* **2009,** *326*, 1509–1512.

Bogdanove, A. J.;Voytas, D. F. TAL Effectors: Customizable Proteins for DNA Targeting. *Science*, **2011,** *333*, 1843–1846.

Carroll, D. Genome Engineering with Zinc-Finger Nucleases. *Genetics* **2011,** *188*, 773–782.

Cathomen, T.; Joung, J. K. Zinc-Finger Nucleases: the Next Generation Emerges. *Mol. Ther.* **2008,** *16*, 1200–1207.

Changxing, L.; Galani, S.; Hassan, F. U.; Rashid, Z.; Naveed, M.; Fang, D.; et al. Biotechnological Approaches to the Production of Plant-Derived Promising Anticancer agents: An Update and Overview. *Biomed. Pharmacother.* **2020,** *132*, 110918.

Chen, K.; Gao, C. TALENs: Customizable Molecular DNA Scissors for Genome Engineering of Plants. *J. Genet. Genom.* **2013,**. *40*, 271–279.

Davies, J. P.; Kumar, S.; Sastry-Dent, L. Use of Zinc-Finger Nucleases for Crop Improvement. *Prog. Mol. Biol, Transl. Sci.* **2017,** *149*, 47–63.

Dey, A. CRISPR/Cas genome Editing to Optimize Pharmacologically Active Plant Natural Products. *Pharmacol. Res.* **2020,** 105359.

Durai, S.; Mani, M.; Kandavelou, K.; Wu, J.; Porteus, M. H.; Chandrasegaran, S. Zinc Finger Nucleases: Custom-Designed Molecular Scissors for Genome Engineering of Plant and Mammalian Cells. *Nucleic Acids Res.* **2005,** *33*, 5978–5990.

Gabriel, R.; Lombardo, A.; Arens, A.; Miller, J. C.; Genovese, P.; Kaeppel, C.; et al. An Unbiased Genome-Wide Analysis of Zinc-Finger Nuclease Specificity. *Nat. Biotechnol.* **2011,** *29*, 816–823.

Gordaliza, M. Natural Products as Leads to Anticancer Drugs. *Clin Transl Oncol.* **2007,** *9*, 767–776.

Greenwell, M.; Rahman, P. K. S. M. Medicinal Plants: Their Use in Anticancer Treatment. *Int. J. Pharmaceut. Sci. Res.* **2015,** *6*, 4103.

Guilinger, J. P.; Pattanayak, V.; Reyon, D.; Tsai, S. Q.; Sander, J. D.; Joung, J. K.; Liu, D. R. Broad Specificity Profiling of TALENs Results in Engineered Nucleases with Improved DNA-cleavage Specificity. *Nat. Meth.* **2014,** *11*, 429–435.

Händel, E. M.; Alwin, S.; Cathomen, T. Expanding or Restricting the Target Site Repertoire of Zinc-finger Nucleases: the Inter-domain Linker as a Major Determinant of Target Site Selectivity. *Mol. Ther.* **2009,** *17*, 104–111.

Hejazi, M.; Baghbani, E.; Amini, M.; Rezaei, T.; Aghanejad, A.; Mosafer, J.; et al. MicroRNA-193a and taxol combination: A New Strategy for Treatment of Colorectal Cancer. *J. Cell. Biochem.* **2020,** *121*, 1388–1399.

Ho, C. K.; Chang, S. H.; Lung, J.; Tsai, C. J.; Chen, K. P. The Strategies to Increase Taxol Production by using Taxus Mairei Cells Transformed with TS and DBAT Genes. *Int. J. App. Sci. Eng.* **2005,** *3*, 179–185.

Holkers, M.; Maggio, I.; Liu, J.; Janssen, J. M.; Miselli, F.; Mussolino, C.; et al. Differential Integrity of TALE Nuclease Genes Following Adenoviral and Lentiviral Vector Gene Transfer into Human Cells. *Nucleic Acids Res.* **2013,** *41*, e63-e63.

Huang, Q.; Roessner, C. A.; Croteau, R.; Scott, A. I. Engineering Escherichia Coli for the Synthesis of Taxadiene, a Key Intermediate in the Biosynthesis of Taxol. *Bioorganic Med. Chem.* **2001,** *9*, 2237–2242.

Jabalameli, H. R.; Zahednasab, H.; Karimi-Moghaddam, A.; Jabalameli, M. R. Zinc Finger Nuclease Technology: Advances and Obstacles in Modelling and Treating Genetic Disorders. *Gene*. **2015,** *558*, 1–5.

Jamieson, A. C.; Miller, J. C.;Pabo, C. O. Drug Discovery with Engineered Zinc-finger Proteins. *Nat. Rev. Drug Discov.* **2003,** *2*, 361–368.

Kim, H.; Kim, J. S. A Guide to Genome Engineering with Programmable Nucleases. *Nat. Rev. Genet.* **2014,** *15*, 321–334.

Ku, H. K.; Ha, S. H. Improving Nutritional and Functional Quality by Genome Editing of Crops: Status and Perspectives. *Front. Plant Sci.* **2020,** *11*, 1514.

Li, B.; Cui, G.; Shen, G.; Zhan, Z.; Huang, L.; Chen, J.; Qi, X. Targeted Mutagenesis in the Medicinal Plant Salvia Miltiorrhiza. *Sci. Rep.* **2017,** *7*, 1–9.

Lichota, A.; Gwozdzinski, K. Anticancer Activity of Natural Compounds from Plant and Marine Environment. *Int. J. Mol. Sci.* **2018,** *19*, 3533.

Maeder, M. L.; Thibodeau-Beganny, S.; Osiak, A.; Wright, D. A.; Anthony, R. M.; Eichtinger, M.; et al. Rapid 'open-source' Engineering of Customized Zinc-finger Nucleases for Highly Efficient Gene Modification. *Mol. Cell.* **2008,** *31*, 294–301.

Mahfouz, M. M.; Li, L. TALE Nucleases and Next Generation GM Crops. *GM Crops*. **2011,** *2*, 99–103.

Miettinen, K.; Dong, L.; Navrot, N.; Schneider, T.; Burlat, V.; Pollier, J.; et al. The Seco-iridoid Pathway from Catharanthus Roseus. *Nat. Commun.* **2014,** *5*, 1–12.

Miller, J. C.; et al. A TALE Nuclease Architecture for Efficient Genome Editing. *Nat. Biotechnol.* **2011,** 29, 143–148.

Moon, S. H.; Venkatesh, J.; Yu, J. W.; Park, S. W. Differential Induction of Meristematic Stem Cells of *Catharanthus Roseus* and their Characterization. *C. R. Biol.* **2015,** *338*, 745–756.

Pabo, C. O.; Peisach, E.; Grant, R. A. Design and Selection of Novel Cys2His2 Zinc Finger Proteins. *Ann. Rev. Biochem.* **2001,** *70*, 313–340.

Pavletich, N. P.; Pabo, C. O. Zinc Finger-DNA Recognition: Crystal Structure of a Zif268-DNA Complex at 2.1 A. *Sci.* **1991,** *252*, 809–817.

Pieterse, C. M.; Van Loon, L. C. Salicylic acid-independent plant defence pathways. *Trends Plant Sci.* **1999,** *4*, 52–58.

Puria, R.; Sahi, S.; Nain, V. HER2+ Breast Cancer Therapy: by CPP-ZFN Mediated Targeting of mTOR?. *Technol. Cancer Res. Treat.* **2012,** *11*, 175–180.

Ramesha, A.; Devi, D. N.; Hegde, S. V.; Srinivas, C. Biotechnological Approaches for the Enhancement of Anticancer Secondary Metabolite Production from Endophytic Fungi. In *New and Future Developments in Microbial Biotechnology and Bioengineering*; Elsevier: 2020; pp. 135–155.

Ren, C.; Gao, C.; Li, X.; Xiong, J.; Shen, H.; Wang, L.; et al. The Antitumor Efficiency of Zinc Finger Nuclease Combined with Cisplatin and Trichostatin A in Cervical Cancer Cells. *Anti-Cancer Agents in Medicinal Chemistry (Formerly Current Medicinal Chemistry-Anti-Cancer Agents)*, **2020,** *20*, 2125–2135.

Reyon, D.; Tsai, S. Q.; Khayter, C.; Foden, J. A.; Sander, J. D.; Joung, J. K. FLASH Assembly of TALENs for High-throughput Genome Editing. *Nat. Biotechnol.* **2012,** 30, 460–465.

Shan, Q.; Wang, Y.; Chen, K.; Liang, Z.; Li, J.; Zhang, Y.; et al. Rapid and Efficient Gene Modification in Rice and Brachypodium using TALENs. *Mole. Plant.* **2013,** *6*, 1365.

Shimizu, Y.; Bhakta, M. S.; Segal, D. J. Restricted Spacer Tolerance of a Zinc Finger Nuclease with a Six Amino Acid Linker. *Bioorganic Med. Chem. Lett.* **2009,** *19*, 3970–3972.

Solowey, E.; Lichtenstein, M.; Sallon, S.; Paavilainen, H.; Solowey, E.; Lorberboum-Galski, H. Evaluating Medicinal Plants for Anticancer Activity. *Sci. World J.* **2014**.

Townsend, J. A.; Wright, D. A.; Winfrey, R. J.; Fu, F.; Maeder, M. L.; Joung, J. K.;Voytas, D. F. High-frequency Modification of Plant Genes using Engineered Zinc-finger Nucleases. *Nature* **2009,** *459*, 442–445.

Tupler, R.; Perini, G.; Green, M. R. Expressing the Human Genome. *Nature* **2001,** *409*, 832–833.

Venugopalan, A.; Potunuru, U. R.; Dixit, M.; Srivastava, S. Reprint of: Effect of Fermentation Parameters, Elicitors and Precursors on Camptothecin Production from the Endophyte Fusarium Solani. *Biores. Technol.* **2016,** *213*, 311–318.

Wang, X.; Wang, K.; Xiao, J.; Song, Y.; Li, H. Neferine sensitized Taxol-resistant Nasopharygeal Carcinoma to Taxol by Inhibiting EMT via Downregulating miR-130b-5p. *Biochem. Biophys. Res. Commun.* **2020,** *531*, 573–580.

Wayne, L. L.; Gachotte, D. J.; Walsh, T. A. Transgenic and Genome Editing Approaches for Modifying Plant Oils. *Trans. Plants* **2019,** 367–394.

Yasumoto, S.; Seki, H.; Muranaka, T. Changes and Improvement of Metabolism in Plant by using TALEN Genome Editing. *Seibutsu-kogakuKaishi* **2014,** *92*, 553–555.

Zeevi, V.; Liang, Z.; Arieli, U.;Tzfira, T. Zinc Finger Nuclease and Homing Endonuclease-Mediated Assembly of Multigene Plant Transformation Vectors. *Plant Physiol.* **2012,** *158*, 132–144.

Zhang, Y.; Zhang, F.; Li, X.; Baller, J. A.; Qi, Y.; Starker, C. G.; Bogdanove, A. J.; Voytas, D. F.; Transcription Activator-like Effector Nucleases Enable Efficient Plant Genome Engineering. *Plant Physiol.* **2013,** 161, 20e27.

Zhou, M. L.; Zhu, X. M.; Shao, J. R.; Wu, Y. M.; Tang, Y. X. Transcriptional Response of the Catharanthine Biosynthesis Pathway to Methyl Jasmonate/Nitric Oxide Elicitation in Catharanthus Roseus Hairy Root Culture. *Appl. Microbiol. Biotechnol.* **2010,** *88*, 737–750.

Index

B

C

D

E

F

G

H